PAIN
Management and Nursing Care

PAIN
Management and Nursing Care

Dawn Carroll, RGN

Senior Research Nurse, Oxford Regional Pain Relief Unit,
Churchill Hospital, Oxford; and Nuffield Department of Anaesthetics,
University of Oxford, UK

David Bowsher, MA, MD, PhD, MRCP(Ed), FRCPath

Director of Research, Pain Research Institute, Walton Hospital,
Liverpool, UK; and Honorary Consultant in Pain Relief

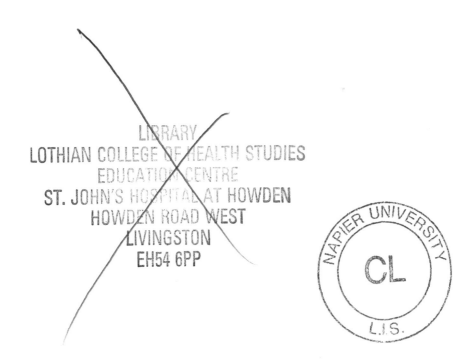

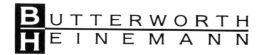

BUTTERWORTH
HEINEMANN

Butterworth-Heinemann Ltd
Linacre House, Jordan Hill, Oxford OX2 8DP

$\mathcal{R}$ A member of the Reed Elsevier plc group

OXFORD LONDON BOSTON
MUNICH NEW DELHI SINGAPORE SYDNEY
TOKYO TORONTO WELLINGTON

First published 1993
Reprinted 1995 (twice)

British Library Cataloguing in Publication Data
Pain: Management and Nursing Care
  I. Carroll, Dawn   II. Bowsher, David
  616.0472

ISBN 0 7506 1588 5

Library of Congress Cataloging in Publication Data
Pain: management and nursing care/[edited by] Dawn Carroll, David Bowsher.
  p. cm.
  Includes bibliographical references and index.
  ISBN 0 7506 1588 5
  1. Pain 2. Nursing. 3. Intractable pain. 4. Analgesia.
  [DNLM: 1. Pain—therapy. 2. Pain—physiopathology. 3. Palliative
  Treatment. WL 704 P1463 1993]
  RB 127.P33234 1993
  616'.0472—dc20
  DNLM/DLC
  for Library of Congress

Phototypeset by Wilmaset Ltd, Birkenhead, Wirral
Printed and bound in Great britain by Martins the Printers, Berwick-upon-Tweed

Contents

Contributors

David Bowsher MA, MD, PhD, MRCP(Ed), FRCPath
Director of Research, Pain Research Institute, Walton Hospital, Liverpool, UK; and Honorary Consultant in Pain Relief

Dawn Carroll RGN
Senior Research Nurse, Oxford Regional Pain Relief Unit, Churchill Hospital, Oxford; and Nuffield Department of Anaesthetics, University of Oxford, UK

Robert A. Charman MCSP, DipTP
Senior Lecturer, School of Physiotherapy, Institute of Health Care Studies, University Hospital of Wales, Cardiff, UK

Peter Davis MA BEd(Hons), Cert Ed, RGN, DN(Lond), ONC
Course Director, Royal National Orthopaedic Hospital Trust, Stanmore, UK

Linda Edgar N., MSc(A)
Assistant Professor of Nursing, School of Nursing, McGill University, Montreal, Canada

Carol Horrigan MSc, SRN, RCNT, DipN(Lond), PGCEA, RNT
Lecturer in Complementary Therapies, Bloomsbury and Islington College of Nursing and Midwifery, and The Royal College of Nursing, London, UK

Debbie Hunter RGN
Acute Pain Control Sister, Anaesthetics Department, York District Hospital, York, UK

Patricia Jacob CertEd, RGN
Staff Nurse, Sir Michael Sobell House, Churchill Hospital, Oxford, UK

Valerie M. F. King RGN, RHV
Primary Nurse, Oxford Regional Pain Relief Unit, Oxford, UK

Jane Latham RGN, DN
Honorary Lecturer, Trinity Hospice, London, UK

Patrick J. McGrath PhD
Professor of Psychology, Paediatrics, Psychiatry and Occupational Therapy, Dalhousie University, Halifax, Canada

Christine Pearce RGN, RNT
St Elizabeth Hospice, Ipswich, UK

Judith Ralphs BSc(Hons), RGN
Sister, Input, St Thomas' Pain Management Centre, St Thomas' Hospital, London, UK

Judith A. Ritchie RN, PhD
Professor of Nursing, School of Nursing, Dalhousie University, Director of Nursing Research, IWK Children's Hospital, Halifax, Canada

Kate Seers BSc, PhD, RGN
Senior Research Fellow, National Institute for Nursing, Radcliffe Infirmary, Oxford, UK

Susan Tempest BPharm, MRPS
Senior Clinical Pharmacist, Palliative and Emergency Medicine, Derbyshire Royal Infirmary, Derby, UK

Anita Unruh MSW, OT(C)
Assistant Professor, Dalhousie University, Halifax, Canada

Janet Walker PhD, BSc, RGN, RM, RHV, CPsychol
Lecturer, Department of Psychology, University of Southampton, Southampton, UK

1

Introduction

Dawn Carroll

Pain is a symptom common to most illness and is often the presenting factor which will prompt the patient to seek medical attention, yet surprisingly until recently pain has been given a low priority by most health professionals. Fortunately this is now changing, and there is an increased awareness for the need and responsibility we have to provide patients with adequate levels of pain control. Pain management has become very fashionable and has been an area of extensive research over the past 10 years, which has lead to much change and development in clinical practice.

As a member of the multi-disciplinary team, the nurse plays a key role in the management of pain. She is the person who spends most time with the patient and is responsible for the administration of analgesic drugs, assessment, monitoring and reporting the effects of given treatments to ensure that an acceptable level of pain relief is achieved. However, the nurse does not always feel able to do this properly, either due to limited knowledge and skills or to lack of awareness of the resources which are available. This can be a particular problem when caring for patients with difficult pain management problems, when the nurse may feel helpless and inadequate as she fails to meet the needs of her patient. It is crucial that the nurse is aware of the pain relieving methods which are available and how and when to use them safely; from the simple nursing interventions such as massage to the high tech more invasive approaches such as epidural infusions of opioids and local anaesthetics.

It is common for analgesic drugs to be prescribed and administered without any consideration for individual patient requirements, particularly in the acute setting. Drugs are often administered with a minimal knowledge of

pharmacology and side effect profile. Formal assessment of pain is frequently neglected, but is vital in order to give the appropriate treatment effectively and safely. The nurse should have a knowledge of the assessment tools which are available and when and how to use them. If a patient is being treated for diabetes or hypertension it is possible to objectively measure the effects of treatment. Such objective measurement is not possible with pain, where we have to rely on subjective measures, namely the patients' report.

Acute pain

Theories that pain is to be 'expected', 'healthy', or that 'a little pain never did any harm' are now fortunately outdated and both attitudes and priorities towards pain have changed. It is now rightly considered that it is 'unacceptable for patients to suffer pain unnecessarily' and that 'patients have a right to no pain'.

The importance of pain control has been long recognised in maternity units by nurses, but it is only recently that this interest has spread to other acute pain settings. The luxury of pre-operative preparation for a potentially painful event should not be restricted to labour pain but available for all patients.

There is an important new theory that pre-emptive analgesia (prevention of pain before it occurs) in the acute setting will play an important role in the future, with implications not only for the immediate post-operative period, but affecting long term outcome and morbidity (McQuay *et al.*, 1988; Wall, 1988). One area of interest is that of phantom limb pain after amputation but as well as the neuropathic pain syndromes, nociceptive pains may be equally important (McQuay, 1992).

There is a current trend towards the use of patient controlled analgesia (PCA) and epidural infusions. The recent report by the Royal College of Surgeons and College of Anaesthetists working party (1990) has highlighted problems relating to the inadequacies of current management in acute pain and recommends that all hospitals should develop an acute pain service. What the report assumes is that all hospitals can afford the high technology which is required to develop the widespread use of PCA and epidural infusions. This is may prove problematic where there are financial restraints such as those currently seen in the UK, where resources are limited and often the high tech interventions are only available for a relatively small proportion of patients; although the portable devices make these interventions more feasible. So what then happens to the majority of patients to whom the acute pain service is not available? The report overlooks and devalues the traditional methods of relief, principally the analgesic drugs, which work well for most patients when prescribed and administered according to the individual patient requirements. It must be remembered that whichever method is applied, high tech or traditional, there must be adequate education and training for the end users, 'the nursing staff', otherwise it will be to the patient's detriment. Too often the high technology is introduced by medical staff, without the provision of adequate training and support networks for those caring for the patients. Although the nurse is keen to extend her role she must have the appropriate training *prior* to implementing changes in practice and *not* after the event.

Chronic pain

Developments in medicine over the past decade and improved surgical techniques have resulted in less invasive surgery; thus less trauma and pain. As a result patients are spending less time in hospital. In contrast, chronic pain is likely to become a growing problem due to the increasing ageing population. Chronic pain sadly receives the least attention and has the most limited resources as is true for most chronic illness. This is so not only for the NHS in the UK, but for countries where private health care is in operation, as people cannot afford to pay for ongoing treatments and insurance companies are increasingly reluctant to pay for ongoing care where curative treatments may be limited.

Pain clinics in the UK were set up in the 1960s by pioneering doctors such as John Lloyd and Sam Lipton, anaesthetists with an interest in pain who recognised that pain generally was not particularly well managed and that a formal service was required. The traditional pain clinics favoured invasive nerve blocking techniques and pharmacological interventions for the management of chronic benign and cancer pain. Today there is a change in trend: nerve blocks are used more selectively and reserved for those patients in whom the pharmacological and less invasive interventions have failed and who obtain long term clinical benefit from them. The use of destructive neurolytic blocks and neurosurgical procedures for pain relief are now largely reserved for those with a limited life expectancy, due to the associated increased morbidity. However, there is much conflict within the speciality and choice of treatment will be influenced by the personal bias of the individual practitioner.

The current approach towards chronic pain has much greater emphasis on both the physiological and psychological implications than previously. The multi-disciplinary approach is thought to be the most effective one and many pain clinics today are looking towards or already have an established multi-disciplinary team. A multi-disciplinary team could comprise anaesthetists, nurses, physiotherapists, psychologists, psychiatrists, physicians, surgeons, oncologists, occupational therapists and social workers, all playing a part in the long term management of a patient with chronic pain.

Chronic pain is an important growing area of research and is often overlooked as with most chronic illness. The cost of chronic pain is high, for both the sufferers and the health care systems; quality of life versus financial restraints.

Cancer pain

Cancer pain attracts much publicity and is an emotive topic. Today it is possible for cancer pain to be generally well managed in western societies, thanks to the work of the hospice movement, World Health Organisation (WHO), and charitable organisations who have been responsible for the development of international education programmes. In the third world patients are less fortunate due to limited resources, political and economic restrictions which affect the availability of drugs and other interventions, but much is being done to improve the situation. The incidence of cancer pain is commonly over estimated by the general public, who often associate cancer with an inevitable painful death and believe that all patients with cancer suffer pain. Many patients who may have previously required specialist advice for management of pain can now be very well looked after in the community by their general practitioners and community services, due to the well publicised principles of cancer pain management (i.e. the analgesic ladder). Those patients whose pain cannot be controlled by straightforward pharmacological interventions may need specialist advice and intervention, which can be obtained from pain clinics or continuing care units. In the majority of cases cancer pain is less difficult to manage than some of the non-malignant pain conditions.

Professional bodies

The International Association for the Study of Pain (IASP) is a multi-disciplinary organisation which has attracted an increasing number of nurses over recent years. Members receive the journal *Pain* and a regular update of international research findings and meetings. The society holds its congress every 3 years. The invited speakers for this are internationally renowned and attract many people world wide; there are usually special sessions for nurses. Most countries have their own chapter of IASP and there are also a number of European Societies which are developing to meet the needs of this growing speciality. The nursing interest in pain is reflected by the increasing number of study days at both national and local levels, which are usually over subscribed. The small but growing number of specialist nurses throughout the country are inundated with requests for advice on clinical and educational aspects of pain management. Many nurses are now familiar with standard pain assessment

techniques, but they are not implemented widely as part of everyday clinical practice.

The Pain Society for Britain and Ireland, which is a multi-professional body, encourages nurse membership and is a useful resource. The annual meeting of the society has formal scientific presentations, free presentations, poster sessions and workshops and is an opportunity for individuals to meet other professionals working in the speciality.

The Pain Research Focus group (RCN Pain Forum) has been established for 2 years and it now has around 100 members. The founder members recognised the need for a Pain Society for nurses, to provide both professional and educational resource support. It received formal recognition as as an RCN subgroup in 1992. The group holds an annual conference and workshops on selected topics throughout

Table 1.1 Problems pertaining to the role of the specialist nurse

Define areas of responsibility – acute, chronic, cancer pain?
Problems – The workload is generally too vast for one nurse to cover all areas. Concentrate on one specific area.
Accountability/responsibility – nursing vs medical? – conflicts – expectations of role.
Support networks – personal and professional – often working in isolation in a new speciality.
Role and function
a. Educational
    personal professional development – availability of resources and training.
    keep updated with current research and development within the area.
    education of nursing colleagues – to be a resource herself – formal education programmes and informal.
    extended role of the nurse – special pain relieving interventions, e.g. PCA, epidurals.
b. Clinical role
    own patient workload.
    standard setting and policy development.
    pain assessment – implementation of tools in clinical areas.
    liaison between medical and nursing colleagues.
    awareness of specific areas which need development.
    implementation of research findings into clinical practice.
    resource for nursing colleagues and patients.
c. Research
    adequate record keeping and documentation.
    audit and evaluation – can the role be justified – patient satisfaction, other colleagues, do they benefit?
    own research and monitoring of current levels of practice.
    advising others on research projects relating to pain.

the year. The committee is working on setting standards and a national curriculum for pain.

The specialist nurse

There is a growing number of nurses in 'clinical specialist' roles in the UK and pain is one of these specialist areas. There are problems with this, as many nurses go into the role with an interest in pain, but have had no previous specialist training and are expected to have specialist knowledge and skills. There is currently no set standard for the specialist nurse in the pain setting and many nurses find that they have to develop their own role, working in isolation, with little support or infrastructure from their nursing and medical colleagues. They often have to depend on external resources, i.e. nurses in similar posts elsewhere, and study days. Pain is too broad a field for a nurse to become specialist in all areas, i.e. acute, chronic and cancer pain, as this would require years of experience, and therefore others' expectations of the specialist nurse are sometimes set too high. It would be more realistic to concentrate time and skills into one particular area.

The clinical nurse specialist has several roles to fulfil: clinical, educational and research. The clinical and educational responsibility is for patients, herself and colleagues. It is important that she is up to date with current developments and research and applies them to her own clinical areas and to be a resource for others. In order for her to function effectively it is important that she is given an adequate infrastructure, personal and professional support, training and resources. The problems with self developed

roles such as these is that they often lead to inter-professional conflicts as to what her role actually is, particularly with regard to the extended role of the nurse. It is important to clarify this at an early stage (See Table 1.1).

This book aims to provide nurses working in the clinical setting with a broad background knowledge of the pain management methods currently available, how they work and when to use them. The nurse plays a central role as a member of the multi-disciplinary team and it is important that she is aware of her role and responsibility for the safe implementation of pain relieving measures, in order to provide her patients with the highest level of care and comfort to hasten recovery. A common problem is the lack of knowledge about available resources, both for clinical advice and education, and each chapter has a list of resources and further reading for those who wish to read about specific areas in greater detail where applicable.

References

McQuay, H. J., Carroll D. and Moore R. A. (1988) Post-operative orthopaedic pain; the effect of opiate pre-medication and local anaesthetic blocks. *Pain*, **33**, 291–295

McQuay, H. J. (1992) Pre-emptive analgesia. *British Journal of Anaesthesia*, **69** (1), 1–3

Report of the Working Party on pain after surgery (1990) *Commission on the Provision of Surgical Services*. Royal College of Surgeons of England and The College of Anaesthetists

Wall, P. D. (1988) The prevention of post-operative pain. *Pain*, **33**, 289–290

2

Pain management in nursing

David Bowsher

Size and nature of the problem

In nursing and medical practice, we are concerned largely with a division between *acute* and *chronic* pains. Acute pain is an immediate consequence of the injury/trauma (including operation – i.e. post-operative pain) and of many acute, particularly inflammatory, illnesses. Nobody knows how much acute pain there is in any community, because it is either unreported or dealt with (rightly) as part of the causative condition. However, it *is* known that pain is the symptom which is responsible for about one third of all family practitioner (GP, primary care) consultations, which is a very large number.

Chronic pain is defined (not very satisfactorily) as pain, of constant or intermittent nature, which has persisted for 3 months or more. Several surveys have been done, in several countries, on the prevalence of chronic pain in the population as a whole. The most authoritative is probably the one conducted for *WHICH? Way to Health* in early 1990 (Rigge, 1991). This survey of just over 1000 people took account of age, sex, socio-economic status, and geographical distribution so as to reflect the population as a whole. Their overall figure (which is very close to that arrived at in smaller and more restricted surveys in Canada and Sweden) is 7%, i.e. just over 1 person in every 14 of the adult population of the UK has been in pain for 3 months or more. This is an enormous number, and shows what an important problem chronic pain is. As might be expected, the prevalence of chronic pain increases with age. Between the ages of 15 and 24, only 4% of people are in pain; between 25 and 34, 5%; from 35 to 44, 7.5%; from 45 to 54; nearly 10%; and over 55, 20% and upward. Since the UK,

like most other Western countries, has an ageing population, the size of the problem can be expected to increase.

Furthermore, 70% of the survey subjects who were in pain stated that they were taking 'painkillers' (unspecified); since, despite this, they were still in pain, it does not say much for most of the treatments currently being handed out for it! For specific conditions, it has been shown that there were 330 000 referrals to hospital for back pain in the UK in 1985. These patients make up 26% of referrals to pain clinics. Another quarter of pain clinic referrals suffer from pain due to nerve dysfunction, and 25% of the UK's 1 000 000 diabetics are reckoned to suffer from chronic pain as a result of this disease (Chan *et al.*, 1990).

Definitions

The International Association for the Study of Pain (IASP) is the official world body dealing with the subject; its membership includes nurses, doctors, physiotherapists, social workers, psychologists, and anyone else with a professional interest in pain and its relief. The IASP (1986) defines pain as:

An unpleasant sensory and emotional experience associated with actual or potential tissue damage, or described in terms of such damage.

Many professionals are not very happy with this definition, which was produced by a committee; however, as all different groups are *equally* unhappy with it, it is accepted.

It is common among lay people to say things like 'Mr Jones has a lower pain threshold than

Mrs Brown', and unfortunately many doctors and nurses go along with this, and do the same. IASP defines *pain threshold* as

The least experience of pain which a subject can recognise.

The original definition, which was: 'the least intensity of stimulation which a subject calls painful', is another way of saying the same thing. If a large number of volunteers are tested, to see *how* hard a clamp must be applied to a finger, or *how* hot a probe applied to the forearm needs to be for the subject to say that it is painful, then it is found that *pain threshold* is in fact fairly constant from one normal person to another, within the usual biological limitations. In terms of temperature, (the easiest to measure) it is usually about 44°C. The catch is, of course, that in medical practice we do not see subjects at the moment they experience the *least* degree of pain. If a pin or a hot object comes into contact with some part of the body, we remove that part of the body from the offending stimulus.

What of course *does* differ between Mr Jones and Mrs Brown is *pain tolerance level* – defined as the greatest level of pain which a subject is prepared to put up with. Pain tolerance level is a far more important concept in medicine than is pain threshold, for it is usually when pain has gone *beyond* tolerance level that a person seeks professional help.

The very important concept of pain tolerance level (which it might have been better to call pain *in*tolerance level) explains a number of observations which are a matter of everyday experience in nursing practice, and therefore often overlooked in terms of theoretical importance. Because pain tolerance level, unlike pain (or any other) threshold, can be influenced (or, to use the technical term, *modulated*) by a large number of factors, pain tolerance level in any single individual can vary from one day to another. It can also vary under different circumstances, so that, for example, most of us have a very low tolerance level for gratuitously inflicted pain, such as someone treading on the toe; but would have a very *high* tolerance level if it were necessary to rescue a child from a burning building. So it might be more convenient to think of pain tolerance level as the greatest amount of pain that a person is able to put up with *at that particular moment and in those particular circumstances.*

Types of pain

The most obvious division of pain is into acute and chronic. The patient who arrives in the A & E Department with a fractured tibia or arrives in the ward with acute appendicitis, is obviously in *acute* pain, as, perhaps a little less obviously, is the patient who comes back from operation to recover from extensive surgery. On the other hand, the patient who has had osteoarthritis for years, or the long term cancer sufferer, are equally obviously suffering from chronic pain.

But we need to define these terms and to try to distinguish the differences as well as the similarities between them. Of course an acute pain often goes on to become chronic, and this poses the problem of *when* this happens. By 'official' definition, chronic pain is pain which has lasted continuously or intermittently for 3 months or more. However, nursing and medical common sense often allow us to to predict much earlier when a pain is likely to become chronic – in the rheumatological clinic, it is conceivable that a patient may be seen within a few weeks of developing rheumatic pains – but we know perfectly well that the pain is going to last.

While keeping in mind the 'official' definitions, it is most practical to adopt a behavioural or psychological description. Acute pain is that pain which is accompanied by *anxiety* on the part of the patient, who is distinctly worried about it. What is the cause? What is going to happen? Does the pain betoken something dreadful? What can be done about it, either by the sufferer or the caring professional?

However, when the pain has been present for some time, the patient begins to accept it as part of life, and becomes *depressed*, which is perhaps the best behavioural definition of chronic pain. Of course there are many individuals in whom depression can only be diagnosed by the expert or the unusually perspicacious person (i.e. the good nurse). 'Much suffering, nobly borne' is no more admirable than little suffering strongly resented – it all depends on the individual's basic psychological makeup. Much depends on the nurse's expectation, and it is not right to expect male human beings to put up with more pain than females. Indeed, biologically (and in very general terms), while men may be better (i.e. more stoical) at handling acute pain, they are usually less good than women when it comes to coping with chronic pain. It is not for members of the caring professions to pass judgement in these matters, but to accept that any patient has as much pain as he/she says he/she has.

Patients' attitudes to, and therefore expression of, chronic pain depend very much on the diagnosis, not necessarily the true diagnosis, but what the patient, correctly or otherwise, believes to be the cause of his/her pain. In many cases, for instance, the pain of cancer is not particularly severe, but the patient with malignant disease, aware of its probable fatal outcome, may (quite understandably) be *more* depressed than a patient with a more severe pain due to a benign cause.

However, there are certain common features in almost every individual's emotional reaction to pain. When pain first strikes, the patient displays *anxiety* – what is causing it, what will happen next, is it serious, am I going to die? When pain continues, i.e. is becoming chronic, sufferers become *depressed* – an extra and apparently inescapable burden has been added to life, and it seems as though nothing is going to change it. As opposed to the mental and perhaps physical hyperactivity of anxiety, depressed patients may become extremely passive and inactive. It is very important for nurses to understand and make allowance for these emotional changes which accompany acute and chronic pain. Patients cannot be reasoned out of anxiety or jollied out of depression. Occasionally, professional psychiatric help is needed, often on the advice of nursing staff who observe the patient over longer time periods than other members of the caring professions.

Attempts have been made to correlate acute and chronic pain with the first and second pain of physiology (see below), but they are not really the same thing at all. Acute and chronic pain can really only be defined clinically; the importance of recognising the difference is that they should be treated differently, particularly when it comes to the attitude to be adopted by the nurse.

Pain measurement

When patients are asked about their pain, they are very keen to try and express how *bad* it is. This is where the nurse has to establish rapport, so that the patient knows that the nurse accepts that the pain *is* bad, and does not need persuading. It is of course necessary to know where a pain *is* – and to determine this, the patient may have to be asked to indicate it with *one finger*, as there is a too frequent tendency to pass the hand vaguely and at a distance over extensive regions of the body. To overcome this, it may be useful to present the patient with a body chart or silhouette and ask them to mark the painful area. One also needs to know whether pain is constant or intermittent; and if it comes intermittently, how often, and how long does each episode last.

However, the most important thing which the health professional needs to know is:

What does the pain feel *like*?

The answer to this question is frequently of great importance in determining the *kind* of pain from which the patient is suffering, and thus, in some cases, the sort of treatment which should be given. There are two ways in which the nature or quality of the pain can be established. One is simply to ask the question. However, we cannot be certain that a word chosen spontaneously by the patient means the same thing to him/her as it does to the nurse: 'aching' or 'burning' are obvious enough; but what does someone else mean by 'galvanic', or even 'electrical'? One way round this is to use a forced-choice paradigm, whereby the subject is obliged to choose a word or words from a list which is put in front of her/him. There are a number of such lists, but the one most used in pain work is the *McGill Questionnaire* (Melzack, 1975) (Figure 2.1). The patient is asked to encircle or underline not more than one word in any group which appears to describe his/her pain. The patient must also be told that it is not necessary to choose a word from every one of the 20 groups, but *only* those words applicable to the pain felt at this moment.

In addition to its diagnostic value, the McGill Questionnaire can be used to quantify the *intensity* of pain for any given patient. The simplest way to do this is to give the score 1 to the first word in any group, 3 to the third, and so on. The score for the whole questionnaire is added up, and divided by the number of words chosen. This makes scores comparable between patients who have chosen words from four or five groups and those who have chosen words from all 20. If the McGill Questionnaire is administered to the same patient on different occasions, scoring makes it possible to assess progress.

However, this is rather cumbersome, and the

Name ....

Address ....

....

McGILL PAIN QUESTIONNAIRE

DIRECTIONS: Look carefully at the twenty groups of words. Choose any ONE word in any group that applies to YOUR pain, and circle it – but do **not** circle more than ONE word in any group, even if more than one *seems* to apply; in that case, circle the one that is *most* applicable. In groups where NO words apply to your particular pain, leave the whole group blank.

1	2	3	4	5
Flickering	Jumping	Pricking	Sharp	Pinching
Quivering	Flashing	Boring	Cutting	Pressing
Pulsing	Shooting	Drilling	Lacerating	Gnawing
Throbbing		Stabbing		Cramping
Beating		Lancinating		Crushing
Pounding				

6	7	8	9	10
Tugging	Hot	Tingling	Dull	Tender
Pulling	Burning	Itching	Sore	Taut
Wrenching	Scalding	Smarting	Hurting	Rasping
	Searing	Stinging	Aching	Splitting
			Heavy	

11	12	13	14	15
Tiring	Sickening	Fearful	Punishing	Wretched
Exhausting	Suffocating	Frightful	Gruelling	Blinding
		Terrifying	Cruel	
			Vicious	
			Killing	

16	17	18	19	20
Annoying	Spreading	Tight	Cool	Nagging
Troublesome	Radiating	Numb	Cold	Nauseating
Miserable	Penetrating	Drawing	Freezing	Agonizing
Intense	Piercing	Squeezing		Dreadful
Unbearable		Tearing		Torturing

Figure 2.1 The McGill Pain Questionnaire.

Make a mark on the line underneath, to indicate how far your pain is between NO PAIN and the WORST PAIN YOU EVER EXPERIENCED IN YOUR LIFE (whatever that was – it doesn't matter for this):

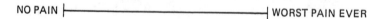

NO PAIN ├──────────────────────────────────┤ WORST PAIN EVER

Figure 2.2 The Visual Analogue Scale.

main use of the McGill Questionnaire is for pain diagnosis when a patient is seen for the first time. The quickest and most effective way of measuring pain intensity is by the Visual Analogue Scale (Figure 2.2) (Bond and Pilowsky, 1966). Essentially, the scale consists of a 10 cm scale, one end of which is marked 'No pain' and the other end 'The worst pain I ever felt'. The patient is asked to mark the line at the point which represents her/his pain *at that moment*; the distance along the line is subsequently measured. It can be done, of course,

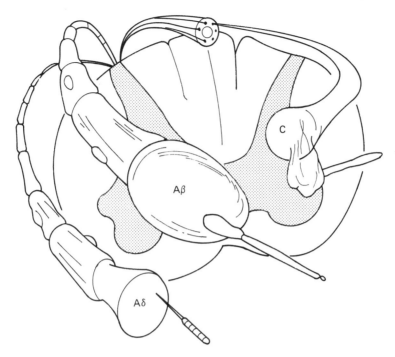

Figure 2.3 Primary afferent fibres from skin to spinal cord. The largest ($A\beta$) and most rapidly conducting myelinated fibres are activated by light touch (illustrated by a cotton bud); these are the fibres which are activated by TENS and vibration. Smaller, more slowly conducting ($A\delta$) myelinated fibres are activated by pinprick, and are involved in acupuncture stimulation. The smallest and slowest fibres (C) are unmyelinated, and are excited by tissue damage, here illustrated by a lighted match; they are often called *nociceptors*.

with strips of paper; but most nurses find it convenient to use a plastic scale* with a slider and a ruler on the back (which the patient cannot see).

Individual patients are remarkably consistent in their scores. The visual analogue scale (VAS) can be used, for example, every time TPR is measured, to assess whether a patient's pain is getting better or worse, or staying the same. Such frequent measurement may be used to evaluate postoperative pain. In chronic pain, however, measurements are made at much less frequent intervals.

Mechanisms of pain sensation

Specialised nerve endings recognise light, giving rise to the sensation we call vision; other specialised nerve endings are sensitive to sound, responsible for hearing, and yet others

to mechanical deformation of the skin, which we call touch. Equally, there are specialised nerve endings which recognise tissue damage; they are called *nociceptors* (Figure 2.3). When impulses from these nerves reach consciousness, we call it *pain*. It is most important to understand that pain results from the excitation of these specialised nerve endings, and *not* from the 'overstimulation' of other nerve endings. Normal touch nerves when stimulated can *never* give rise to any sensation other than touch, just as rods and cones when stimulated can never give rise to any sensation other than that of light 'stars in front of the eyes' when the eye is injured.

What the nerve endings recognising tissue damage are actually stimulated by is some chemical substance which is released or formed as a result of cell disruption. A number of substances are involved in this process, including prostaglandins. Some drugs interfere with these chemical processes, notably aspirin and the group known as 'non-steroidal anti-inflammatories' (NSAIDs). Such drugs act as pain-

*Plastic VAS rulers are available from the Pain Relief Foundation, Walton Hospital, Liverpool L9 1AE.

killers by (partially, at least) preventing the generation of 'pain' messages in the specialised nociceptor nerve endings.

Mention has been made earlier of the difference between pinprick sensation and true pain, in the context of pain perception threshold and pain tolerance level. In fact there are other specialised nerve endings which are sensitive to pinprick and/or sudden, pricking, heat – the kind of stimulus that warns of danger and makes you withdraw *before* tissue damage occurs. It is these nerve endings, or receptors, which are evaluated in measuring what is called 'pain perception threshold', while tissue damage receptors are responsible for pain tolerance level. So in fact physiology tells us that pain perception threshold and pain tolerance level are two entirely different phenomena, as different from each other as sight and hearing, mediated by two different kinds of receptor and nerve. At least two important practical observations can only be satisfactorily explained by the existence of two different and independent types of nerve ending (Bowsher, 1982):

1. As mentioned above, the reflex response to pinprick or to the a sudden encounter with something hot is to *withdraw before* tissue damage occurs; even, in fact, to try and prevent tissue damage from occurring. The response to tissue damage, once it has happened, is to keep still. This is often brought about by the tonic (i.e. long-term) contraction of muscles in *spasm*, *rigidity*, or *guarding*. A moment's thought reveals that this reflex could not possibly share the same circuit as the almost opposite reaction of sudden withdrawal.
2. Pain perception threshold (pinprick threshold) varies very little, either from time to time in the same person or from one person to another. But pain tolerance level varies enormously, both from one individual to another and in the same person at different times and under different circumstances. For example, a normal individual would soon say 'Stop' if someone else is inadvertently treading on their toe; but would hardly notice the pain (at the time) when rescuing a helpless patient from a burning ward.

   In dealing with sick patients, it is of course pain tolerance level which matters, and which we seek to alter with nursing care and medical or surgical treatment. It is pain tolerance level which is measured by the visual analogue scale, which is why it is such a valuable tool. If performed at the same time as TPR, it can be used as a record of the patient's progress towards the goal of pain relief. If the score does not get less over time, then it means that the pain-relieving treatment being used is not effective, and should be changed. Pain perception threshold is irrelevant to nursing care and medical care.
3. Narcotic analgesics such as morphine usually abolish tissue-damage (nociceptive) pain; but they have very little effect on pain perception threshold, i.e. pinprick sensation. Every nurse knows this, but may fail to grasp its importance. If a patient in pain from trauma is given an injection of morphine, the pain may disappear, as does the muscle spasm surrounding any resulting fracture. But if the patient is then give an injection of antibiotic, he/she is as aware of the needle as a normal individual. The practical importance of this is that you don't test pain tolerance level (true tissue-damage pain) with a pin; what you test with a pin is pinprick sensation.

Just as consideration of the reflex differences between reactions to pinprick and to tissue damage reveals that they must activate different segmental spinal circuits, so the difference between the effects of narcotics on tissue-damage pain and pinprick reveals that the pathways in the central nervous system by which these two stimuli become conscious must be different. The central pathway conveying pinprick stimuli to consciousness is relatively insensitive to morphine, while the pathway conveying messages generated by tissue damage is highly sensitive to narcotics.

Pain mechanisms in the spinal cord

When the peripheral nerve fibres carrying impulses generated by painful stimuli enter the spinal cord, they end in the *dorsal horn* of the spinal grey matter by passing through the *dorsal root* of the spinal nerve (Figure 2.3). As the motor nerve fibres supplying muscles leave the cord through the *ventral root* of the spinal nerve, it is possible for surgeons to relieve pain without producing muscle paralysis by cutting all the dorsal roots carrying nerve fibres from the part(s) of the body involved by damage or disease. However, this is not often done nowadays, because the dorsal root carries fibres subserving all sensations, not just pain; so a patient whose dorsal root(s) have been cut by the operation of *dorsal rhizotomy* lose all sensations, not just pain. They also lose messages from muscles telling the central nervous system about their state of contraction, so although not paralysed, they have no control over muscle contraction, which is almost as bad.

However, fibres carrying different types of sensation end at different levels in the dorsal horn of the spinal grey matter. Pain fibres end most superficially of all, while fibres conveying information about muscle contraction end most deeply. So it is sometimes possible for the neurosurgeon to damage the *superficial grey matter* of the dorsal horn without damaging deeper parts, thus hopefully abolishing pain sensation and little else. This operation is known as *Dorsal Root Entry Zone* (DREZ) destruction (Nashold and Ostdahl, 1979).

When a nerve fibre ends, it is involved in a *synapse*, in which the nerve message is chemically transmitted to the next nerve cell and its fibre. It is at synapses that modulation occurs and drugs act. An example of modulation is *accommodation*, whereby the nervous system gets used to certain stimuli such as the pressure of clothes on the body, so that we cease to take any notice of them. A more active form of modulation would be *inhibition*, whereby, for example, another *distracting stimulus* may make someone 'forget' about an ongoing painful stimulus. As we shall see later, this mechanism can be exploited therapeutically.

Many different chemical substances are involved in transmission at different synapses. However, no one transmitter substance is confined to a single functional system, so that, for instance, the transmitter called 'Substance P' which is found in many peripheral pain fibres, is also found in some fibre systems in the central nervous system which have nothing to do with pain; worse still, there are *some* pain fibres in the periphery whose transmitter substance is *not* Substance P but some other chemical.

The sensitivity of a synapse to any given drug depends on the ability of the drug in question to imitate or oppose the action of the natural transmitters at that particular synapse. Now it

happens that morphine, and drugs like it (narcotics), imitate an *inhibitory transmitter* (i.e. one which prevents further transmission) at the synapses in the spinal cord where peripheral pain fibres end. This of course is why morphine and other narcotics are such powerful weapons in the fight against pain. But morphine also acts at other synapses which have nothing to do with pain, such as the brain systems which control respiration (which are inhibited) and vomiting (which are excited). Thus morphine given systemically, by mouth or by injection, which becomes distributed via the bloodstream throughout the whole nervous system, not only reduces pain, which is desirable, but also depresses respiration and may produce nausea and/or vomiting, which are undesirable.

By a happy accident, as explained above, pain fibres are the ones which terminate most superficially in the spinal cord, i.e. nearest to its outer surface. So if a morphine-like drug is introduced into the space just outside the spinal cord, it seeps into the surface of the cord and acts only on the nearest synapses, i.e. those where pain fibres end, and does not reach the respiratory and vomiting centres in the brain. Thus pain relief without unwanted side effects can be produced by the technique of subarachnoid or epidural drug infusion.

The gate control theory

The mechanisms described above, and much else, can all be explained in terms of the *Gate Control Theory*, first put forward by Melzack and Wall in 1965. Many subsequent versions and modifications of the theory have been published, but essentially what it says is illustrated in Figure 2.4.

Imagine the central nervous system (spinal cord and brain) as a field surrounded by a fence which can be entered through a gate. Pain enters through the gate from outside; the more pain, the wider the gate opens. There are two ways in which the gate can be closed: it can be pulled to from the outside or pushed to from the inside. Pulling to can be brought about by the action of large peripheral nerve fibres carrying impulses generated by light mechanical stimuli such as touch. An example of this is 'rubbing a pain better'. This instinctive action activates large cutaneous nerve fibres which prevent (inhibit) some of the pain impulses from enter-

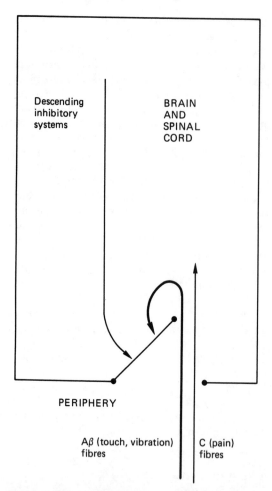

Descending inhibitory systems

BRAIN AND SPINAL CORD

PERIPHERY

Aβ (touch, vibration) fibres

C (pain) fibres

Figure 2.4 Gate control. This shows how thin (tissue damage responding) fibres force open the 'gate' into the central nervous system, bringing pain to consciousness. The gate can be pulled to from the outside, reducing pain, by the activation of large Aβ fibres (see Figure 2.3). by rubbing/massage, TENS, or vibration. The gate can also be pushed to from inside the CNS by various inhibitory systems descending from the brain; some of these inhibitory systems are activated by acupuncture, others by drugs.

ing the spinal cord. A more effective way of activating a greater number of large peripheral fibres is to stimulate them electrically by the technique of *transcutaneous nerve stimulation* (see Sjölund and Eriksson, 1980) or by *vibration* at particular frequencies.

Pushing the gate to from inside is brought about by messages descending from higher centres in the brain. We have already mentioned *distraction*. Another method may be *relaxation*. Finally, stimulating electrodes may be inserted into the fibres descending from the

brain which close the gate, and pain relief brought about by *deep brain stimulation*.

Opioids, enkephalins and endorphins

Opium, or its chemically pure form *morphine*, has been used for centuries as a painkiller, without its mechanism of action being understood. The really remarkable thing about morphine is that the only sensation with which it interferes is pain; it has no effect on touch or temperature sensation, or even on pinprick (see p. 10).

Considerations like this made scientists realise that morphine must be imitating some naturally-occurring *inhibitory* transmitter substance, i.e. one which prevents nerve impulses being generated in a neurone when a message is received (see Fields and Basbaum, 1989). This led to the discovery of the *enkephalins*, two naturally-occurring inhibitory transmitters which act like morphine in the spinal cord. The small *interneurones* which use enkephalin transmitters are in the grey matter near the surface of the spinal cord, and they synapse with the neurones which receive impulses from peripheral nociceptors (nerve fibres activated by tissue damage), preventing further messages being sent onwards by inhibiting them. As stated above, morphine (and drugs with a similar action, the *narcotics*) infused into the epidural or subarachnoid space can seep into the superficial part of the spinal cord and suppress pain transmission by imitating the action of the enkephalins.

But there are at least two ways of suppressing pain by the natural activation of enkephalin-containing interneurones. One of these is through the excitation of fine myelinated peripheral fibres which are set off by pinprick stimuli. This is the mechanism of pain suppression by *acupuncture*. In acupuncture, the needle is used to stimulate small myelinated nerve fibres by twiddling manually or exciting electrically two or three times a second (2 or 3 Hz), i.e. at a *low frequency*; but because pinprick requires considerably more energy than touch, at a (relatively) *high intensity*. Compare acupuncture with transcutaneous nerve stimulation, where the electrical stimulus is delivered at a *high frequency* (50 Hz or more), but a *low intensity*, equivalent to rubbing or touching very lightly.

Because acupuncture activates enkephalin-containing interneurones within the spinal cord, it should, in terms of gate control theory, be considered as one of the methods of slamming the gate from inside – though only just inside!

Shortly following the discovery of the enkephalins in the spinal cord, *beta-endorphin* was found in and near the pituitary gland in the brain. This is also a naturally-occurring morphine-like substance which can act both as a transmitter substance in the brain and as a *neurohormone* – a substance which, when released, may circulate within the nervous system and act at synapses which are sensitive to it. Beta-endorphin pathways run close to the thalamus in the forebrain and on down to the midbrain. It is at these points that neurosurgeons sometimes insert stimulating electrodes (deep brain stimulation – see above) to excite beta-endorphin release and so suppress pain – an example of gate-closing from a more distant point.

Under normal circumstances, beta-endorphin release is brought about by commands from the prefrontal region of the cerebral cortex. This is the brain area largely concerned with emotion, and explains why pain can be suppressed by the stress of, for example, rescuing someone else from danger, or by one's own fear or excitement – or even distraction.

Ascending pain pathways (Figure 2.5)

Pain is of course actually experienced, or consciously appreciated, in the brain, not in the spinal cord. So some consideration has to be given to the pathways by which impulses generated in the body by tissue damage reach the brain, where they are interpreted as pain sensation.

We have already seen how and where these impulses get into the spinal cord, and what may happen to them there. In the normal course of events, the messages pass through several synapses within a very short distance in the spinal grey matter, and thus are transmitted from the superficial grey matter of the spinal cord to the deeper layers in the same segment, and on the same side. From the deep grey matter of the spinal cord, long nerve fibres cross over to the other side of the cord and run up to the brain in the *anterolateral column* (or *funicu-*

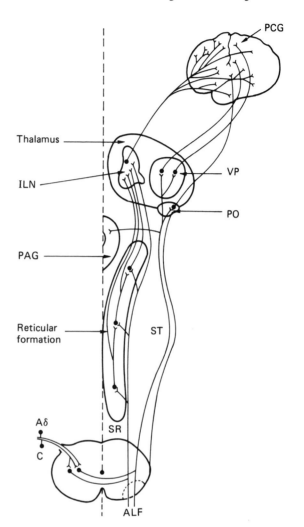

Figure 2.5 Central pain pathways. The anterolateral funiculus (ALF) of the spinal white matter contains two kinds of long ascending fibres; spinothalamic (ST) axons, principally activated by Aδ (pinprick) peripheral afferents, and spinoreticular (SR) axons, activated mainly, but indirectly, by C (tissue damage) peripheral afferents. Above the spinal cord, ST fibres remain on the lateral border of the brain stem and, after giving off collaterals to the periaqueductal gray (PAG) in the midbrain, terminate in the ventrobasal thalamus. The ventrobasal thalamus has two parts: the ventroposterior nucleus (VP), which projects point-to-point to the first somatic sensory area in the postcentral gyrus (PCG), and the posterior group (PO) of cells, which project to the second somatic sensory area in the region of the insula and parietal operculum. In the brain stem, SR fibres swing medially and end at various levels of the reticular formation; the longest SR axons reach the intralaminar nuclei (ILN) of the thalamus. The reticular formation also projects to the ILN, which gives rise to the so-called "diffuse" thalamocortical projection. This projection reaches all areas of the non-primary cortex, although with prefrontal predominance.

lus) of the spinal white matter (Bowsher, 1986) are near the surface of the cord (at between 4 and 5 o'clock, if you consider the spinal cord as a circle), and it is possible to cut or destroy them by the operation of *anterolateral cordotomy*, which can be performed by open operation at any spinal cord level, or in the neck by the insertion of a coagulating needle *percutaneously* between the vertebrae. Anterolateral cordotomy abolishes pain on the opposite side of the body below the level of operation.

There are two important points about cordotomy which everyone should understand and take account of. The first is that 'pain fibres' are not the only ones to run in the anterolateral funiculus: ascending fibres carrying messages about temperature and pinprick also ascend in the anterolateral funiculus, so that those sensations are also abolished (on the opposite side of the body) by anterolateral cordotomy. This means that it is easy to test the effectiveness of cordotomy by seeing if pinprick sensation is abolished in the part of the body where it is desired to get rid of pain; but it does not mean that pain and pinprick are the same thing, simply that the fibres carrying messages generated by them run together in the spinal cord.

The second important point about cordotomy is that after a time, usually from about 6 or 9 months upwards, the effects of cordotomy wear off. Nobody really understands this process, since once nerve fibres are cut or destroyed within the central nervous system they cannot be repaired; but it is assumed that the functions of the damaged fibres are taken over by other, undamaged, fibres – the theory of 'alternative pathways'. The practical implication of this is that anterolateral cordotomy is only used for pain when the duration of life is expected to be short, i.e. in malignant disease. Cordotomy is not used nowadays for non-malignant pain.

When the fibres in the anterolateral funiculus of the spinal cord reach the brain, they undergo further synaptic relays. The impulses are eventually distributed in a very diffuse manner to most of the cerebral cortex, where they become conscious. Because the messages are so widely distributed, it is not (unfortunately) possible to remove a small piece of cortex and thereby abolish pain, in the way that (for example) touch sensation may be abolished by a stroke damaging a relatively small area of cortex. However, it is sometimes possible to block the access of pain messages to the cortex by *hypnosis* (Hilgard and Hilgard, 1975).

Impulses generated by touch and vibration reach the brain by passing up the *posterior* or *dorsal* columns of the spinal cord white matter, on the same side as that on which they enter. This makes it possible to gain the same effect as from transcutaneous nerve stimulation by placing a stimulating electrode on or over the dorsal columns (*dorsal column stimulation*, DCS); but of course DCS is a form of high-frequency low-intensity stimulation which reaches a far greater number of fibres than does TNS.

Neurogenic pain

Neurogenic pain is defined as pain arising from peripheral nerves along their course or from the central nervous system, due to abnormal functioning (malfunction or dysfunction) *without involving the excitation of specific pain receptors (nociceptors)* (Bowsher, 1991). Everything that has been said in this chapter so far has been about pain caused by tissue damage, and the excitation of specialised nerve endings by chemical processes resulting from tissue damage, which is not involved in neurogenic pain (although of course there may be tissue damage, and therefore tissue-damage (nociceptive) pain as well). Neurogenic pain includes the categories commonly called *neuropathic pain* (usually involving peripheral nerves), deafferentation pain (often involving physical lesions of the nervous system) and *central pain* (usually applied to pain arising from central nervous system damage such as stroke), and it differs in a number of important respects from tissue-damage pain.

First, because neurogenic pain does not involve 'pain nerves' in the peripheral or central nervous system, none of the drugs (including morphine) or surgical procedures which suppress tissue damage pain have any really effective action on this type of pain.

Some neurogenic pains are quite common: for example, postherpetic neuralgia following shingles; painful diabetic neuropathy; trigeminal neuralgia; reflex sympathetic dystrophy following fracture; causalgia following nerve injury; some cases of phantom limb pain; and central post- stroke pain ('thalamic syndrome') which follows some 2% of all strokes. In addition, there are mixed tissue damage and neurogenic pains. For example, a herniated intervertebral disc causes tissue-damage pain in the back and neurogenic pain in the leg (sciatica) by compressing a nerve root; and many tumours may compress nerves or even the spinal cord in addition to causing tissue damage. In none of these cases does any tissue-damaging process excite specific 'pain' nerve endings in the way described above.

There are a number of ways in which neurogenic pain can be recognised. The pain is frequently (but not always) described as *burning* and/or *shooting*, in addition to any other words used. If the 'burning' is described in terms of scalding or ice-burn (like holding one's hand in iced water), the diagnosis is even more likely.

People with neurogenic pain suffer from instability of the autonomic nervous system, so that their pain is frequently made worse by emotional or physical (cold, fatigue) stress; and is relieved by relaxation, so that the patients are able to fall asleep normally despite their pain (they may wake in pain, or be woken by it).

But the most characteristic feature of neurogenic pain, which is *never* seen in tissue damage pain, is allodynia. This is pain triggered by a non-painful stimulus such as a light touch or even a puff of wind. While patients may describe this as 'tenderness', it differs from the tenderness of inflammation in that firm pressure is rarely painful.

A number of manoeuvres, such as blockade of sympathetic ganglia, are reputed to be helpful in some forms of neurogenic pain. Transcutaneous or dorsal column stimulation may be helpful in some cases, because high-frequency low-intensity stimulation does not act through an enkephalin or endorphin mechanism. Acupuncture, on the other hand, which is so useful in some tissue damage pains of musculoskeletal origin, is of no help in neurogenic pains because it acts by releasing the morphine-like enkephalin which exerts its influence only on the classical tissue-damage pain pathways; and these are not implicated in neurogenic pain.

The mainstay of treatment for neurogenic pain at the present time, however, is *amitriptyline* (Watson *et al.*, 1982). This is a drug normally used as an antidepressant, but which has a separate and specific action on neurogenic pain. Amitriptyline is not the ideal treatment for neurogenic pain, but at the present time it is the best available. The important thing about it, from a practical point of view, is that the sooner it is administered, the more effective it is. This is why it is important to be able to recognise neurogenic pain, and not to waste time trying (unsuccessfully) to alleviate it with conventional analgesics before turning to amitriptyline.

References

Bond, M. R. and Pilowsky, I. (1966) The subjective assessment of pain and its relationship to the administration of analgesics in patients with advanced cancer. *Journal of Psychosomatic Research*, **10**, 203–207

Bowsher, D. (1982) A note on the distinction between first and second pain. In *Anatomical, Physiological, and Pharmacological Aspects of Trigeminal Pain* (ed. B. Matthews and R. G. Hill), Excerpta Medica, Amsterdam, pp. 3–6

Bowsher, D. (1986) Pain mechanisms in man. *Medical Times*, **114**, 83–96

Bowsher D. (1991) Neurogenic pain syndromes and their management. *British Medical Bulletin*, **47**, 644–666

Chan, A. W., MacFarlane, I. A., Bowsher, D. *et al.* (1990) Chronic pain in patients with diabetes mellitus: comparison with a non-diabetic population. *The Pain Clinic*, **3**, 147–159

Fields, H. L. and Basbaum, A. I. (1989) Endogenous pain control mechanism. In *Textbook of Pain*, 2nd edition (ed. P. D. Wall and R. Melzack), Churchill Livingstone, Edinburgh, pp. 206–217

Hilgard, E. R. and Hilgard, J. R. (1975) *Hypnosis in the Relief of Pain*. William Kaufmann, Los Altos, California

International Association for the Study of Pain (1986) Classification of chronic pain. Descriptions of chronic pain syndromes and definitions of pain terms. *Pain*, **Supplement 3**

Melzack, R. (1975) The McGill Pain Questionnaire: major properties and scoring methods. *Pain*, **1**, 277–299

Melzack, R. and Wall, P. D. (1965) Pain mechanisms: a new theory. *Science*, **150**, 971–979

Nashold, B. S. and Ostdahl, R. H. (1979) Dorsal root entry zone lesions for pain relief. *Journal of Neurosurgery*, **51**, 59–69

Rigge, M. (1990) Pain. *WHICH? Way to Health*, **April**, pp. 66–68

Sjölund, B., Eriksson, M. (1980) *Relief of Pain by TENS*. John Wiley & Sons, Chichester

Watson, C. P. N., Evans, R. J., Reed, K. *et al.* (1982) Amitriptyline versus placebo in postherpetic neuralgia. *Neurology*, **32**, 671–673

Woolf, C. J. (1989) Segmental afferent fibre-induced analgesia: transcutaneous electrical nerve stimulation (TENS) and vibration. In *Textbook of Pain*, 2nd edition (eds P. D. Wall and R. Melzack), Churchill Livingstone, Edinburgh, pp. 884–896

3

Pain assessment

Dawn Carroll

Pain assessment is the most important part of the nurse's role when caring for the patient in pain, for which there are many tools readily available. It is not yet possible to measure pain objectively in the clinical setting as we would measure a blood pressure; instead we have to rely on subjective verbal methods. This chapter will describe the principles of pain assessment and a selection of the available assessment tools and their application in the clinical and research setting.

Basic principles of pain assessment

1. Subjective rating to be made by the patient.
2. Believe what the patient says about his pain.
3. Act promptly if pain is at unacceptable level.
4. Frequent evaluation of any interventions.

Communication

Good communication and observational skills are important for effective pain assessment.

Non-verbal communication (NVC)

Non-verbal communication is an important part of pain assessment, but is not the primary measure, except in those patients where verbal communication is impaired, e.g. the unconscious patient. NVC is a way in which people communicate information about themselves to others through non-verbal signal, e.g. body language. Speech can be used in combination with NVC. It should be noted that there are gender and cultural differences in the type of displays used. The nurse should be aware of the way in which people can display signals to indicate that they are in pain.

Visual displays of pain

Body movement – limited or restricted movement, guarding of parts of the body, abnormal postures and changes in stature.

Visual – eye contact increased/decreased, tears, facial expression – grimacing, muscle tension.

Vocal signals – sighing, crying, unspontaneous noises, change in pitch, impaired speech fluency.

Distance – patients can become physically withdrawn.

Emotion – anger, sadness, changes in mood.

Physical signs of pain

Changes in physiological signs can support the patient's report of pain, but should not be used as the sole measure (except in the unconscious patient where subjective verbal measurement is not possible).

Examples of physical signs of pain

Physiological – relative changes in blood pressure, pulse respiration rate, sweating.

Physical – in chronic pain there may be changes in limb size due to lack of use and muscle wasting, neurological abnormalities, change in temperature and skin colour (as in reflex sympathetic dystrophy) muscle spasm.

When to use non-verbal assessment of pain

1. *Primary measure* – patients with verbal communication problems, e.g. the elderly or very young, unconscious, mental retardation and psychological disturbance.
2. *Secondary measure* – all pain conditions.

Verbal communication

This should be the primary method of assessment unless no other method is possible. This chapter will concentrate on the verbal methods of assessment in adults (also refer to Chapters 9 and 10).

Patient expectations and information giving

Good communication is the starting point towards both pain assessment and effective pain management. It is important to establish the patient's expectations, not only directly related to pain but indirectly about what is going to happen to him.

Verbal communication – aims

– to provide information for the patient.
– to obtain information from the patient.

It is very important that we let the patient know what is happening to him at all times, e.g. informed consent, ethical issues are to be considered.

Acute pain

It is well documented that anxiety and pain are related (Chapman, 1985) and that it is important to alleviate fear as much as possible prior to surgery as this can reduce post-operative pain. This can be done simply by providing patients with adequate information about what is going to happen to them. The level of information given is crucial, as too much technical information can overwhelm the patient and lead to increased anxiety and pain and too little information can be equally detrimental. The level of information should be clear and concise and tuned towards each patient's needs. Ideally this should be presented both verbally and in written form, as patients often need time to digest information. It is important that this is done in a quiet relaxed atmosphere without interruption and the nurse should not appear hurried as this will restrict the patient.

Acute pain information

Indirectly related to pain

1. Operation details, duration of stay, planned schedule of events.
2. How the patient will feel after operation? How long will he be in bed? Will he have a drip? Ward routine, e.g. meal times, visiting.
3. Long term outcome and recovery, future hospital visits.

Directly related to pain

Will pain occur – when will it occur – how bad will it be – how long will it last – what can be done about it – how can he communicate his pain to others – what choices are there – what if pain relief is unsatisfactory – what does the pain mean.

What are the patients' expectations? Are they realistic?

Many patients have misconceptions about pain; some may not have considered the possibility of pain at all. It is important to discuss the possibility of having pain as it can be very disturbing for patients to awake from the anaesthetic in pain; they often feel that something has gone wrong, which can lead to unwarranted fear and increased anxiety. Other patients may expect to have a lot of pain; this may be based on previous personal experience or on information given by members of the general public, which can often be quite inappropriate. The nurse should identify the patient's expectations in order to allay unnecessary fears and anxiety and provide more accurate informed advice. It is important to emphasise that if pain occurs it will be treated promptly. Patients often do not know what to do if they have pain or who to report it to, or what measures will be taken to relieve it.

What will happen if the patient suffers pain?

As a general rule, pain after surgery is at its worst for the first few days and then declines. There are many factors which affect post-operative pain but the main predictors are the type and duration of surgery as well as individual variations (see Chapter 5). Some patients have an aversion to taking drugs of any kind and may express that they do not wish to take any medication. These feelings may be due to fears of addiction or concern about adverse effects or due to an unpleasant previous experience. It is important to keep the door open, as patients often change their minds if pain occurs. Another common fear is that of injections; it should be explained that there are other methods available. It can be useful to warn patients if there is a possibility of having a nerve blocking procedure as part of the anaesthetic. It can be very alarming for a patient to wake up and feel no sensation in a limb, as they often attribute this to surgical error or that something has gone wrong. It is also important to explain what may happen after the block has worn off, i.e. no pain at all, gradual onset of pain, or sudden onset of severe pain.

Communication with other health care professionals is vital for continuity of care, e.g. patient, nurse, doctor, family and other health professionals who may be involved in care.

Chronic pain

It is important that the patient's expectations related to the disease and treatment are established before any treatment is given.

What are patient's expectations in relation to treatment and outcome?

Patients with chronic pain frequently have illogical, unrealistic expectations relating to treatment and often seek a diagnosis and a cure. They often feel that surgical intervention is the answer to their problems and end up receiving differing opinions from many specialists and a multitude of treatments with limited benefit. In many cases cure is unattainable and the aim is to control the symptom in order to improve the quality of life. It is sometimes difficult to come to an agreed medical diagnosis or label; some labels are more acceptable than others and blame is often placed on the medical profession. All patients should be given a proper explanation when possible of what is causing the pain, what it means and what can be done about it. It often helps to inform the patient about what is not the cause, for example life threatening disease such as cancer. Chronic pain can be extremely disabling and can have a devastating affect on normal family life.

Pain documentation and choosing an assessment tool

How to take a pain history

Taking and recording a well detailed pain history is important to help determine possible cause of pain and to plan an appropriate treatment regimen. The following are useful points to use as guidelines.

Site of pain – where is the pain(s)?
Character of pain – what does the pain feel like?
Frequency of pain – how often does it occur?
Aggravating and relieving factors – what makes the pain worse/better?   ADL's?
Disability – how does pain affect every day life?
Duration of pain – how long has it been present?
Response to current/previous treatments – how effective/ineffective?

Site of pain – where is the pain?

A body chart is an effective tool used to record the site of pain. These are commonly used in hospices and pain clinics and may vary in detail. A basic body chart is a simple diagram on which the patient marks the areas which correspond to his pain. If a patient has more than one pain these can be coded using different colours or symbols. They can be used either independently or be incorporated into a more detailed pain chart. The chart illustrated in the figure (Figure 3.1) includes dermatome levels and levels of sensory impairment.

Type of pain – what does the pain feel like?

This can be done by simply asking the patient to describe his pain in his own words, e.g. a dull, nagging, aching. Or this can be approached using a more formal assessment such as the McGill Pain Questionnaire (Figure 3.2) (Melzack, 1975, 1983). This can be used in both the acute and chronic setting and has now been validated in several languages (e.g. French, Spanish, German, Italian).

The questionnaire consists of 78 descriptors which are placed in rank order into 20 groups. Each of the groups describes the affective, sensory, and evaluative nature of pain. Patients are asked to choose the word from each group (if any) which best describes their pain. The simple scoring methods are to sum the number of words chosen (1–20) and the sum of the

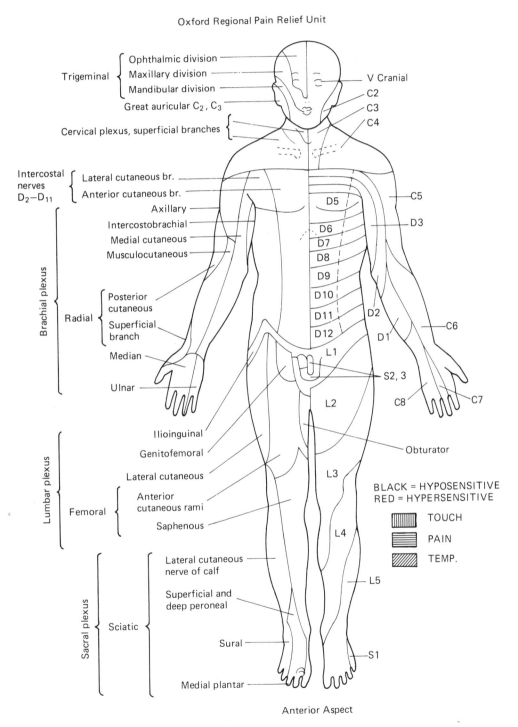

Figure 3.1 Oxford Regional Pain Relief Unit Body Chart

McGill Pain Questionnaire

Some of the following words describe your present pain. Circle the **one word in each group** that best describes it. Mark only one word in each group. Skip the groups that do not apply.

1	2	3	4	5
flickering	jumping	pricking	sharp	pinching
quivering	flashing	boring	cutting	pressing
pulsing	shooting	drilling	lacerating	gnawing
throbbing		stabbing		cramping
beating		lancinating		crushing
pounding				

6	7	8	9	10
tugging	hot	tingling	dull	tender
pulling	burning	itching	sore	taut
wrenching	scalding	smarting	hurting	rasping
	searing	stinging	aching	splitting
			heavy	

11	12	13	14	15
tiring	sickening	fearful	punishing	wretched
exhausting	suffocating	frightful	gruelling	blinding
		terrifying	cruel	
			vicious	
			killing	

16	17	18	19	20
annoying	spreading	tight	cool	nagging
troublesome	radiating	numb	cold	nauseating
miserable	penetrating	drawing	freezing	agonising
intense	piercing	squeezing		dreadful
unbearable		tearing		torturing

Total number of words chosen:
McGill Score:

Guidelines

Dimension	Groups
Sensory	1–10
Affective	11–15 and 20
Evaluative	16
Miscellaneous	17–19

Figure 3.2 McGill Pain Questionnaire

ranked value of words chosen from the 20 groups of descriptors, a total of 78 words. Patients can also grade the severity of each chosen descriptor.

The McGill pain questionnaire is used most commonly in the research setting and specialised pain centres, particularly in the USA. Even the shortened version can take some time to complete (approximately 5–20 minutes) depending on the individual patient ability. This may have drawbacks in the immediate post-operative setting and those chronic pain patients who are in a highly anxious state may

be unsuitable for this lengthy assessment, although it is generally useful in the assessment of chronic pain. The major advantage of the McGill Pain Questionnaire is that it considers the character and quality of the pain as well as the overall intensity. The clinical application of the McGill Pain Chart remains controversial (Gracely, 1992; Holroyd et al., 1992), but nurses should be familiar with this tool as it provides a useful guideline to the wide range of descriptors which may be used by their patients and which may aid accurate diagnosis and treatment.

Frequency of pain. How often does the pain occur?

Not all pain is constant. Intermittent pain which may occur only several times a day can be equally debilitating for the patient. Attacks can last seconds, hours or days and can affect the patient's ability to function normally, e.g. migraine, facial pain. For example, a patient may have a constant pain in the back with associated intermittent leg pain; the mechanisms of the two pains may be very different and need different approaches.

Aggravating or relieving factors – what makes the pain better or worse?

It is important to identify the factors which aggravate and those which relieve the pain, e.g. heat, cold, exercise, rest, movement. This is important not only for diagnostic purposes, but can give clues as to which treatments may be beneficial. These may vary widely between patients, from simple movements to heavy physical exercise brought on by both work and leisure related tasks.

Some patients may have pain which is related to movement or rest and may have to perform a specific task before the pain occurs; it is important to consider this when undertaking assessment. In the research context patients may be asked specifically about the 'maximum pain position' and may be questioned about 'pain on rest' or 'pain on movement' separately. In postthoracotomy pain it is common to ask patients about the 'pain on coughing', which may be more informative than 'pain on rest'.

Disability – how does the pain affect the patient?

Chronic pain is frequently associated with disability and it is important to assess what is the major problem for the patient; the disability or the pain, as this will affect the treatment to be prescribed. Formal disability assessments are commonly used in rehabilitation and orthopaedic centres. They are useful in conditions such as rheumatoid arthritis and pain following trauma as an outcome measure. It is important to appreciate that when an intervention is applied there may be no overall change in pain levels but activity levels may increase. Improv-

ing function alone is of great importance to the patients' quality of life.

Duration of pain. How long has the pain been present?

In chronic conditions pain may have been present for many years, in the acute setting it may only be minutes or hours in duration. It is important when treating patients with chronic pain to find out whether the pain has changed at all since the original onset, as this may indicate disease progression or a new causative factor. In acute pain it is normal for pain to decline over a short period of time. If it does not and the pain either escalates or does not resolve as expected, it must then be further investigated as prolonged pain can be an indication that there is an underlying physical cause, such as infection.

Response to current and previous treatments. What drugs/treatments has the patient had in the past and how effective were they?

Patients with chronic pain may have received a multitude of treatments over a period of time. It is important that all previously tried pain relieving interventions, as well as those being currently used, are documented in the patient's records and kept up to date; this will help to prevent wasting time and effort in the future. Useful information to record includes; the name of drug/treatment; dose; when it was given; how long was it used for; how often was it used; how effective it was and why was it stopped; if adverse effects occurred then what were they.

Patients, particularly those who are elderly, or those who are taking a selection of tablets, often get confused about their medication schedule. It is important that the nurse ensures that patients are aware which tablets they are taking and the reason they are being prescribed. A drug diary is one method to improve patient compliance; all prescribed medications are listed and the times that they are to be taken recorded, any special points can be included in the diary. The patient should keep the card with him and take it to all clinic attendances that he may have so that all changes can be recorded. Any discontinued medications can be simply deleted.

Medication diary					
Patient name: David Bowsher					
Tablet name	**Dose**	**No. of tablets to be taken**	**Time**	**Comments**	**Date**
ibuprofen	400 mg	1 (capsule)	3 times a day am, 2 pm, 10 pm	for pain relief take with food	1.3.91
amitriptyline	75 mg	1 (capsule)	before going to bed	for pain relief	2.6.92

Choosing a pain assessment tool

Practical tips

- Choose a simple tool which is quick and easy to use.
- Use a tool that has been validated and shown to work.
- Adapt existing tools if necessary.
- Ensure that those who are to use the tool understand them.
- Use one tool in each clinical setting.
- Try out a selection of different charts to find one which is most suitable.
- Find out from other users what they think – pros and cons.
- Make sure that assessment and evaluation is done regularly.
- Act promptly on results shown from patient assessment.

Who does the assessments? Patient or nurse?

There is much research evidence to say that professionals frequently underestimate the patient's level of pain, one of the contributing factors responsible for this are the attitudes of medical and nursing staff (Donovan, 1983; Kuhn *et al.*, 1990; Lavies *et al.*, 1992). In addition, following surgery there is inadequate prescribing and administration of analgesic drugs (Mather and Phillips, 1986; Royal College of Surgeons Report, 1990); these findings emphasise the need to implement formal assessment.

Pain assessment tools subjectively measure the patient's unique experience of pain and assessment should ideally be done by the patient and evaluated by the nurse, who is present at each assessment time. The classic analgesic study method uses a single nurse observer technique to reduce bias. However, this is unrealistic in the clinical setting. There is no reason why a patient cannot complete assessments independently and indeed they often do, following initial supervision and guidance, with choice of an appropriate tool. The success of pain assessment does, however, depend on the frequency that the charts are evaluated by nursing and medical staff. It is pointless for the patient to make the effort to complete a pain chart if no-one takes the trouble to review it regularly and take necessary appropriate action. In the outpatient/community setting patients complete pain diaries and do this well. Patients find the charts beneficial and the assessments are not intrusive on their time. Those who use pain charts find them beneficial. It enables patients and their families to make a contribution to their care and have a better understanding of the pain, and they feel that health care professionals are taking more interest. Diaries make the evaluation of treatment much easier from the medical point of view and are often more reliable than the patients' retrospective recollection. Pain assessment is crucial for accurate dose titration of morphine in cancer pain management and pain diaries help in the precision of dose selection.

Frequency of pain assessment

Regular re-evaluation is necessary in all pain settings. The frequency of assessment should be judged according to the individual patient needs and situation. As a rule, the following guidelines may be useful:

Acute pain. Frequent initial assessments to be done according to individual patient needs, at least hourly in the immediate post-operative period and then less often as the pain decreases over time. Assessment will be affected by time restraints, but these should not be used as an excuse to avoid assessment, no matter how busy the ward situation.

Chronic pain. Often concerned with long term outcome and assessment is done less frequently than in the acute setting, this may be in terms of days and weeks rather than hours. When introducing new treatments i.e. change in drug

class or dose it may be appropriate to increase the frequency of assessment.
Cancer pain. This will depend on the level of pain control which has been obtained. If poorly controlled it may be necessary to do at least hourly assessments as in the acute setting, but the interval can be increased once the pain level is at a more stable and acceptable level.

Which assessment tool to choose

The easiest way to find out if a patient is in pain is to ask him: 'Have you got pain – yes or no?' However, this is too simplistic and provides no information about either the quality or quantity of the pain, which is important when making a decision as to which treatment to give, or when evaluating the overall effect of a previously given treatment. Therefore a more formal tool is required for effective assessment and it is in the patient's best interest if this is done in the form of written documentation which is incorporated into the individual care plan. There are no rules as to which pain assessment tool is the best for clinical use and there are many to choose from. The important issue is that an attempt is made to formally assess pain rather than it being ignored. Nurses should have a background knowledge of available assessment tools; which one is most suitable for a particular patient group, and that the benefits of formal assessment are recognised. It can be useful to find out what assessment tools other colleagues are using and what they like or don't like about the charts which they may be using. Pain assessment should be approached with a positive attitude and not be seen as being yet another form to fill in.

Categorical verbal rating scales

Pain intensity – how bad is the pain?
severe (3)
moderate (2)
mild (1)
none (0)

Pain relief – how much relief has the treatment given?
none(0)
slight (1)
moderate (2)
good (3)
complete (4)

Categorical verbal rating scales were originally designed as a research tool (Wallenstein and Houde, 1975) and are the traditional scales used in single dose studies. The patient is asked at each assessment time 'how bad is your pain at the current time?' The observer should not suggest or emphasise words to the patient as it will bias his report, e.g. '*is* the pain still severe?' The same is done for pain relief: 'how much relief have you got from XXX at the current time?'. These scales work well and are quick to use and simple, being suitable for most pain settings. Critics claim that there is not enough choice or scope within the categories; however, they remain one of the most reliable, sensitive and reproducible scales. The diagram shows a 4-point pain intensity scale and 5-point pain relief scale, but there are other similar scales with more points which are commonly used. The concept of 'current' pain intensity is relevant to the acute setting but always so for chronic pain and where pain levels fluctuate. In chronic pain it may be sometimes more relevant to ask about 'typical' pain intensity or relief over a given period of time, e.g. 'how bad has the pain been over the last week/day' rather than 'how intense is the pain at the present moment in time?' The manner in which the assessments are presented to the patient by the assessor is crucial to the answer which is obtained.

Global rating scales

These scales are used to evaluate the overall efficacy of treatment: 'How effective was the treatment?' The example shown below is a 5-point scale.

poor = 0
fair = 1
good = 2
very good = 3
excellent = 4

The Oxford Pain chart (McQuay, 1990)

The Oxford Pain chart is an example of how categorical scales have been incorporated into a pain diary (Figure 3.3). This was originally developed as a tool for use in chronic pain, but could be easily adapted for other situations.

OXFORD PAIN CHART

Name_____   Treatment Week _____

Please fill in this chart each evening before going to bed. Record your pain intensity and the amount of pain relief. If you have had any side-effects please note them in the side-effects box.

	DATE								
Pain Intensity How bad has your pain been today?	severe								
	moderate								
	mild								
	none								
Pain Relief How much pain relief have the tablets given today?	complete								
	good								
	moderate								
	slight								
	none								
Side effects Has the treatment upset you in any way?									

How effective was the treatment this week? *poor fair good very good excellent* Please circle your choice.

Figure 3.3 Oxford Pain Chart

Make a mark on the line underneath, to indicate how far your pain is between NO PAIN and the WORST PAIN YOU EVER EXPERIENCED IN YOUR LIFE (whatever that was — it doesn't matter for this):

NO PAIN |———————————————————————| WORST PAIN EVER

Figure 3.4 Visual Analogue Scale

Visual analogue scales (Figure 3.4)

The concept of a linear scale has been popular for a long time and visual analogue scales are another sensitive and reproducible research tool which are popular in the clinical setting (Scott and Huskisson, 1976; Huskisson, 1983). Despite controversy over the design of these scales, e.g. should the lines be vertical or horizontal; should they have end markers or not; should they incorporate numerical or verbal descriptors at regular intervals, the crucial issue is whether or not the patient is able to use them and are they reproducible? All scales should be both reliable and reproducible and the visual analogue scales are, when used correctly. In the research context the visual analogue scales appear to be more sensitive than the categorical scales, as they are capable of measuring smaller changes. However, when taken into an uncontrolled setting there is more room for loss of sensitivity, particularly when there are multiple users involved. There are specific problems when using visual analogue scales for certain patient groups; the very young, in the immediate post-operative period and with those with impaired vision. Visual analogue scales can also be used to measure pain relief, mood, sleep and disability and are easily adapted.

Burford Pain Thermometer (Burford Nursing Development Unit, 1984)

This chart is well received by nurses, because it is simple to use and works well (Figure 3.5). It incorporates both numerical and verbal scoring

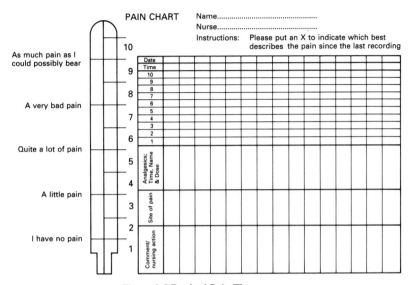

Figure 3.5 Burford Pain Thermometer

values which are presented on a thermometer. The patient after looking at the words selects the number which correlates best to his pain level and records it on the chart. The chart allows for flexible timings of reassessment. The chart works well in the clinical and research setting, despite the disparity between the end markers of numbers and word descriptors. In this adapted version the nurse can record her comments and action taken at the time of assessments.

A major disadvantage with the Burford Pain Thermometer, as with many other pain assessment charts, is that it only measures pain intensity and does not consider pain relief. Pain relief scores are often found to be more sensitive than those of pain intensity in the research setting. A pain relief score is particularly important in the management of chronic pain where there is a changing baseline level of pain intensity and when a new treatment has been introduced. In this case a change in pain intensity (higher or lower scores) may be attributed to the new treatment, when in fact it may be due to other factors, e.g. patient was not at work, therefore pain at lower level than usual.

London Pain Chart

Another popular assessment chart is the London Hospital Pain observation chart (Figure 3.6) (Sharpe, 1986) which uses a body chart and pain rating scales. There is a facility to record nursing and pharmacological interventions and any relevant comments.

Tools used in assessment of paediatric pain

These are discussed in the chapter on paediatric pain.

Non-pain related assessments

In the chronic pain setting other factors are as important as the pain itself such as sleep, mood and depression. If any of these are improved then there may be an effect on the patient's coping ability and the pain itself. Methods used to assess sleep and mood are similar to those used for pain, either using visual analogue scales or verbal rating scales. Depression can be assessed using more complex validated psychological tests such as the Beck or Hamilton Depression Scales.

Outcome of pain assessment

Nursing research since the 1970s has highlighted the benefits attained from the use of pain assessment which is simple to implement; patients receiving higher quality pain relief, nursing staff developing their knowledge and

THIS CHART records where a patient's pain is and how bad it is, by the nurse asking the patient at regular intervals. If analgesics are being given regularly, make an observation **with** each dose and another **half-way between** each dose. If analgesics are given only 'as required', observe two-hourly. When the observations are stable and the patient is comfortable, any regular time interval between observations may be chosen.

TO USE THIS CHART ask the patient to mark all his or her pains on the body diagram below. Label each site of pain with a letter (i.e. A, B, C, etc.)

Then at each observation time ask the patient to assess:

1   the pain in each separate site since the last observation. Use the scale above the body diagram, and enter the number or letter in the appropriate column.

2   the pain overall since the last observation. Use the same scale and enter in column marked OVERALL.

Next, record what has been done to relieve pain:

3   note any analgesic given since the last observation stating name, dose, route and time given.

4   tick any other nursing care or action taken to ease pain.

Finally, note any comment on pain from patient or nurse (use the back of the chart as well, if necessary) and initial the record.

Excruciating	5
Very severe	4
Severe	3
Moderate	2
Just noticeable	1
No pain at all	0
Patient sleeping	5

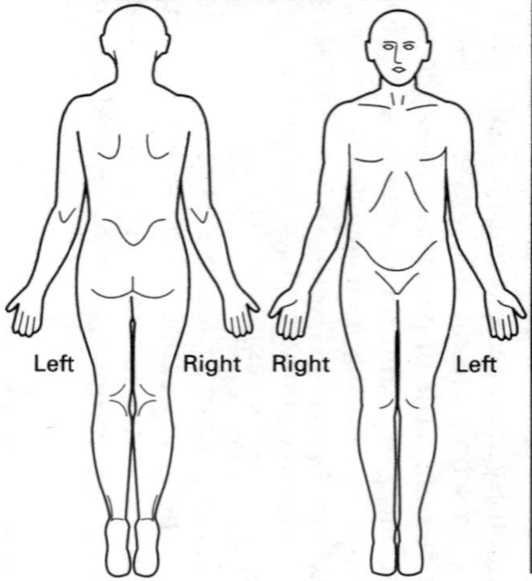

PAIN OBSERVATION CHART

PATIENT IDENTIFICATION LABEL

DATE _____

SHEET NUMBER _____

TIME	PAIN RATING			ANALGESIC GIVEN (Name, dose, route, time)	MEASURES TO RELIEVE PAIN								COMMENTS FROM PATIENTS AND/OR STAFF	Initials
	IN SITES		OVER ALL		Lifting	Turning	Massage	Distracting activities*	Position change*	Additional aids*	Other*	Specify where starred	
	A B C D E F G H													

Left   Right   Right   Left

Figure 3.6 London Hospital pain observation chart

obtaining greater satisfaction, greater prescribing flexibility. Despite this evidence pain assessment is still not widely used and is excluded from standard patient care plans. Nursing responsibilities include continual re-assessment of pain, the administration and evaluation of pain relieving interventions to provide the optimum effect, safely. Pain assessment is a method used to formally document a patient's unique experience of pain, which then can be treated promptly and effectively. Our own attitudes and beliefs should not affect the patient's right to pain relief.

References

Burford Nursing Development Unit (1984) Nurses and Pain. *Nursing Times*, **18**, 94

Chapman, C. R. (1985) Psychological factors in post-operative pain. In *Acute Pain* (eds G. Smith and B. G. Covino) Butterworths, London

Donovan, B. D. (1983) Patient attitudes to post-operative pain relief. *Anaesthesia and Intensive Care*, **11**, 125–129

Gracely, R. H. (1992) Evaluation of multi-dimensional pain scales. *Pain*, **48**, 297–300

Holroyd, K. A., Holm, J. E., Keefe, F. J. *et al.* (1992) A multi-centre evaluation of the McGill pain questionnaire: results from more than 1700 chronic pain patients. *Pain*, **48**, 301–311

Huskisson, E. E. (1983) Visual Analogue scales. In: *Pain Measurement and Assessment* (ed. R. Melzack), Raven Press, New York, pp. 33–37

Kuhn S, Cooke, K., Collins, M., Jones, J. M. and Mucklow, J. C. (1990) Perception of pain after surgery. *British Medical Journal*, **300**, 1687–1690

Lavies, N., Hart, L., Rounsefell, B. and Runciman, W. (1992) Identification of patient, medical and nursing staff attitudes to post-operative opioid analgesia: stage 1 of a longitudinal study of post-operative analgesia. *Pain*, **48**, 313–319

Mather, L. E. and Phillips, G. D. (1986) Opioids and adjuncts: principles of use. In *Acute Pain Management* (eds Cousins and Phillips) Churchill Livingstone, Edinburgh

McQuay, H. J. (1990) Assessment of pain, and effectiveness of treatment. In: *Measuring the Out-* comes of Medical Care (eds A. Hopkins and D. Costain)

McQuay, H. J. (1992) Pre-emptive analgesia. *British Journal of Anaesthesia*, **69** (1), 1–3

McQuay, H. J., Carroll, D. and Moore, R. A. (1988) Post-operative orthopaedic pain; the effect of opiate premedication and local anaesthetic blocks. *Pain*, **33**, 291–295

Melzack, R. (1975) The McGill Pain Questionnaire: major properties and scoring methods. *Pain*, **1**, 277–299

Melzack, R. (1983) The McGill Pain Questionnaire. In *Pain Measurement and Assessment* (ed. R. Melzack) Raven Press, New York, pp. 41–48

Royal College of Surgeons of England and College of Anaesthetists (1990) Report of the working party on pain after surgery

Scott, J. and Huskisson, E. C. (1976) Graphic representation of pain. *Pain*. **2**, 175–184.

Sharpe, S. (1986) The use of the London Hospital Pain observation Chart. *Nursing*, **11**, 415–423.

Wall, P. D. (1988) The prevention of post-operative pain. *Pain*, **33**, 289–290

Wallenstein, S. L. and Houde, R. W. (1975) The clinical evaluation of analgesic effectiveness. *Methods of Narcotic Research* (eds S. Ehrenpries and A. Needle), Marcel Decker, New York

Further reading on pain assessment and pain research methodology

Max, M. B., Portenoy, R. K. and Laska, E. M. (eds) (1991) Advances in pain research and therapy. *The Design of Analgesic Clinical Trials*. Raven Press, New York

Further reading on non-verbal communication

Argyle, M. (1990) *The Psychology of Interpersonal Behaviour*, 4th ed. Penguin, London

Goffman, I. (1971) *Relationship in Public*. Allen Lane

Morris, D., Collett, P., Marsh, P. and O'Shaughnessy, M. (1979) *Gestures, Their Origins and Distribution*. Cape

4

Pain in the nursing curriculum

K. Seers and P. Davis

'Freedom from pain should be a basic human right limited only by our knowledge to achieve it.' Liebeskind and Melzack (1987)

Introduction

Pain is something we all experience, and caring for those who are in pain is a fundamental part of nursing. Pain is often part of the experience of illness and an understanding of pain and its relief is thus a basic and essential part of nursing.

Research has demonstrated that pain relief in adults and children is not ideal (Marks and Sachar 1973; Cohen 1980; Weiss et al., 1983; Mather and Mackie 1983; Donovan et al., 1987; Seers, 1989). Large numbers of people continue to suffer poorly controlled pain. Nurses appear to lack knowledge about pain and its relief (Cohen, 1980; Watt-Watson, 1987) and generally do not accurately assess pain (Hunt et al., 1977; Seers 1989) or its relief (Choiniere, 1990). In addition, Owen et al. (1990) found that patients did not have the necessary knowledge about pain relief to contribute effectively to their own pain management.

So, although research over several years has shown that pain is not well controlled, recent studies suggest the situation is slow to change. This results in many people in our care suffering pain, a large part of which may well be avoidable and thus unnecessary. At least part of the reason for this seems to be a lack of knowledge. Teaching about the care of people in pain is important for pain sufferers. Sofaer (1984, 1985) demonstrated that a ward based teaching package about pain and its relief produced some significant improvements in patient outcomes. Nurses are therefore in the fortunate

position of having the potential to improve the pain relief of people in their care.

Pain relief has often been overlooked as a subject in its own right, perhaps partly because it spans so many areas of care. However, this approach does not appear to have resulted in an adequate coverage of pain in the curriculum. Watt-Watson (1987) found that nurses expressed frustration with difficulties in pain assessment and inadequate pain relief for patients. Pain is a complex phenomenon, requiring a systematic and comprehensive approach to its teaching. Of course, learning about pain does not guarantee an automatic improvement in pain management. However, it can be argued that creating a learning environment in which the complex nature of pain and its management can be appreciated and related to practice, will facilitate such an improvement.

Project 2000

The pain component of a curriculum for nurses was developed specifically with Project 2000 in mind, but basic concepts would apply equally to any nurse education programme.

Teaching about pain is important at two levels:

a) Actual content and its implications for nursing care.
b) Developing the processes involved in understanding and applying this content:

   i) The analytical skills outlined by the United Kingdom Central Council for Nursing, Midwifery and Health Visiting (UKCC) (1988) (sections 5.1, 5.2).
   ii) Achieving learning outcomes (UKCC, 1988, section 6.2).

Decisions about content and process should be founded on what is basic and essential rather than merely relevant and interesting.

Common Foundation Programme (CFP)

Caring for people in pain draws on all of the areas taught in the CFP. It is envisaged that pain would be used as a thread through all areas. Specific teaching would be in life sciences, social and behavioural sciences but within a nursing framework. This learning, and aspects from all CFP areas, would be applied during supervised care of people in pain. This is crucial in bridging the gap between theory and practice. Ways of facilitating the integration of theory and practice are important when devising a pain curriculum.

Branch programmes

The major input of teaching of pain in the curriculum would be in the branch programmes. It is not enough to say pain is implicitly covered by other content areas. Research suggests this approach has been hit and miss and patients in pain are not receiving adequate pain relief. A specific pain component of the curriculum is necessary.

All aspects of the CFP, including communication processes and social/behavioural sciences, would be utilised and built on in the branch programme. The concepts taught in the CFP would be applied specifically to pain, thus drawing on and integrating CFP skills, enabling students to apply them in theory and in supervised practice, promoting their analytical, problem solving skills with people in all types of pain. Caring for people in pain is a balance of many skills. Basic skills such as assessment, acting on that assessment towards an agreed goal and evaluating progress towards this goal, involving the person with pain whenever possible, are essential and basic skills for all aspects of nursing.

The ability to apply knowledge to practice is important and can be expected to facilitate the attainment of a dynamic knowledge base from which clinical decisions can be made and which will grow with added experience gained in practice as well as with continued theoretical learning.

Most teaching about pain management is perhaps appropriate for the adult and child branches, although this does not preclude its importance in mental health and mental handicap, where comparatively little research on pain and its relief has been undertaken.

Post-registration education

a) Whilst these curricula are intended for Project 2000 courses, many qualified nurses may recognise that they could benefit from it, and elements of it could be incorporated into a programme according to their needs.
b) Aspects of these curricula could be extended for practitioners who are competent in the theory and practice of the basic curriculum, for example, developing additional skills in complementary methods of pain relief, addressing specific problems with specific groups of patients relevant to their practice.

These would need to be linked to English National Board (ENB) and higher education frameworks in order to obtain professional and academic credibility. They would be in the form of modular programmes and each module would accumulate credits towards a recognised qualification.

Since pain is so central to nursing, we would expect modules in pain and its management to be central to the continuing professional development of the nurse.

Some, but not all, nurses would develop pioneering and innovatory roles, acting as a resource for colleagues. It would seem entirely appropriate that Masters Degree level study, specifically addressing pain and its management, should be developed. It is expected that appropriately qualified nurses will continue to pursue PhD level study in this field.

The following section was developed from initial work of the RCN Pain Forum and discussions of a 1-day workshop group (Davis and Seers, 1991).

The current situation

The teaching and nursing management of pain is changing and hopefully developing for the better. Currently nurses are playing a major role in bringing about change. To maximise the beneficial changes and developments, those involved with the changes need to identify and understand in their own situation factors that may promote progress and that may hinder progress. Examples of these factors would be:

Factors promoting the teaching of pain

- Students are receptive and eager to learn about this topic.
- Pain as a topic matches the general trend of health promotion and the individual's control of their life.
- Pain is being taught in present curricula in an increasing proportion and more systematically.
- There is a growing number of nurses interested in pain management and an increased body of nursing research based knowledge and skills on pain which also encourages an ethos of research application generally.
- At present, pain and its relief have a high profile and nurses are more aware of and perceive it as a priority.
- There is a more general awareness of the diversity of methods of pain relief for use by nurses, e.g. complementary therapies.
- As nursing is increasingly understood in an holistic context, pain is viewed as an integrated phenomenon.
- Good examples exist of multi-disciplinary collaboration.
- The topic provides a good opportunity to link theory with practice.
- The present situation of flux, in both the development and organisation of nursing, provides an ideal opportunity for making changes.
- Pain and its management provide an ideal vehicle to aid, in all areas, the professional development of nurses.
- The increasing initiatives to develop and use standards of care are useful for the initial teaching of students by providing a helpful structure.
- Pain management demands an ethical commitment by nurses.

Factors hindering the teaching of pain

- Students and teachers have existing beliefs that need challenging.
- The teaching of nursing management of pain is still ad-hoc, fragmented, inadequate and tagged on and these problems are not recog-

nised, leading to the problem being reflected in practice.
- There is a lack of understanding and skills shown by teachers and practitioners in accessing and using a knowledge base and thus there are no suitable role models.
- The teaching of pain is seen as a low priority without ethical implications.
- There is a lack of an holistic approach to persons in pain both in teaching and practice, e.g. this produces routinised care and single method approaches.
- There is little time and resources to develop the professional capabilities of nurses.
- The development of standards may restrict and stifle a creative and individualised approach to pain management.

Standard, kind and content of pre- and post-registration nurse education

Patient and client needs should form the starting point and foundation of any care to ensure adequate management of an individual's pain. To ensure that there is clarity about what is adquate, standards of practice should be developed and achieved. To facilitate the achievement of standards of practice, adequate education is a prerequisite for pre- and post-registration nurses (see Figure 4.1).

Outcomes

Outcomes will be dependent on the level to be achieved at specific times in a programme or course, e.g. diploma level for Project 2000 courses, and will need to take account of prior experience and future professional development possibilities. The student should progress from novice to competent practitioner but would

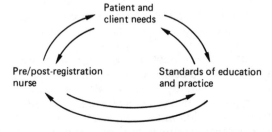

Figure 4.1 Relationship between client and standards of nursing.

not be expected to be an expert as a first level nurse. Progression to expert, as nursing at an advanced level was sought, should be appropriate to the nurse's role, needs and ability.

Outcomes may be identified as those related to attitudes of the nurse and patient, assessment of pain, nursing interventions and evaluation of the care given. For example in the Project 2000 course these may be:

Attitudes

The nurse will need to reflect on and discuss the following attitudes towards pain and its management:

- Pain is real, regardless of cause.
- The person's pain is theirs.
- Pain is an integrated, complex phenomena.
- Pain can and should be managed.
- A 'partnership', between sufferer and carer, should exist.
- The person with pain is believed.

Assessment

Knowledge and skills should include:

- General types and characteristics of pain, intensity, duration and so on.
- Relationship with person in pain.
- Existing skills and strategies used by patients, e.g. coping strategies.
- Impact of pain on activities of living.
- An understanding of resources and their access.
- Side effects of therapy.

Intervention

Knowledge and skills should include:

- Patient and family education.
- Assessement of pain and prioritising interventions.
- Ability to individualise pain regime.
- Administration of analgesics and side effects.
- Communication and working with other health care professionals.
- Awareness of complementary methods.
- Basic nursing methods to promote comfort, e.g. positioning.
- Supporting patients' existing strategies, e.g. self-medication programmes.

Evaluation

Knowledge and skills should include:

- Ability to document all elements of nursing process.
- Review outcomes of interventions and take appropriate action.

To achieve these outcomes the following may act as a core or guidelines but not as a rigid prescription of content and process.

Content

Content should progress from the nurse's prior experience of pain and health and move to concepts and models of pain eventually relating to specific practice, as within a branch.

A syllabus containing components as, for example, by Pilowsky (1988) or IASP (1991), but modified to reflect a nursing perspective, may be useful, for example, as in the IASP Pain Curriculum for Basic Nursing Education (1993). However, areas of importance such as developing skills in communication, advocacy, assertiveness and self-empowerment must also be considered.

It is recommended that pain management be an assessed component of the programme.

Process

Development of communication skills is an essential element of the teaching of pain in the curriculum. These skills may be developed as themes across the whole programme or course, as they are applicable to many aspects of nursing and not just pain management. Acquisition of knowledge, skills and attitudes may be facilitated in a variety of ways and settings, for example:

Knowledge and attitudes about pain and experience
- Reflection on their own experience.
- Discussions with patients.
- Laboratory induced pain experiences.
- Lectures/discussions.

Skills of assessment and management
- Develop communication skills.
- Care studies, project work.
- Critical incident analysis.
- Focused clinical experience.
- Developing negotiation, advocacy,

integration, prioritorising action through, e.g. role play.

Selection preparation and development of teachers

The location and context of teaching are important as is the support for this teaching. All competent nurses should be responsible for teaching about pain and its management. These initiatives should:

- Be nurse led so that theory is related to nursing practice.
- Use other health care professionals and the patient and relatives as appropriate within a nursing framework.
- Require a motivated, experienced teacher or one willing to acquire knowledge.

Nurses teaching in the clinical area:

- Will require continual professional development.
- Will require facilitators in practice areas such as nurse researchers, clinical nurse specialists and nurse teachers.

Support for teaching requires:

- Resources supported by management.
- All concerned to appreciate the complexity and dynamic nature of all aspects of pain management and its legitimacy as a subject in its own right.
- The support of colleagues so that attitudes and beliefs are shared.
- An understanding that as it is a relatively new and expanding area of teaching, individuals may feel isolated.
- National and local networks available and accessible to provide information, teaching and support, e.g. RCN Pain Forum.

Conclusions

Pain has been identified as an important and legitimate subject in its own right. The underlying principle must be to improve the care of people who are in pain. Research has consistently shown this care is inadequate and that we lack an adequate knowledge base. Teaching about pain and its management as a subject in its own right is a prerequisite for fulfilling the basic human right of freedom from pain. We contend that it is our professional responsibility to ensure we are not limited from fulfilling that right purely by our failure to utilise available knowledge. To enable people to exercise their right to freedom from pain, a duty is implied. The exact balance of responsibility in executing that duty will be between those involved in care. This is likely to include a variety of health care professionals, the person in pain and others important to the sufferer. The nurse has a key role in assessing and achieving that balance.

Many of those involved in practice, education, research and management are working either in isolation or together to address these issues and there are pockets of excellence. However, it must be unprofessional to allow people in pain to take such pot luck in the relief of their pain. As we are accountable for our care, failure to address the issue of pain and its management could lead to litigation by those suffering from pain. Indeed Meinhart and McCaffery (1983) say:

'Failure to treat pain is inhumane and constitutes professional negligence.'

It is the responsibility of all nurses, practitioners, educators, researchers and managers, to ensure we are not negligent.

References

Choiniere, M., Melzack, R., Girard, N. *et al.* (1990) Comparisons between patients' and nurses' assessment of pain and medication efficacy in severe burn injuries. *Pain*, **40** (2), 143–152

Cohen, F. (1980) Postsurgical pain relief: patients' status and nurses' medication choices. *Pain*, **9**, 265–274

Davis, P. and Seers, K. (1991) Teaching nurses about managing pain. *Nursing Standard*, **5** (52), 30–32

Donovan, M., Dillon, P. and McGuire, L. (1987) Incidence and characteristics of pain in a sample of medical-surgical inpatients. *Pain*, **30**, 69–78

Hunt, J. M., Stollar, T. D., Littlejohns, D. W. *et al.* (1977) Patients with protracted pain: a survey conducted at the London Hospital. *Journal of Medical Ethics*, **3**, 61–73

International Association for the Study of Pain (1991) Core curriculum for professional education in pain. IASP, Seattle

International Association for the Study of Pain

(1993) Newsletter, September – October 1993. Technical corner: Pain curriculum for basic nurse education. Edited by C. B. Berde, pp. 4–6

Liebeskind, J. C. and Melzack, R. (1987) The international pain foundation: meeting a need for education in pain management (editorial). *Pain*, **30**, 1–2

Marks, R. M. and Sachar, E. J. (1973) Undertreatment of medical inpatients with narcotic analgesics. *Annals of Internal Medicine*, **78** (2), 173–181

Mather, L. and Mackie, J. (1983) The incidence of postoperative pain in children. *Pain*, **15**, 271–282

Meinhart, N. T. and McCaffery, M. (1983) *Pain. A Nursing Approach to Assessment and Analysis.* Appleton Century Crofts, Norwalk

Owen, H., McMillan, V. and Rogowski, D. (1990) Postoperative pain therapy: a survey of patients expectations and their experiences. *Pain*, **41** (3), 303–307

Pilowsky, I. (1988) An outline curriculum on pain for medical schools. *Pain*, **33**, 1–2

Seers, K. (1989) Patients' perceptions of acute pain. In: Wilson-Barnett, J. & Robinson, S. (ed.) *Directions in Nursing Research: Ten Years of Progress at London University*. Scutari, London, pp. 107–116

Sofaer, B. (1984) *The Effect of Focused Education for Nursing Teams on Postoperative Pain of Patients*. Unpublished PhD thesis, University of Edinburgh

Sofaer, B. (1985) Pain management through nurse education. In: *Perspectives on pain. Recent Advances in Nursing 11*, Churchill Livingstone, Edinburgh, (ed. L. A. Copp) pp 62–74

UKCC (1988) *UKCC's Proposed Rules for the Standard, Kind and Content of Future Pre-registration Nursing Education*. UKCC, London

Watt-Watson, J. (1987) Nurses' knowledge of pain issues: a survey. *J. Pain Symptom Management*, **2** (4), 207–211

Weiss, O. F., Sriwatanakul, K., Alloza, J. L. *et al.* (1983) Attitudes of patients, housestaff, and nurses toward postoperative analgesic care. *Anaesth. Analg.*, **62**, 70–74

5

Acute pain

Debbie Hunter

Introduction

Pain and how it is felt by any particular individual can be seen to vary due to three components; the intensity of the painful stimulus, the individual's previous learning about such stimuli and finally the individual's current mood. The degree of pain felt will vary with changes in any of the these. Pain usually serves a protective function and is a temporary phenomenon, but on occasions it may persist for weeks or much longer, leading to the syndrome described as chronic intractable pain which is dealt with in later chapters. This chapter will deal with the management of acute pain, which can be concisely defined as pain of rapid onset and of short duration (measured in days rather than months). Thus it can be seen that acute pain is not only the pain occurring after surgery but also includes other painful conditions such as renal colic, acute pancreatitis, myocardial infarction and the pain caused by trauma such as fractured ribs. Studies have shown that as many as 58% of patients who attend hospital for both medical and surgical conditions suffer excruciating pain at some time during their stay (Donovan *et al.* 1987) Thus it should be remembered that acute pain is a problem on both medical and surgical units.

Acute pain can serve a protective function, acting as a warning sign to indicate that an injury or other acute insult has occurred. We are therefore alerted to take the necessary action to prevent further damage. An example is the pain occurring with an inflamed appendix. This leads the patient to seek medical assistance. However, once this protective function has been completed, continuing pain can compromise the individual as it is often accompanied by increased heart rate, blood pressure and respiratory rate. These can be deleterious to the patient and there is evidence to suggest that the effective management of acute pain can lead to reduced morbidity (Yeager *et al.*, 1987).

The management of acute pain has been ignored and not recognised as a problem in hospital practice for many years. One of the major problems with acute pain has been the delegation of responsibility for its management to those who are least experienced – the junior doctors, who are not adequately prepared in their undergraduate training for this responsibility. However, the major worries of causing addiction and respiratory depression are shared both by medical and nursing staff and lead to under-prescribing and under-utilisation of prescribed analgesics.

Principles of nursing management of acute pain

The management of the patient at ward level is on a day-to-day basis and carried out by the nurse looking after the patient. Advice and support is available from the acute pain team for individual fluctuations in the patient requirements and the concept of balanced analgesia is introduced. With the use of specialised techniques such as patient controlled analgesia (PCA) or epidural infusions the introduction of concomitant medication for breakthrough pain may be necessary. Therefore the following are important:

assessment – problem of definition – planning – intervention – evaluation

The process shown above should be followed in order to manage the patient's pain correctly.

1. Assessment

The various methods of assessments have been widely discussed and the importance of assessment is that it should become routine in the management of acute pain. It should be quick and easy to achieve and involve the patient at all times and be recorded in a systematic way.

2. The problems of definition

The problem should be identified and it should be considered as a multi-disciplinary problem. The practitioner should also be aware of their limitations and involve 'experts' where possible for advice and support.

3. Planning

Planning the patient's acute pain management programme should involve the patient and the members of a multi-disciplinary acute pain team and the patient's primary nurse. They should be based on relevant and recent published research and also on clinical experience.

4. Intervention

In the acute pain setting most interventions would be on a drug-related basis, where the choice of the route of drug administration should be considered, depending on patient assessment. The use of alternative methods of intervention such as relaxation, comfort measures and psychological aspects should not be overlooked.

5. Evaluation

Continuous evaluation of the suitability of the choice of drug used in the management of the patient's pain will be ongoing and the regular assessment will highlight the effectiveness of the pain management programme being followed.

Increasing the awareness of acute pain through education and practice would enable nurses and practitioners to set their standards of management of the patient in acute pain.

Current problems in the management of acute pain

1. No formal pain assessment.
2. No account of individual patient variations in level of pain experienced or amount of analgesia required.
3. Inflexible prescribing and inappropriate administration of analgesic drugs.

Preoperative assessment

The management of acute pain, such as that occurring postoperatively, should begin where possible with the preoperative assessment of the patient. This may take the form of a formal questionnaire or more usually by informal discussions between the patient, his anaesthetist and nursing staff. One of the main aims of the preoperative assessment should be to alleviate patients' anxiety regarding what will happen to them and the amount of pain they will experience following their operation. Open questioning techniques should be used to ascertain the patients' previous experience and expectations of pain, and their normal coping strategies should be discussed with them.

Counselling

The aim of counselling according to the British Association of Counselling, and their basis for working is:

'The task of counselling is to give the client an opportunity to explore and discover and clarify ways of living more resourcefully and toward a greater well-being'.

Preoperative counselling in the management of postoperative pain takes the form of a one-to-one discussion between the nurse and her 'client', by giving advice and answering questions about pain. Anxiety is universal in all preoperative patients, and is influenced by the uncertainty of impending surgery, past experiences of surgery, and the suggestions or experience of family members, friends or even other patients.

The use of preoperative visits, giving reassurance and encouragement, has been shown to reduce both anxiety (Fell *et al.*, 1986) and reduce opioid requirements postoperatively (Leigh *et al.*, 1977); hospital stay may also be shortened. In a recent study (McCleane and Cooper, 1990) the most common fear felt by patients following surgery is the fear of postoperative pain, and in fact 50% of the patients interviewed postoperatively still expressed their highest anxiety as postoperative pain, stressing that their pain was not treated sufficiently.

Pain is a subjective experience and is influenced by the emotional state of the patient; because of this the use of music to reduce postoperative pain has been explored (Locsin, 1981). The basis behind the use of music in the intraoperative or postoperative period is that it may reduce anxiety, therefore reducing postoperative pain. It has also been shown that music may reduce blood pressure and pulse rate, and patients may use less opioid or other medications during the postoperative period. The argument for the use of music is far from clear, however, as the study quoted is one of only a few on the subject and only examined a small surgical population.

Pain assessment

In order to improve the management of acute pain we must first be able reliably to assess patients' pain. Pain is a personal experience that causes an individual to suffer. The amount of suffering is influenced by the patient's emotional status and can only be described subjectively by the individual involved. It results in characteristic signs mediated by the autonomic nervous system such as sweating, tachycardia and tachypnoea. These are signs of very severe pain and serve little use in the assessment of acute pain. The degree of suffering can be assessed in many ways as described elsewhere (see chapters on pain assessment, paediatric pain and cancer pain).

In an attempt to quantify their pain, patients can be asked to express its severity according to a simple linear scale. Choice of scale will depend on various factors such as the patients age and the amount of detail required by the assessor. The simplest method would be to ask the patient whether he has pain or not. However, if the answer is affirmative this does not provide information as to the character or severity of the pain. Therefore more detailed scales have been developed for the assessment of pain in both adults and children, and these are described in other chapters. It is important to remember when making the choice of scale that they are easy to use and easily understood by the patient.

Visual analogue scales may be used in children over the age of 7 and the verbal scales were introduced for use in adolescents by Melzack (1975). Neonates in pain are very difficult to assess using any form of measurement scale, but an indication as to the presence and degree of pain can be made indirectly from facial expressions, body movements, heart rate and the character of their cry. Assessment tools for children include facial expression scales (Wong and Baker, 1988), the Eland colour scale (Eland, 1981) and the Hester Poker Chip Scale (Hester, 1979). Facial expression scales have also been demonstrated to be successful in adults, where there are language problems or mental impairment (Frank et al., 1982).

Pain assessment tools for adults tend to be more complex and often provide more information about the severity and character of the pain, e.g. the McGill Pain Questionnaire (Melzack, 1975). This is useful in the management of chronic pain, but is less appropriate in the routine assessment of acute pain as it can take 10–20 minutes to complete. Other scoring methods include verbal rating scales and visual analogue scales. A variation of the visual analogue is a slide rule which is presented to the patient and which allows the investigator to read off the back of the ruler (Thomas and Griffiths, 1982). Observer scoring systems often have poor correlation with the patient's assessment of pain, and should be avoided. The patient's individual subjective rating of pain is important and should be formally assessed. Pain charts can be used for repeated assessment and charting of results allows changes in amount of pain experienced to be recorded and promptly acted on. In acute pain it is useful to assess pain on movement rather than on rest (such as coughing or twisting of the trunk) (see Table 5.1).

Table 5.1. Nurse pain score

Score 0	no pain at rest no pain on movement
Score 1	no pain at rest slight pain on movement
Score 2	intermittent pain at rest moderate pain on movement
Score 3	continuous pain at rest severe pain on movement

Whichever form of pain assessment is chosen, it is vital to formally assess the patient in pain, and record their pain scores as the first stage in improving the management of acute pain.

Methods of administration of analgesics

Intravenous analgesia

Several routes of administration are available, including:

1. Intermittent boli of opioid by clinician or nurse.
2. Continuous infusion of opioid.
3. Patient controlled analgesia.

Intermittent boli of opioid

This technique is commonly used in theatre by anaesthetists and in recovery rooms by both anaesthetists and recovery staff. The patient is given small boli of diluted opioid, which has been prescribed by the anaesthetist, until the pain is under control. During the intravenous administration of the opioid the nurse monitors the patient's response to the opioid; pain relief, respiratory rate, conscious level and blood pressure. This is a very effective method of providing analgesia quickly in this situation and has been shown to improve the patient's impression of their pain management throughout the postoperative period. However, it requires a nurse to be present with the patient during the injection and therefore this could not be easily extended to the general ward situation.

Intravenous infusions of opioid

This technique is commonly used in Intensive Care Units, High Dependency Units and on some appropriately staffed and trained general wards (paediatric and adult) in the UK. It involves the continuous delivery of the opioid drug in a dilute solution to the patient's circulation through an intravenous canula. The infusion can be provided by a mechanical (e.g. clockwork syringe driver) or electronic infusion device (e.g. syringe pump or intravenous infusion device). The common availability and relative cheapness of these devices has made this a popular technique to those dissatisfied

with conventional analgesic regimes, particularly in paediatrics where it removes the need for repeated intramuscular injections. There are disadvantages that need consideration:

A. It takes several hours of continuous infusion before the patient reaches a steady state where the plasma concentration of the drug is stable. During this phase the plasma concentration may well be too low to provide effective analgesia. This phase can be shortened by providing intravenous boli but this has to be done where there are the necessary staffing levels to monitor the patient.
B. Patients respond to opioid drugs differently: the infusion rate required to provide analgesia in one patient may cause another to stop breathing and become unconscious. Indeed this technique has been shown to cause significant periods of apnoea in postoperative patients (Catling *et al.*, 1980). It is difficult for the clinician to judge the infusion rate necessary for the patient due to this variability of response. To overcome this, it is vital to closely monitor the response of the patient to the infusion and adjust the infusion rate as necessary. In most postoperative general surgical wards this degree of nursing care is difficult to provide and this is the major reason why the technique is not more widely used.

Patient controlled analgesia

Background

The principles of Patient Controlled Analgesia (PCA) using intravenous analgesia drugs were established over 20 years ago (Sechzer, 1968), when it was used as a research tool to provide an objective measurement of the severity of postoperative pain. As in current systems, early units involved the patient pressing a button when in pain. This rang an alarm which called a nurse to come and administer the analgesic intravenously. This manual administration was gradually replaced by increasingly sophisticated infusion pumps, but the size and expense of these prohibited their more general use. Until 1984 there were only two suitable PCA pumps available in the UK. However, advances in computer control of medical equipment have now provided hospitals with a large choice of PCA pumps ranging from sophisticated units

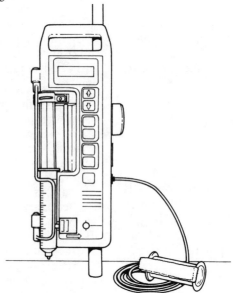

Figure 5.1. The Graseby PCAS

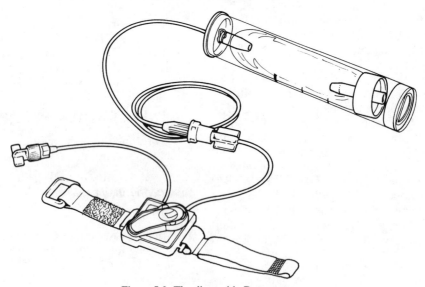

Figure 5.2. The disposable Baxter system

such as the Graseby PCAS (Figure 5.1) to the disposable Baxter system (Figure 5.2).

Technique

PCA works by giving the patient responsibility for the control of their own pain. Under normal circumstances a patient receiving intramuscular analgesia in a busy ward waits until he feels pain before asking the nursing staff for analgesia. The delays inherent in this system are shown in Figure 5.3.

Further problems occur due to the natural variability in the amount of analgesia patients require, even following the same operation. Intramuscular analgesia is usually written up as a fixed dose given 3–4 hourly. Studies have shown that patients can have a 5–10 fold difference in analgesic requirements over any given 24-hour period. Thus with the traditional system many patients will not be receiving the dose of analgesia they require whilst others will be receiving too much.

PCA, however, removes medical and nursing

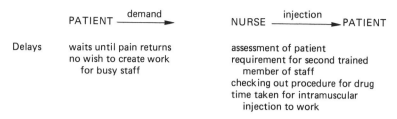

Figure 5.3 Delays occurring with conventional intramuscular analgesia

staff from the equation and the patient has direct control over their analgesia (Figure 5.4).

Worries about patients overdosing themselves with opiates from these pumps have proven unfounded; however, most pumps allow the clinician to limit the maximum dose the patient can receive.

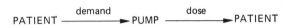

Figure 5.4 PCA system

How the pumps work

Most PCA pumps currently available utilise 30 or 50 ml syringes which are filled with the analgesic of the operator's choice. The simplest units allow the operator to set the size of the bolus dose and the lockout time. The bolus dose is the amount of drug or the volume of fluid that the patient will receive each time he presses the button. The lockout time is the period after a dose has been received by the patient during which the machine will not administer a further bolus. This is used because drugs such as morphine administered intravenously take considerable time to take effect. Thus the enforced delay (often set at 5 minutes) prevents the patient taking more doses than may be necessary. Most units also provide the option of giving a background infusion of the opioid independent of patient demands. Units now available also offer the facility of providing loading doses and may have the ability to monitor the dose the patient has received which is then compared to an hourly or 4 hourly maximum that cannot be exceeded.

Pumps are connected to the patient by a dedicated intravenous line or to the intravenous line already present via a one-way valve. This valve is required to prevent reflux of the analgesic up the intravenous line towards the drip chamber in the event of the cannula becoming blocked. If not prevented by the presence of the one-way valve this could cause a large bolus to be administered to the patient following removal of the blockage.

Oral ingestion of opioids

Most opioids can be given orally and this route is commonly used in patients following surgery where the abdomen has not been disturbed, e.g. limb surgery. It is most popular, however, in the control of chronic pain in the terminally ill. The drug needs to pass down through the stomach into the small intestine to be absorbed, hence patients who have had abdominal operations, are vomiting or have an ileus following surgery are not suitable for this technique. It should also be noted that relatively large doses of opioids will be necessary, as opioids such as morphine are metabolised in the walls of the intestine and by the liver, through which they must pass before entering the general circulation of the patient. This route of administration is popular in the period following the return of the patient to oral intake.

Sublingual and buccal administration of opioids

Opioids can be administered in a tablet form which is then inserted under the tongue or beside the gum. The drug is then absorbed through the mucous membrane into the bloodstream at a rate that is slower than intravenous but faster than intramuscular injections. The dose of drug required is less than with the oral route, as the drug avoids the breakdown that occurs in the bowel wall and the liver (see above). The tablet is also easily removed if overdosage occurs. Buprenorphine and morphine can be given in this way. This route has not proven popular due to the incidence of poor analgesia, nausea, vomiting and sedation.

Subcutaneous infusions of opioids

This technique is similar to giving an intravenous infusion of opioid. A cannula is inserted just below the skin, in the subcutaneous fat and a continuous infusion of diluted opioid is administered through the cannula. The drug then diffuses through surrounding tissues into the bloodstream from where it can get to the central nervous system. It will be obvious that this slows down the response to changes in the infusion rate and therefore has several disadvantages whilst offering no advantage over intravenous infusions in the management of postoperative pain. However, it should be noted that the avoidance of cannulation of a vein makes it popular in the control of pain in the terminally ill where rapid changes in infusion rates are not necessary.

Transdermal opioids

Transdermal drug delivery depends on the absorption of an opioid through the skin into the tissues and bloodstream from a patch applied to the skin. This technique has been used with success for the provision of the ante-anginal drug GTN. The absorption of the drug depends on many factors including the design of the patch, the solubility of the drug used and the blood flow to the region where it is applied. Currently a patch containing a synthetic opioid called fentanyl is undergoing clinical trials. Again this technique is similar to providing a continuous intravenous infusion of the opioid but without the requirement for an infusion pump. However, it is not possible to control the absorption rate and hence control the dose given to the patient. It also takes longer to reach the analgesic level in the plasma due to the tortuous route of administration. This can be overcome by applying the patch prior to surgery. Another problem is that it takes a considerable time for the plasma concentration to fall following removal of the patch; this could be a problem if the patient has received an overdose. This method of analgesia has yet to be fully evaluated and its place in the control of postoperative pain to be determined.

Rectal Administration of opioids

Absorption through the mucous membrane of the rectum is as rapid as buccal or sublingual administration. Several preparations of opioid for rectal administration are available. However, they are seldom used in the UK.

Local anaesthetic techniques

Local anaesthesia was introduced by the Austrian surgeon Karl Koller, who used topically applied cocaine for eye surgery in 1884. The use of preoperative local anaesthetic techniques by themselves or in combination with general anaesthesia has become increasingly popular during the last decade. Local anaesthetic drugs block the conduction of impulses along a nerve, therefore if the drug is injected close to nerves carrying painful stimuli to the brain it will provide analgesia. The commonest local anaesthetic drugs used in the UK are lignocaine, bupivacaine and prilocaine. These can be used in: topical application, local infiltration, nerve blocks, plexus blocks, caudals, epidurals and spinals.

Topical application

This is frequently used in paediatric wards when EMLA Cream is applied to children's hands prior to venepuncture. EMLA is a mixture of prilocaine and lignocaine which is absorbed by the skin results in anaesthesia. This cream has also been used to provide postoperative analgesia following such procedures as circumcision. Bupivacaine is now frequently applied topically by surgeons simply by spraying it on the wound before skin closure. Bupivacaine is chosen due to its long duration of action. This has been shown to provide effective analgesia for several hours after procedures such as hernia repair and orchidopexy.

Local infiltration

This is another simple technique and does not require any special skill or experience. The area around the wound is infiltrated with local anaesthetic (usually bupivacaine). Some surgeons worry about there being an increased risk of infection following the use of the topical or infiltration technique, though there is no evidence to support this. The technique can only be used as an adjunct to other analgesic therapy, as the effect wears off after a period of hours. Some clinicians have extended the duration of action by inserting catheters around the wound and giving infusions of local anaesthetic into these.

Nerve blocks and plexus blocks

Some operations are performed in a region supplied by only one or two nerves. The anaesthetist who has knowledge of the route these nerves take can inject local anaesthetic around them and thus prevent the painful stimuli being transmitted centrally. Examples of these include the use of sciatic nerve blocks for operations on the big toe and side of the foot, and ilioinguinal and iliohypogastric nerve blocks for hernia operations.

Similar knowledge is required to perform plexus blocks where a group of nerves can be anaesthetised with a single injection. An example of this is the brachial plexus block, which can provide preoperative and postoperative analgesia for arm surgery. A catheter can be inserted near the plexus of nerves and the analgesia prolonged by the use of infusions of local anaesthetic. Where nerves carry both motor and sensory nerves the local anaesthetic will cause loss of muscle function in those muscles supplied by the nerve blocked. This can be advantageous during an operation but can decrease mobility if prolonged into the postoperative period.

Further examples of nerve blocks and plexus blocks are shown in Table 5.2.

Caudals, epidurals and spinal blocks

Epidurals and spinals will be dealt with later in the chapter. Caudal local anaesthetic blocks are another approach to the epidural space. In fact, the first epidurals performed were introduced by this route. To perform a caudal the anaesthetist injects the local anaesthetic into the epidural space through the sacral hiatus which is situated at the base of the spine. This reliably provides analgesia for areas supplied by the sacral nerves such as the anus, rectum, vagina and part of the legs. It can also provide analgesia for the lumbar nerves if sufficient volume is injected; however, this is not so reliable except in children where caudal analgesia can be used for a wide variety of procedures such as hernia repairs, circumcision and orchidopexy. The duration of the block depends on the concentration and volume of local anaesthetic used. It can last for many hours (6–12 hours) and during

Table 5.2 Nerve and plexus blocks

	Areas of analgesia/ indications
Head and neck	
Retrobulbar block	intraocular surgery
Upper limb	
Brachial plexus block	major area of arm and hand
Ulnar nerve block	fifth metacarpal and little finger
Median nerve block	palmar aspect of hand and of first two fingers
Digital nerve block	allows simple operations on fingers/toes
Body/trunk	
Intercostal nerve block	area of thorax and abdomen supplied by each nerve, useful in fractured ribs, thoracotomy and following cholecystectomy
Paravertebral block	another approach to intercostal nerves, similar uses
Lower limb	
Sciatic nerve block	lateral aspect of limb below knee and whole of foot, useful in ankle and bunion surgery
Femoral nerve block	anterior aspect of thigh and knee, useful in pain relief of fractures of femur and in supplementing sciatic block for knee surgery.
Lateral cutaneous nerve of thigh block	lateral aspect of thigh, useful in hip surgery and in combination with previous two blocks

this period the patient's legs will be numb and weak. Retention of urine can also be a problem.

Other techniques

Transcutaneous nerve stimulation

This involves the application of electrodes to the skin of the patient around the area that requires pain relief. A small electrical current is passed between the electrodes and stimulates the sensory nerves. The current is supplied by a small battery powered box which allows the patient to control the frequency and the strength of the stimulus. This technique has proven to be useful in the treatment of chronic pain but is seldom used in the management of acute pain. It may decrease requirements for opioid analgesics but is not suitable as the sole analgesic method following major surgery.

Inhalational analgesia

The most common agent used for inhalational analgesia is Entonox, a mixture of 50% nitrous oxide and 50% oxygen. This is often administered by midwives to women for the management of pain in labour. It is also useful to facilitate physiotherapy in postoperative patients, those with fractured ribs and for analgesia during changing of wound dressings. It is a potent analgesic while it is being administered but it is not possible to administer it for long periods. This is due not only to the possibility that it may have an effect on bone marrow function of the patient but also because there may be significant exposure of nursing staff to the agent as it is difficult to prevent it polluting the ward. It also tends to give the patient a dry mouth because it is supplied as a dry gas with no humidification.

Spinal administration of opioids and local anaesthetic drugs

These can be injected into the fluid that surrounds the spinal cord, i.e. the cerebrospinal fluid, or into the epidural space. The distinction between the effects and administration of these two techniques is large, though anatomically they are only separated by the dura mater. The dura mater surrounds the spinal cord and contains the cerebrospinal fluid. The epidural (extradural) space lies between the dura mater and the bone and ligaments of the spinal canal. Catheters can now be inserted into both areas; however, those for inserting into the CSF have only recently become available and the usefulness of these has yet to be established. Opioids injected into both these areas act on receptors found in the spinal cord itself that modulate the pain messages being transferred to the brain. Due to the differences in the techniques the use of spinal and epidural drugs for postoperative analgesia will be covered separately.

Spinal analgesia

Prior to the recent arrival of spinal catheters, spinal anaesthesia and analgesia was a one-shot technique. The anaesthetist injected local anaesthetic to provide anaesthesia for the oper-

ation and this lasted for 3–4 hours at the most. The inclusion of an opioid such as morphine in this injection can prolong the analgesia provided for up to 24 hours. The dose of morphine required to achieve this length of analgesia is extremely small (0.1–0.2 mg). The quality of analgesia has been shown to be superior to conventional intramuscular techniques in several studies. However, it should be noted that there are problems with the technique. There is large variability in the response of patients to the drug and some may have incomplete analgesia. Nausea, vomiting and pruritus are problems as is the incidence of urinary retention which can necessitate catheterisation. The most important complication, however, is respiratory depression which may present many hours after the spinal. It should be noted that the incidence of this occurrence is increased if additional opioids are administered to the patient by any other route, and therefore this must be avoided.

Epidural analgesia

Epidural analgesia has been used in anaesthesia for many years, particularly in the provision of analgesia for women in labour. Its use has gradually extended to the general surgical population, as anaesthetists and surgeons have come to recognise the potential benefits of this technique. However, its use for the provision of good quality postoperative analgesia has been limited due to the necessity to nurse these patients on Intensive Care or High Dependency Units. There are four main forms of providing epidural analgesia. The original technique as used on most labour wards with an epidural service is by providing bolus doses of local anaesthetic (usually bupivacaine) when the patient requires analgesia. Concentrations of 0.25% or 0.5% bupivacaine are usually used for these 'top-ups' which are usually required every 1–2 hours. This technique has several disadvantages for both staff and patient. It requires a member of staff (usually medical) to provide the regular top-ups, following which the patient's blood pressure must be closely monitored. If there is any delay in the top-up the patient quickly becomes uncomfortable. The local anaesthetic causes marked loss of motor function in the lower limbs and the patient is unable to move, often to the extent of being unable to turn in bed. This can lead to problems with the development of bed sores unless the patient is turned regularly. The patient will also not be aware of their bladder and will require catheterization. However, the major problem with this technique is the risk of causing marked hypotension after the epidural has been topped up. This is due to the blockade of the sympathetic nerve supply to the lower limbs, causing vasodilation and therefore a decrease in the blood pressure. These problems have confined the use of this technique to areas such as the labour ward, ITU and HDU where there is the staffing level and equipment to look after these patients.

The second method is to provide a continuous infusion of local anaesthetic which removes the need to perform repeated 'top-ups' of the epidural. The concentrations and infusion rates of the local anaesthetic (again usually bupivacaine) used for this technique vary tremendously. The degree of loss of motor function will depend on both the concentration used and the rate of infusion; however, it is usually enough to prevent mobilisation. Again the patient will require catheterisation. Hypotension can still be a problem and the fluid balance of the patient must be observed carefully. This technique is seldom used outside the specialised operational areas mentioned above, though some clinicians have used the technique on a specific ward where there are sufficient numbers of trained staff.

The third technique involves the provision of bolus doses of opioid drugs such as diamorphine diluted in saline (typical dose 2.5–5.0 mg in 10 ml of saline). This has also been shown to provide satisfactory analgesia after major surgery, with each top-up lasting between 5 and 12 hours depending on the drug used and the patient. This prolonged action has made it more popular with clinicians but this method also has problems. As with all these techniques, siting the epidural is time consuming and it can be difficult to find the time required during a busy list unless assistance is available to the anaesthetist. Postoperatively the top-ups are provided by medical staff (usually the on-call anaesthetist) and in a busy hospital this can add an appreciable workload to a service that is already stretched. Delays in the top-ups lead to breakthrough pain and this decreases patient satisfaction with the technique. Furthermore, there are certain people in whom the technique does not appear to work: these may be due to

technical failures such as misplacement of the epidural or other problems. Nausea, vomiting and pruritus can be a problem, particularly during the first 24 hours, and may require treatment. Urinary retention is again common and most patients will require catheterisation. Finally, the complication of respiratory depression which can occur many hours after the injection of the opioid drug has tempered enthusiasm for this technique. However, this method is more popular in the UK (Semple and Jackson, 1991).

Finally, clinicians have started to look at the use of infusions of very weak solutions containing small amounts of opioids and local anaesthetic agents to provide a more balanced analgesic technique. This has been termed epidural infusion analgesia (EIA). The local anaesthetic agent is usually bupivacaine at a concentration between 0.008 and 0.15%. The opioid drug chosen varies, with some units using fentanyl and others morphine or diamorphine. A typical combination is 0.15% bupivacaine and 0.005% diamorphine (equivalent to 2.5 mg diamorphine in 50 ml saline). This is infused via the epidural at a rate of between 4 and 8 ml an hour, so the patient actually receives a very small dose of both the local anaesthetic and the opioid. This removes the problem of loss of motor function, allowing most patients to move about in bed and mobilise when allowed. Hypotension can still be a problem if the fluid balance of the patient is not carefully observed and they are allowed to become hypovolaemic from blood or other fluid loss. Respiratory depression is less of a problem than with bolus doses of epidural opioids, but must still be considered. This technique is now used in some hospitals in the labour ward, the ITU, the HDU and even on general wards. However, the staff on these wards must have been provided with suitable training and have the immediate back-up of named members of medical staff (usually anaesthetic), and the patients require to be reviewed on a regular basis. This can only be safely achieved by the provision of an Acute Pain Service.

Acute pain services

The recent report from the Royal College of Surgeons and College of Anaesthetists Working Party, 1990 starts with the statement

'The treatment of pain after surgery in British hospitals has been inadequate and has not advanced significantly in recent years.'

This situation is a sad reflection on the level of resources and training given to this subject. Additional problems involve the lack of responsibility for pain management by any one individual and the shortcomings of traditional analgesic regimes. The report makes several recommendations which include the establishing of an Acute Pain Service (APS) managed by an Acute Pain Team (APT) in all major hospitals. The use of an APS was pioneered in the USA in 1988 (Ready et al., 1988), with the first teams in the UK being operational in 1989 (Wheatley et al., 1989).

The aims of an Acute Pain Team (APT) should be:

1) To provide supervision of the management of postoperative pain.
2) To apply and advance new analgesic methods.
3) To support and educate both medical and nursing staff, in the use of new techniques.
4) To monitor and improve the service.

Developments in technology and clinical practice have for some time allowed the provision of more complete analgesia in specialised units such as Intensive Care Units (ICU). High Dependency Units (HDU) and on labour wards. Extension of these advanced techniques such as PCA or EIA to general surgical wards can only be safely achieved by controlled introduction with the supervision and responsibility for the management of these patients by named individuals such as an APT.

How an acute pain service works

Patients should be assessed preoperatively by the anaesthetist and the optimum analgesic technique decided upon following discussion with the patient and the surgical and nursing staff. Following surgery the patient is commenced on either PCA or EIA. Treatment is initiated in recovery by the anaesthetist and nursing staff. Several important observations are carried out in recovery and are recorded on a pain chart (Figure 5.5). This chart is designed to promote regular assessment of the patient, thus contributing to patient safety. The pain chart contains the patient's details and the monitoring instructions and includes the para-

meters to be recorded such as respiratory rate, pain score, sedation score, and the amount of drug used. These observations are recorded at 15-minute intervals in recovery and are then recorded as the other routine postoperative observations (hourly for 4 hours then 4 hourly if the patient remains stable).

Patient details are also entered onto a board in the anaesthetic office. This information, including name, ward, operation and analgesics technique in use, facilities the regular review of the patients by the APT. Ward rounds take place once or twice daily when medical, nursing, physiotherapy and pharmacy staff visit all the patients admitted to the service. During the ward round the APT assess the patient's pain using appropriate pain scoring systems such as a VAS. The analgesic technique being used is discussed with the patient and nursing staff, and modifications to their treatment made if necessary to optimise their analgesia. The team ensure the pain charts are correctly filled in, as they are used on a monthly basis to audit the service.

It is important that nursing and junior medical staff can call on a member of the APT if problems such as inadequate analgesia are encountered. It is the responsibility of the APT to decide when the patient's analgesic technique is to be altered, including the decision to terminate treatment by the intravenous or epidural route. This usually occurs when the patient can be commenced on oral analgesia.

Admission to the service

Most patients will be admitted to the APT by their anaesthetist following surgery. However the facility for referrals from surgeons, physicians, nursing staff and physiotherapists concerning patients who are not receiving adequate analgesia should be available. This is necessary as some patients who are in severe pain are admitted with non-surgical conditions.

Structure of the APT

An APS requires a multidisciplinary team selected from the medical, nursing and pharmacy staff. Most teams are formed from nursing and anaesthetic staff, as postoperative patients are the main users of the service. Anaesthetic staff also provide a trained pool of

Patient Controlled Analgesia (PCA) – for further information see over

Patient Details
Reg. No
Name
Age
Sex
Weight
Ward
Date
Operation
Anaesthetist
Surgeon

Surgery			**Incision**	
General	1		UAB	1
Gynae	2		LAB	2
GU	3		Peripheral	3
Ortho	4		Thor	4
Trauma	5		Thor/abdo	5
Obstetric	6		UAB/LAB	6
Other	7			

ASA   1   2   3   4   Elective   Acute
Comment

Drugs
Perioperative Opioids (Drug + Dose)
Preop ....
Perop ....
Recovery ....
Antiemetic ....

Local Anaesthetics

Spinal	1		Other	6
Epidural	2		NSAID's	7
Caudal	3			
Intercostal	4			
Ilioinguinal	5			

Infusion

Analgesic Drug – Morphine
Concentration – 1 mg/ml
Bolus Dose   – 1 mg
Lockout time   – 5 minutes
Antiemetic

	Date	Time	AMOUNT DISCARDED	Initials
Start				
Refill				
Refill				
Refill				

Total Volume Infused   =   mls

Nursing Checks – Recovery every 15 mins   **Ward** hourly for 4hrs, then 4hrly
(PLEASE NOTE – THE INFORMATION ON THE BACK OF THIS SHEET WILL HELP YOU FILL THIS SECTION IN CORRECTLY)

Date	Time	Respiratory Rate	Pain Score	Sedation Score	IV Site	Tries/ Good	Dose	Volume	Initial

Figure 5.5 A pain chart

Pain Team To Fill In

	Nausea	Vomiting	Itching
First 24hrs	Y/N	Y/N	Y/N
Next 24hrs	Y/N	Y/N	Y/N

Other side effects

How would you describe your satisfaction with the treatment of your pain?

Poor	Fair	Adequate	Good	Excellent
1	2	3	4	5

Which of the following words best describes the severity of pain you experienced?

Absent	Mild	Discomforting	Distressing	Excruciating
1	2	3	4	5

Would you consider having this type of pain control again?

Definately	Probably	Possibly	No
1	2	3	4

Would you recommend this technique to a friend?

Definately	Probably	Possibly	No
1	2	3	4

24 Hour Pain Score (VAS 0–10) .....   **24 Hr Pain On Movement Score (VAS 0–10)** .....

Time to comfort .....   **Duration of treatment** ..... **hrs**

Total Pain Score .....   **24 Hour Opiate Dose** ...... **mgs**

Average Pain Score .....   **Duration of catheterisation** ... **hrs**

Comments

Figure 5.5 A pain chart *continued*

staff who are familiar with the problems and management of modern analgesic techniques.

The provision of this expertise as part of their 24 hour hospital cover, thus supplying readily available backup for the ward staff, must be regarded as the ideal standard for any APS. The appointment of a senior nursing position in acute pain, such as an acute pain sister, is also a fundamental requirement. This post facilitates the setting up of in-service training programmes and provides a valuable link between nursing and medical staff.

Practical points about advanced analgesic techniques

PCA and EIA should only be introduced to a ward situation where there is support from senior medical and nursing staff. Training should be provided in the use and management of the pumps and in the monitoring of the patients. The time saved by nursing staff not having to check and administer intramuscular injections should be reinvested in the patients, monitoring their pain and degree of sedation. The use of a sedation score has proven useful in several centres. Patients appear to become progressively more sleepy and unrousable prior to developing respiratory depression. Experience has shown that 50 ml syringes will require changing once or twice daily. The safety and speed of this process can be increased by enlisting the help of the hospital pharmacy. They can prepare batches of syringes under sterile conditions on a monthly basis which can then be frozen and ordered when needed. The availability of prefilled syringes in the ward also

Nursing Checks

1. **RESPIRATIONS**
   If respiratory rate is less than 10/min – inform Maternity Anaesthetist
   If respiratory rate is less than 8/min – **STOP PUMP**
                                             bleep and inform Maternity Anaesthetist

2. **PAIN SCORE**: Score 0 = No pain at rest
                                  No pain on movement (see below)
                    Score 1 = No pain at rest
                                  Slight pain on movement
                    Score 2 = Intermittent pain at rest
                                  Moderate pain on movement
                    Score 3 = Continuous pain at rest
                                  Severe pain on movement

   Movement = Patient attempt to touch the opposite side of bed with hand
   If pain relief is inadequate encourage patient to press the button, and check IV site
   Inform Maternity Anaesthetist if continuing inadequate pain relief

3. **SEDATION SCORE**
                    Score 0 = None (patient alert)
                    Score 1 = Mild (occasionally drowsy; easy to arouse)
                    Score 2 = Moderate (frequently drowsy; easy to arouse)
                    Score 3 = Severe (somnolent; difficult to arouse)
                    Score S = Sleep (normal sleep, easy to arouse)

4. **IV Site** – check for leaks, obstruction of tubing or tissuing – **inform houseman**

5. **Tries/good** } this information obtained from screen display, if unsure how to
   Dose   use pump display – **Please Ask**

6. **Volume** = amount remaining in syringe

   PROBLEMS
   If there are any problems with PCAS please contact the Maternity Anaesthetist, Dr Madej, Dr
   Wheatley, Dr Jackson or Sister Hunter.

   PLEASE NOTE
   All wards have copies of the document PCA written by ourselves, this should be read by any Nurse
   or Junior Doctor who has not previously met this system of pain control. We will be delighted to
   answer any questions about this technique during our daily ward visits.

   AT END OF TREATMENT
   1 **Please fill in comment as appropriate**
   2 **Please return pump and this form to theatre reception as soon as possible**

Figure 5.5 A pain chart *continued*

facilitates the changing of syringes by nursing staff. If both PCA and EIA are being used in a hospital it is better that the infusion pumps and prefilled containers be completely different. This decreases the possibility of the wrong drug being connected.

Summary

In order to challenge the traditional attitudes and methods of treating postoperative or acute pain, there must be a responsible and account-able team to provide advice, education, and support to both medical and nursing staff. If advanced methods of pain relief are introduced by a team of specialists, then the fear of safety on the general surgical wards become minimised.

The presence of an APT can not only ensure the safe introduction of these techniques, but serves to increase the awareness of acute pain, causing the nursing and medical staff to question the use of traditional methods in alleviating postoperative pain.

Recent developments in the management of acute pain

The recent report by the Working Party on Acute Pain (Royal College of Surgeons Report, 1990), has highlighted the inadequacies of its current management and has identified priorities for the future, it states that:

'the treatment of pain after surgery in British hospitals has been inadequate and has not advanced significantly for many years.'

The working party highlights several ways that pain relief can be improved which include:

1. Improved education and training – to change attitudes of medical and nursing staff.
2. Implementation of routine formal pain assessment – for all patients.
3. Introduction of new methods of pain relief – for safer and more effective pain relief.
4. Provision of Appropriate facilities and resources – acute pain team, high dependency units.
5. Standard policy on pain relief.
6. The use of counselling and psychological methods.
7. Research.
8. Audit.

Pre-emptive analgesia

There is evidence to support the theory of pre-emptive analgesia: the blocking of pain pathways before the stimulus occurs, to prevent the pain occurring. This idea involves the use of nerve blocking procedures and analgesic drugs before surgery (Wall, 1988; McQuay and Dickenson, 1990).

Day surgery

The concept of day surgery has evolved from improved surgical techniques and recent developments in anaesthesia. The introduction of day surgery has obvious benefits for both the patients (spending less time in hospital) and hospital resources (cost effective). Patient selection is important and should consider not only the surgery type, but individual patient factors such as age, general health status and home situation. Patients undergoing day sur-

gery procedures have special requirements which influence the choice of pre-medication, anaesthetic and pain relieving techniques, as they will all affect the ability for patients to be discharged on the same day of surgery. As a general rule opioids are avoided and less sedative analgesic drugs are used (such as the non steroidal anti-inflammatories, e.g. ibuprofen). Many procedures are performed under local anaesthesia, which may be preferable to general anaesthesia. Patients may experience severe pain, despite undergoing relatively minor surgery and should have the pain treated appropriately before discharge is considered; if necessary, arrangements to stay overnight should be made. It is also important that patients are given adequate supply of analgesic drugs on discharge, with instruction relating to appropriate administration; it may be difficult for the patient to get to the chemist immediately so supply availability should be checked.

Summary

Pain relief in the acute pain patient has been a low priority in the past. Mortality due to inadequate pain relief has not been publicised however. Badly managed pain leads to mortality from chest infection, myocardial infarction and deep vein thrombosis due to lack of mobility.

The nurse is the primary care team member who spends most time with the patient, therefore nurses are the ideal day-to-day managers of the patient suffering from acute pain. Time may be limited due to a busy ward schedule and therefore the nurse must implement the following plan:

1. Identify the patient's need on an individual basis.
2. Obtain a prescription for those needs.
3. Carry out treatment.
4. Evaluate the effectiveness of treatment.
5. Implement any changes required.

A patient's pain is subjective and they should be believed at all times, while the nurse is involved directly in pain assessment and pain management. Whichever approach to pain management is utilised within the hospital the nurse along with other health care professionals must continue to have adequate education and in-service training, as new methods of analgesia become available.

The treatment of postoperative pain remains the core of APT work. Development of the service to include any acute pain situation may be referred and dealt with by the team. An example of this is the provision of epidural infusion of analgesia, preoperatively to a patient who is to undergo amputation. The acute pain team is involved several days before the patient attends theatre by siting the epidural, establishing an adequate sensory block which postoperatively is used to prevent the occurance of phantom limb pain. The epidural is also used in theatre during the operation and therefore cuts down the requirement for either a general anaesthetic or a lighter anaesthetic. Also, the provision of pain relief to patients undergoing extra-amniotic termination of pregnancy, who are managed on busy gynaecological wards, may not be adequate, and provision of PCA by the acute pain team is helpful for both the physical and psychological aspects of the traumatic experience.

References

Catling, J. A., Pinto, D. M., Jordon, C. and Jones, J. G. (1980) Respiratory effects of analgesia after cholecystectomy: comparison of continuous and intermittent papaveretum. *British Medical Journal*, **281**, 478

Donovan, M., Dillon, P. and McGuire, L. (1987) Incidence and characteristics of pain in a sample of medical-surgical inpatients. *Pain*, **30**, 69–78

Fell, D., Derbyshire, D. R. Maile, C. J. D. *et al.* (1985) Measurement of plasma catecholamine concentrations: an assessment of anxiety. *British Journal of Anaesthesia*, **57**, 770–774

Frank, A. J. M., Moll, J. M. H. and Hort, J. F. (1982) A comparison of three ways of measuring pain. *Rheumatology and Rehabilitation*, **21**, 211–217

Leigh, J. M., Walker, J. and Janaganathan, P. (1977) Effect of preoperative anaesthetic visit on anxiety. *British Medical Journal*, **2**, 987–989

Locsin, R. (1981) The effect of music on the pain of selected postoperative patients. *Journal of Advanced Nursing*, **6**, 19–25

McCleane, G. J. and Cooper, R. (1990) The nature of preoperative anxiety. *Anaesthesia*, **45**, 153–155

Melzack, R. (1975) The McGill Pain Questionnaire: major properties and scoring methods. *Pain*, **1**, 277–299

Ready, L. B., Oden, R., Chadwick, H. S. *et al.* (1988) Development of an anesthesiology based postoperative pain management service. *Anesthesiology*, **68**, 100–106

Sechzer, P. H. (1968) Objective measurement of pain. *Anesthesiology*, **29**, 209–210

Semple, P. and Jackson, I. J. B. (1991) Postoperative analgesia: survey of current practice. *Anaesthesia*, **46**, 1074–1076

Thomas, T. A. and Griffiths, M. J. (1982) A pain slide rule. *Anaesthesia*, **37**, 960–961

Yeager, M. P., Glass, D. D., Neff, R. K. and Brinck-Johnson, T. (1987) Epidural anesthesia and analgesia in high-risk surgical patients. *Anesthesiology*, **66**, 729–736

Further reading list

The publications listed combine to offer interesting and varied reading with more detailed references well listed:

1. Nursing Now Series (1985) Pain. Springhouse Corporation, Philadelphia Various contributors.
2. Melzack, R. (1985) (Ed) Pain Measurement and Assessment. Raven Press, New York
3. Hasking, J. and Welchen E. (1985) Post-operative pain: understanding its nature and how to treat it. Faber & Faber Ltd., London
4. McCaffery, M. (1979) Nursing the Patient in Pain (2nd Edn) J. B. Lippincott Co., London
5. McCaffery, M. and Beebe, A. (1989) Pain – clinical manual for nursing practice. The C.V. Mosby Co., Missouri
6. World Health Organization Guidelines (1986)
7. Clinical Journal "Pain" Available monthly
8. Latham, J. (1987) Pain Control. Austen Cornish Publishers/Lisa Sainsbury Foundation, London. (2nd edition 1990)
9. The Royal College of Surgeons of England and College of Anaesthetists Report on the Working Party: Pain After Surgery, 1990

6

Chronic pain

J. Latham

Introduction

Clinicians and researchers involved in the field of pain have been trying for many years to give the ultimate definition of what 'chronic pain' actually is. The result has been a spectrum of concepts which have encompassed issues such as time-scale, specific clinical syndromes and related behavioural/life-style changes.

Collins Concise English Dictionary (eds McLeod and Hanks, 1987) has some interesting definitions of both the words 'chronic' and 'pain':

'Chronic'

i) Continuing for a long time; constantly recurring.
ii) (Of a disease) developing slowly or of long duration.
iii) Inveterate; habitual.
iv) Very bad/serious.

'Pain'

i) The sensation of acute physical hurt or discomfort caused by injury, illness etc.
ii) Emotional suffering or mental distress.
iii) 'On pain of . . .' – subject to the penalty of . . .
iv) Also called: 'pain in the neck' or thing that is a nuisance.

These definitions start to give us an insight into how very complex the subject of chronic pain is, and this chapter aims to look at some of the key issues involved in it.

The nurse's responsibility to the patient with chronic pain

'Pain is whatever the experiencing person says it is, existing whenever he says it does . . .' (McCaffery, 1972). This is perhaps one of the most famous statements in nursing literature on pain, and highlights the fact it is only relatively recently that nurses have started to recognise the philosophy that each patient's pain should be treated as an individual experience without pre-conceptions of how each patient should respond and thus be treated in a particular clinical situation.

It is, however, important to think beyond this statement because it is actually what we *do* with the information that the patient gives us about their pain that will ultimately lead to the incurable or the cured. To enable this to occur effectively the nurse has to have a sound knowledge base of communication skills, the physiological and psychological mechanisms that are involved in chronic pain and the resultant therapeutic alternatives which may be available. This concept in itself can prove to be a major challenge to nurses because patients with chronic pain have such individual experiences. Inherently this indicates that the nurse has to be aware of a wide range of therapeutic needs, for example, there may be different responses from patients to the same drug so the dose of that drug may vary considerably from one patient to another. It is also important to be aware of what are realistic as opposed to unrealistic goals and also which options the patient is likely to comply with and what they will not – failure to comply and meet anticipated goals means failure to cure. Nurses should recognise that while they are coping with the complex individual needs of each chronic pain patient, the situation can be extremely mentally exhausting and appropriate support systems should be available to discuss related problems.

It is essential to realise that chronic pain patients frequently require the expertise of the whole multi-disciplinary team and the nurse not only gains her support from this team, but also plays a key role in recognising when referral is appropriate to another member of the team for specialist support. Nurses also need to have the confidence to realise that 'good nursing can reduce the patient's tension and anxiety which in turn dissipates panic and increases the patient's tolerance of pain, the patient then feels more comfortable and once again more in control of himself.' (Williams, 1987, 1991).

The vicious cycle of chronic pain

A painful experience leads to physical and behavioural reactions and responses which, if not interrupted at an appropriate and/or an early enough stage, will lead to a chronic pain syndrome developing. The longer these reactions and responses are allowed to occur unabated, the more likelihood there is that an entrenched, intractable self-perpetuating cycle of pain will develop, making it more and more difficult for the cycle to be interrupted (Figure 6.1).

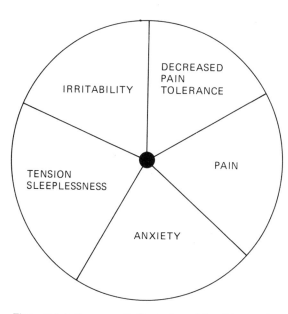

Figure 6.1 A diagrammatic illustration of the vicious cycle of chronic pain

Onset of chronic pain

A key area of debate which is likely to continue as more becomes known about the physiological mechanisms involved in pain is when does pain become chronic as opposed to acute? Whilst initially it was felt that chronic pain was pain lasting for 6 months or longer, this time-scale has now shortened considerably, for example, the International Association For The Study Of Pain (IASP) presently defines it as pain that lasts continuously or intermittently for 3 months or more. It is quite possible in the future that this time-scale will shorten even more.

Chronic pain – implications for the patient and society

As discussed on pages 50–51, chronic pain all too often encompasses every aspect of a persons' life, and the longer it is allowed to continue the more intractable the problem becomes. It is therefore important that we are aware of the key actual/potential implications for patients suffering with chronic pain and the resultant moral, social and financial implications for society.

Illness behaviour

When patients initially present with pain they are usually seen to be physically ill, therefore recognised patterns of illness behaviour are allowed, and indeed generally accepted by the therapeutic team, carers and family/friends. This is appropriate when a physical cause and resultant treatment can be identified, even if, as with so many chronic pain syndromes, the correct diagnosis and treatment often take some time to be identified. In the majority of these cases, once the pain has been successfully treated, a return to normal life-style occurs and any behavioural changes associated with their illness eventually resolve.

Problems arise with this scenario when the pain is subsequently found to have non-physical components. The patient will inevitably have developed behavioural patterns in keeping with a physical illness which may well have been positively reinforced by all involved in their care. In these cases, once the underlying problem has been identified, positive life-style therapy in conjunction with the appropriate psychological/psychiatric treatment is essential to re-establish the patient in society as a 'physically well' person.

Interpersonal relationships

Inevitably a patient with chronic pain requires a great deal of care, attention, understanding and patience. This in turn can place extra demands, physical and/or psychological, on all relationships in the patient's life, which can include the spouse, next-of-kin, family, colleagues and carers. Additional nursing, medical, paramedical and social support may be required not only for the patient themselves, but also for the carers to enable them to provide an appropriate level of long-term care without putting themselves under intolerable levels of stress.

The change in emphasis in interpersonal relationships may lead to the patient's role in society changing, which they may or may not welcome. It is essential, if a chronic pain patient wishes to maintain their independence as much as possible, that these wishes are respected and encouraged with positive reinforcement from all involved. A perceived loss of identity and/or status, real or not, when involved in interpersonal relationships, can swiftly lead to a loss of self-esteem and therefore a negative influence on recovery. It is also equally important to recognise that some people positively welcome the secondary gain of additional attention and support from spouse or next-of-kin, family, friends, and colleagues. In these cases, it is important to be aware that this could influence the course of recovery as they may feel that if the pain and/or its cause are cured then the increased support will end.

Social isolation can play a key factor in how patients cope or not cope with chronic pain, and can either be a predisposing or a resultant factor due, for example, to unemployment or family/peer group stress. If this is identified as a problem then behavioural/life-style therapy will have an important role to play in treatment.

Financial implications

It is not uncommon for patients with chronic pain to experience changes in their financial situation. Unemployment or retirement can occur due to chronic illness and the resultant time off work, especially in times of recession. This in turn can lead to a lower standard of living if a regular salary is lost and the patient has to depend on unemployment benefits and/or disability pensions. Loss of self-esteem as a result of financial hardship and thus lack of previous status and interests is not uncommon with chronic pain patients.

It is important to be aware when assessing a patient with chronic pain that change in financial status can in itself be one of the contributing causes towards chronic pain syndromes. In these cases social and psychological support is essential if self-esteem is to be restored and recovery made.

A chronic pain syndrome that has developed as a result of modern society and has direct financial implications for both the patient and society is 'litigation syndrome'. In these cases patients are unlikely to have their chronic pain cured until their financial claim is settled, because pain to them is continuing evidence of their problem. If the patient has unreasonable expectations of the outcome of the situation, or using the situation for secondary gain, either personal or financial, then the syndrome is unlikely to resolve, and the patient is in turn likely to suffer worse financial hardship as a result of the more long-term effects of 'chronic disability'.

Types of chronic pain

It is important to identify that there are three main types of chronic pain which can present:

1. Recurrent acute pain that occurs regularly or irregularly over a prolonged period of time – even a life-time. There will be periods of total or comparative relief between these acute episodes, e.g. migraine, pancreatitis, sickle-cell crisis.
2. Chronic acute pain that is time limited and will resolve when the condition causing the pain is cured or controlled, or when the patient dies, e.g. carcinoma, burns, end stage vascular disease.
3. Chronic benign (non-malignant) pain that can range from a mild to severe intensity pain occurring almost daily due to a non-life-threatening cause. It may be present for the rest of the patient's life, as response to currently available methods of treatment is variable and often disappointing, e.g. arthritis, osteoporosis, myofascial pain, peripheral neuropathies, life-style disorders, psychiatric syndromes.

Common syndromes associated with chronic pain

Relationships between disease processes and chronic pain

Arthritis ⟶ back and/or
Osteoporosis   localised joint
                  pains, fractures,
                  contractures
Carcinoma ⟶ depending on the
                  sites of the disease –
                  visceral, bone,
                  neurogenic, central
                  pain
Peripheral vascular ⟶ Ischaemia,
disease   gangrene,
                  amputation
Diabetes ⟶ neuropathy,
                  vascular ischaemia,
                  infection,
                  amputation
Cerebrovascular ⟶ thalamic pain,
accident   contractures
Cardiovasular ⟶ angina
disease
Chronic obstructive ⟶ chest pain,
airways disease   secondary
                  osteoporosis
Herpes zoster ⟶ post-herpetic
                  neuralgia
Falls/trauma ⟶ myofascial pain,
                  fractures, resultant
                  secondary pain
                  syndromes, e.g.
                  Colles fracture –
                  reflex sympathetic
                  dystrophy, facial
                  trauma – atypical
                  facial pain
Surgery ⟶ chronic post-
                  surgical nerve
                  injuries/
                  entrapments,
                  inflammatory
                  syndromes,
                  adhesions
Life events, e.g. ⟶ exaggeration of
bereavement, isolation, other physical pain
marital problems, symptoms, lack of
dependence, litigation success in
Depression   treatment, 'total
                  body pain
                  syndrome' etc.

Specific chronic pain syndromes

Chronic back pain

Chronic back pain is one of the commonest problems presented to a wide sphere of clinicians including those in general practice, rheumatology, orthopaedics, neurology, psychological medicine and pain clinics. Approximately 25% of patients referred to pain clinics with chronic benign pain suffer from chronic back pain (McQuay, 1989) and it remains one of the most intractable causes of social and financial distress to both the individual and society. The implications for society can also be seen to be changing with modern trends, for example increasing numbers of medico-legal cases now occur where problems such as arachnoiditis are claimed to be secondary to injury/accident or medical intervention. A major contributing factor is the problem of achieving an accurate diagnosis when there may be so many possible physical and psychological components: it has been suggested that as few as 20% of patients with back pain have their pain source accurately diagnosed (Kirwan, 1989). Inherently the problem of achieving an accurate diagnosis leads to the problem of achieving an appropriate treatment plan with realistic outcomes and expectations which may include an improvement in the existing lifestyle or complete cure. All too often patients who have had multiple invasive procedures such as surgery get referred to pain clinics as a last resort, often worse than before they had the invasive procedures. Undoubtedly early appropriate treatment leads to a higher chance of total cure.

Chronic back pain can be identified as belonging to three main categories (McQuay 1989):

i) Pain as a result of malignant disease.
ii) Pain which has failed to respond to appropriate conservative measures.
iii) Pain which has failed to respond or recurs following surgery.

Symptoms that present can be divided into two main categories (Waddell 1982):

i) Pathological, e.g. a disease process which involves the spine such as tumours, infections and ankylosing spondylitis. In these cases symptoms involving other systems may also be present, which portray a picture of general ill-health, and relief is not classically obtained by rest.

ii) Mechanical, e.g. recurrent episodes of pain exacerbated by activity and eased by rest.

Causes of chronic back pain include osteo-arthritis, osteoporosis, spinal or related malignancy, prolapsed intervertebral disc, facet joint degeneration, spinal stenosis, muscle spasm, arachnoiditis, surgery and behavioural/lifestyle problems.

Appropriate treatment plans are very much decided on an individual patient basis once all contributing components have been identified. Options include pharmacology, invasive techniques such as nerve blocks, transcutaneous nerve stimulation, acupuncture, physiotherapy, lifestyle/behavioural therapy and complementary therapies such as aromatherapy, massage and reflexology.

Myofascial pain

Myofascial pain refers to the pain caused as a result of trauma/stress to a muscular trigger point involving the fibrous connective tissue which is present in sheets between the muscles.

Unfortunately, whilst acute myofascial pain can be very successfully treated with measures such as freezing the area with a vapocoolant spray and stretching the muscle, local anaesthetic trigger point injections, dry-needling and acupuncture, it is one of the most poorly recognised and inadequately treated musculo-skeletal pains (Travell, 1976). This is felt to be largely due to lack of knowledge about specific referred pain patterns of individual muscles (Simons and Travell, 1989). Chronic myofascial syndromes occur either if inadequate acute treatment has been offered and/or perpetuating factors such as mechanical stresses, nutritional inadequacies, metabolic/endocrine inadequacies, chronic infection and/or emotional stress are present (Simons and Travell, 1989). In these cases effective treatment inevitably involves a combined plan to correct both the primary cause and the perpetuating factors.

Neurogenic pain syndromes

Bowsher (1987) stated that over 25% of patients referred to the Walton Pain Relief Service presented with a neurogenic pain syndrome.

Neurogenic pain occurs as a result of damage to nerves of either a peripheral or central origin. Damage that is peripheral in origin leads not only to spontaneous firing of the affected peripheral nerve fibres but also to spontaneous firing in the posterior root ganglion cells of the damaged nerves (Nathan, 1987). Examples of syndromes that can present include post-herpetic neuralgia, trigeminal neuralgia, causalgia, (including reflex sympathetic dystrophy) and phantom limb/organ pain. Whilst pain involving the central nervous system can be due to impulses arriving in the system from the peripheral network, it can also be due to an insult occurring in the system itself (Nathan, 1987), for example thalamic syndrome as a result of cerebrovascular accident. Neurogenic pain is classically described as a burning, stabbing, shooting pain which may also ache and/or throb. This can be accompanied by incomplete sensory deficit and autonomic deficit in the painful area.

One of the most important factors to remember when deciding on an appropriate treatment plan for patients with these syndromes is that the mechanism causing neurogenic pain is different to that of 'nociceptive' pain, i.e. a pain caused by stimulation of specific receptors. It is therefore unlikely that neurogenic pain will respond to groups of drugs such as opiates. It should, however, also be recognised that some pain syndromes such as peripheral vascular disease and spinal disc lesions may have a combination of both neurogenic and nociceptive pain mechanisms, so a combination of therapies may be indicated.

Treatments for neurogenic pain include antidepressants/convulsants, neural blockade and transcutaneous nerve stimulation.

Psychogenic pain syndromes

Chronic pain syndromes can be present as a result of behavioural/lifestyle problems such as bereavement, isolation, marital problems, unemployment, litigation syndrome and depression. Whilst this group of syndromes can be some of the most intractable, and at times frustrating, it is important that all the contributing factors are diagnosed and each component handled sensitively yet firmly by the appropriate member of the team. It is obviously import-

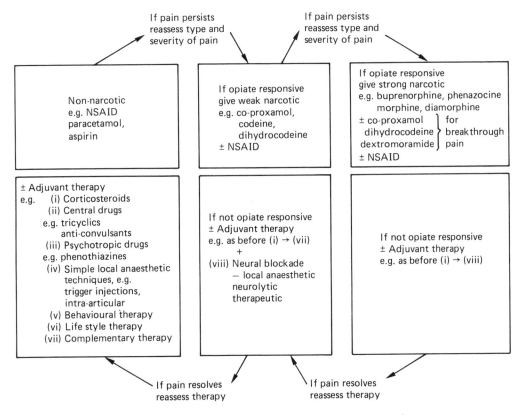

Figure 6.2 An outline of treatment options for chronic pain

ant to communicate to the patient that you believe they have pain, but it is equally important that you discuss the possible causes, and available therapies that may or may not be helpful.

Treatment plans depend very much on the problems identified and patient compliance. It is important to recognise that some patients will respond well to treatment, but others may not actually want to be cured. Treatments may include nonconventional analgesic drugs such as the anticonvulsants and antidepressants, behavioural/lifestyle therapy, complementary therapies and social services support.

The nurse's role with this group of patients is challenging and often multi-faceted, encompassing both direct involvement in treatments and also being a referral or re-referral point to other members of the team, e.g. the psychologist, psychiatrist or social workers, as it is often the nurse that patients will trust with all their problems and worries.

Treatment of chronic pain

The key to effective treatment of chronic pain is to do nothing until an assessment has been made and then the appropriate treatment(s) can be decided for each identified component of the syndrome. The commonest mistake to make when treating chronic pain is to decide on treatment options before an appropriate diagnosis has been made. This will then inevitably lead to the patient's syndrome becoming more intractable, thus lessening the chances of successful treatment in the short/long term. It is also important when assessing pain to identify how drugs and treatments were administered previously, as failure may be due to problems such as inadequate therapeutic doses, too infrequent use and too short a course. Figure 6.2 illustrates the logical approach that should be adopted when considering treatment options for each patient following assessment (adapted from 'Pain Control', J. Latham, 1991).

Pharmacology

There are particular issues that are raised when specifically considering chronic pain, and these are discussed below.

Addiction

Addiction should not occur if the appropriate drug is given for the appropriate pain, and it is adequately monitored. The problem of addiction with patients is a real danger if the wrong drug is given either because of mis-diagnosis or lack of pharmacological know-ledge, and/or if inadequate monitoring or communication occurs. Examples of the first scenario include chronic back patients being inappropriately prescribed long-term opiates and patients being inappropriately prescribed benzodiazepines. Examples of the second scenario include lack of communication between therapeutic teams which may lead to multiple prescribers.

Tolerance

Due to the often long-term use of drugs for chronic pain patients there is a fear amongst some practitioners that the patient may become tolerant to a drug dose and therefore require repeatedly higher doses in an attempt to achieve therapeutic efficacy. Whilst this problem by no means occurs with every patient taking long-term medication, it is wise to be aware that it could be a potential problem with some chronic pain patients. If the dose of drug does require to be increased on a regular basis to try and maintain therapeutic levels, then it is important to also exclude other causes such as a change in the presenting problems or the fact that another route of administration may be more efficacious. In a small number of patients it may be felt that this is a worrying problem that may require changes in the medication regime.

Side effects

It is important when prescribing drugs in the treatment of chronic pain to be aware of poten-tial side effects. This knowledge is essential both if appropriate co-adjuvants are to be given, and if the patient is to be made aware of any potential problems. If a patient is not given appropriate co-analgesics or is not told of potential side effects then the likelihood of compliance with effective long-term treatment is very much reduced. With opiate therapy, for example, it is important to remember to give laxatives and anti-emetics as necessary in con-junction with advice that the patient may feel a little sleepy if the dose is increased. With drugs such as tricyclic anti-depressants, for example, it is important to warn the patient that they may feel sleepy and have a dry mouth when they start the drugs and also when dosages are increased. It is also, however, important to stress in this case to the patient that if they persist with the drugs that these side effects are likely to wear off and the benefits of treatment will be obtained.

Specific groups of drugs used in chronic non-malignant pain

Simple analgesics

This group of drugs, which includes aspirin and paracetamol, are much under-estimated and are useful in the treatment of mild to moderate visceral pain, and musculoskeletal pain.

Non-steroidal anti-inflammatory drugs (NSAIDs)

This group of drugs, which includes voltarol, indocid, naprosyn and feldene, are useful as analgesics and in the treatment of generalised and localised inflammatory conditions. They are also useful specifically in the treatment of bone pain which is thought to be due to excess-ive prostaglandin release, as they are thought to inhibit release of prostaglandins.

Opioid analgesics

This group of drugs are useful in the treatment of opiate responsive (nociceptive) pain which has proved resistant to non-opioid therapy. It is particularly important when treating chronic pain patients to be aware that opioids should not be used when a patient has an opiate non-responsive pain such as neurogenic or psycho-genic pain. Whereas simple analgesics act mainly peripherally, opioids act mainly centrally on perception of pain in the brain.

It is important to be aware that there is more than one pharmacological group of opioid analgesics. For example there are the opioid agonists such as dihydrocodeine, co-proxamol, morphine and diamorphine, and the opioid agonists (or partial agonists) such as buprenorphine. The partial agonist group are thought to antagonise the action of the agonist group if they are given together; however, current research may change our thinking on this in the future.

When treating chronic non-malignant pain with opioids the oral route should always be used in preference to injection. At the present time morphine is the opioid of choice. Pethidine is not felt to be appropriate due to the fact it is so short-acting and also it has potential toxicity problems with components such as norpethidine.

The use of opioids, particularly morphine, in the management of chronic non-malignant pain is a controversial issue. However, the following guidelines are proposed (Glynn *et al.*, 1991).

Guidelines for opioid use in non-malignant pain

1. All other treatments have failed.
2. The pain is shown to be relieved by opioids.
3. The patient, after clear explanations and discussion with family and family practitioner, is willing to take opioids.
4. Other doctors involved in the patient's care agree with opioid prescription.
5. Appropriate follow-up.

Corticosteroids

This group of drugs, including dexamethasone, hydrocortisone and methylprednisolone, are useful in the treatment of generalised and localised inflammatory conditions of the joints such as rheumatoid arthritis and soft tissue inflammatory conditions such as tennis elbow and tendinitis. They are also very useful both orally and in injection preparation in cancer pain (see Chapter 14).

Antidepressant / Anticonvulsant drugs

This group of drugs includes tricyclic antidepressants, such as amitriptyline, imipramine and dothiepin and anticonvulsant drugs such as carbamazepine and sodium valproate. The precise role and mechanism of these drugs is uncertain, but they are clinically useful in the management of neurogenic pain syndromes, where there is nerve damage, particularly that which is burning, shooting, or aching in character. As well as giving pain relief the antidepressants also have an effect on mood and sleep, which is beneficial.

Amitriptyline has been proven to be effective in the treatment of diabetic neuropathy (Max *et al.*, 1987) and post-herpetic neuralgia (Watson, 1982). More recently, research has shown amitriptyline to be effective in more heterogenous pain conditions at lower doses than used for the treatment of depression (McQuay *et al.*, 1992), without having an effect on mood. More detailed information on specific drug groups and individual drugs, including indications and sided effects can be found in Chapter 14.

Neural blockade

Neural blockade can be an effective treatment when the pain is due to nerve irritation or invasion. In the past both neurolytic agents (which can actually destroy the nerves) and local anaesthetic agents have been used in various procedures to treat chronic pain syndromes such as these. In present day practice, however, clinicians have become far more cautious in the use of neurolytic agents, particularly when treating non-malignant disease as more has become known about the potential long-term side effects that can occur with the use of these agents and other less potentially damaging techniques/options have become recognised.

Some of the techniques that are most common in the treatment of chronic non-malignant pain include:

- Epidural injections for back pain.
- Epidural and intrathecal catheters for the administration of opiates and local anaesthetics in end stage vascular disease.
- Lumbar sympathetic block for peripheral vascular disease.
- Lumbar psoas block for hip pain.
- Stellate ganglion block/thoracic somatic paravertebral block for post-herpetic neuralgia.
- Specific joint/trigger point injections for localised painful areas.
- Regional sympathetic block for reflex sympathetic dystrophy syndrome.

More detailed information on specific procedures can be found in Chapter 15.

Adjuvant therapies

Adjuvant therapies can be extremely beneficial and cover a wide range of options that can be carried out by nurses or other appropriate professionals working within the multi-disciplinary team who have had appropriate recognised training. It is important to recognise that these therapies may be considered in conjunction with other treatments, so a balance is required for each patient to achieve their individual needs, preferences and compliance. Therapies that are available include:

Transcutaneous nerve stimulation.
Acupuncture.
Relaxation.
Hypnotherapy.
Reflexology.
Massage.
Imagery.
Lifestyle/behavioral therapy.

Conclusion

Effective treatment of chronic pain patients relies upon the resources of a multi-disciplinary team who are able to offer a comprehensive service to tackle the physical, behavioural, social and financial facets of an otherwise intractable problem.

This inevitably leads to the use of community and/or hospital resources which can often be ill-afforded by the caring teams concerned. Particular concerns encompass the fears that chronic pain patients may not be seen as a priority in future health care plans as they inherently become a long-term user group of many support services and thus have long-term cost implications on the system.

However, as has been shown in this overview of chronic pain, the problem *can* be treated with the appropriate knowledge and support; therefore emphasis should be placed on these positive aspects of care which in the long-term offer a better quality of life to many patients and also prove a more cost-effective option.

References

Bowsher, D. (1987) *Mechanisms Of Pain In Man*, ICI Pharmaceuticals Division

Glynn, C. J., McQuay, H. J., Jadad, A. J. and Carroll, D. (1991) Response to controversy corner: Opioids in patients with non-malignant pain. Questions in search of answers. *Clinical Journal of Pain*, 7, no. 4

International Association For The Study Of Pain Classification Of Chronic Pain (1986) Seattle

Kirwan, E. O'G. (1989) In: *Textbook Of Pain* (eds P. D. Wall and R. Melzack), Churchill Livingstone, Edinburgh, pp. 335–340

Latham, J. (1991) *Pain Control*, Austen Cornish Publishers, London

Max, M. B., Culhane, M., Schafer, S. C. *et al.* (1987) Amitriptyline relieves diabetic neuropathy pain in patients with normal or depressed mood. *Neurology*, 37, 589–596

McCaffery, M. (1972) *Nursing Management Of The Patient With Pain*, J. B. Lippincott, Philadelphia

McLeod, W. T. and Hanks, P. (1987) *The New Collins Concise Dictionary Of The English Language*, Guild Publishing, London

McQuay, H. (1989) In: *Anaesthesia*, Vol. 2. (eds W. J. Nimmo and G. Smith), Blackwell Scientific Publications, Oxford, pp. 1204–1208

McQuay, H. J., Carroll, D. and Glynn, C. J. (1992) Low dose amitriptyline in the treatment of chronic pain. *Anaesthesia*, 47, p. 646–652

Nathan, P. W. (1987) In: *Oxford Textbook Of Medicine*, 2nd edn, Vol. 2, Sections 21.23–21.24 (eds D. J. Weatherall, J. G. G. Ledingham and D. A. Warrell), Oxford University Press, Oxford

Simons, D. G. and Travell, J. (1989) In: *Textbook Of Pain* (eds P. D. Wall and R. Melzack), Churchill Livingstone, Edinburgh, pp. 318–385

Travell, J. (1976) Myofascial trigger points: clinical review. In: *Advances In Pain Research and Therapy*, (eds J. J. Bonica and D. Albe-Fessard) Raven Press, New York, pp. 919–926

Waddell, G. (1982) An approach to backache. *British Journal Of Hospital Medicine*, 28, 187–219

Watson, C. P., Evans, R. J, Reed, K. *et al.* (1982) Amitriptyline versus placebo in postherpetic neuralgia. *Neurology*, 32, 671–673

Williams, M. (1987 and 1991) In: *Pain Control* (ed. J. Latham), Austen Cornish Publishers, London, pp. 38–54

7

The cognitive behavioural treatment of chronic pain

Judith Ralphs

Introduction

Pauline is 39 years old, married with two teenage daughters aged 13 and 16. Bill her husband is a self-employed builder. Pauline has severe pain that started 5 years ago following a car accident when she injured her left arm and back. Although the injury has healed, the pain remains; it is constant but varies in intensity. Doctors have told her that she has nerve damage and some scar tissue. Following two operations and numerous painkilling drugs Pauline has been informed little more can be done and she must learn to live with it.

As she found it was too painful to sit all day and typing was impossible, Pauline has given up her secretarial job. She now spends her days at home alone as Bill works long hours and her children are at school. Housework tends to be done in the morning when her pain level is lower, but she is exhausted when finished. Pauline spends her afternoons resting on the sofa so she has enough energy to cook supper. If the family see she is in pain they will tell her to rest and take her pills. Bill works very hard so is happy to sit on the sofa watching television all evening with his wife. She notices that they are going out less. Recent visits to friends have been a disaster, being 'pure agony' followed by a week in bed to recover. Before the accident, Pauline used to play in the local badminton team, and now misses the exercise and company.

Pauline often gets depressed and believes her life is worthless and hopeless. She feels guilty that she is not a better wife and mother and misses her job and the independence that brought. She is aware she is often short tempered and tearful. She notices that her older daughter spends much of the weekend with friends. Despite these feelings, Pauline sometimes manages to be quite pleased that she does generally keep going in spite of the severe pain.

Six to eight coproxamol tablets are taken daily depending on the pain and occasionally dihydrocodeine if she has to go out or the pain is particularly bad. However, these pills only 'take the edge off' the pain. Diazepam 10 mg nightly seems to help sleep but she notices a drowsy feeling in the morning.

Every 2 months Pauline visits the local Pain Clinic for nerve blocks. These reduce the pain for a couple of days which she uses to rush around catching up with everything and going out more. Unfortunately the pain seems to return even more severely. She likes the contact with the staff and knows the Sister well. Here at least people understand her pain, even though they cannot do much.

About twice a year her pain becomes so bad that Pauline has to be admitted to hospital. The nurses are often confused when the painkillers do not work and she never seems to get better. Some of the nurses are kind and will do things for her; others give her the impression that they think she is a malingerer and hypochondriac.

Pauline believes the future is bleak and does not see how things could improve. She prays that one day there will be a cure and she will be free of pain.

Pauline's story is typical of many who have chronic intractable pain, and illustrates many of the problems that face chronic pain sufferers. These can be divided into various features.

Patients often continue a search for a cure, and find it difficult to accept that the pain may not be curable. Many have undergone numerous unhelpful and even harmful procedures. These patients occupy much health professional time and are often unpopular as they

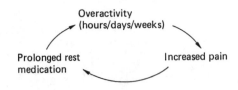

Over time the pattern looks like this:

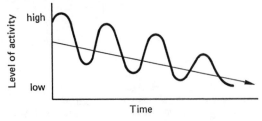

Figure 7.1 The under/overactivity cycle

do not provide clinical success and are often miserable and demoralised people to deal with. Sufferers complain that few believe or understand their pain.

The under/overactivity cycle (Figure 7.1)

Pauline's case is an example of the vicious circle of the 'under/overactivity cycle', common amongst chronic pain patients. When the pain is more bearable Pauline overdoes things by doing all the housework at once which exhausts her and increases the pain. In consequence she then rests all afternoon or longer, leading to underactivity. As time goes on the periods of overactivity become shorter and rest periods become longer. Muscle weakness and a poor fitness level and general disuse often result.

Medication problems

For many chronic pain sufferers drug usage is unhelpful and ineffective. Despite the consumption of many potent drugs that are effective for acute pain, chronic pain remains undiminished or only slightly reduced. In return for only a little pain relief, side effects such as impaired cognitive function, mood, and drowsiness reduce quality of life even further. Frequently drugs are used to allow the overdoing of things; if Pauline goes out she uses pain killers to increase her activity level temporarily but this results in even more pain the following day. Analgesic drugs are often used inappropriately. High dosage, mixing of drugs, irregular use and unwanted side effects are common.

Chronic pain sufferers should not be labelled addicts or weak-willed as drug usage is an understandable method of trying to cope when no other help is offered.

Family involvement

The family is affected by the pain too. Their response to the pain patient may be instrumental in determining the patient's coping, and response to pain. Pauline's family is very solicitous to her pain complaints, paying her attention and encouraging her to rest. Pauline has learnt that displaying pain behaviour – rubbing, moaning, sighing – elicits the attention she wants, which is very reinforcing. She is thus in the habit of rubbing her arms and wincing when her family can see her.

Mood

Changes in lifestyle, deterioration in quality of life, treatment disappointments, and side effects of the drugs contribute to feelings of depression, anxiety and hopelessness which in turn increase the suffering caused by the pain (Figure 7.2).

A new approach to pain

The cognitive behavioural approach focuses on function and changes in quality of life caused by the pain, rather than on the underlying pathology. This approach aims to teach chronic pain sufferers the skills they need to cope better with the pain and therefore reduce the suffering involved. Treatment success is measured in terms of goals achieved, improved mood and quality of life and not primarily a reduction in pain level.

From this perspective, rather than the pain being *caused by* anxiety and depression, the pain *contributes* to these mood changes. The labels 'psychosomatic' and 'psychogenic' are unhelpful since the pain is, as McCaffrey (1979) states, whatever the patient says it is. Moreover, patients with clear-cut organic problems are no less susceptible to the psychological effects of pain than are those with undiagnosed conditions. It should also be remembered that the pain pathways and mechanisms involved are still not fully understood, and many painful conditions once considered to be psychogenic

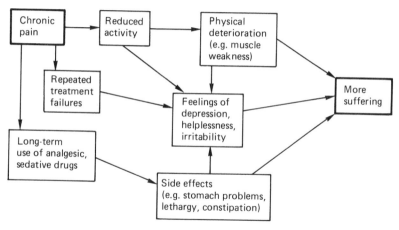

Figure 7.2 Overview of problems caused by chronic pain

have since been proved to have an organic cause.

Theoretical background

Before going further into the practicalities of the cognitive behavioural approach, it is helpful to understand some of the theoretical framework that has been developing over that last 20 years.

Pain behaviour

Activities such as rubbing, moaning and grimacing are signals to the outside world of distress and pain. These behaviours were useful when the pain was in the acute phase as a way of eliciting appropriate assistance, but once in the chronic phase they become unhelpful; encouragement to rest or take pills only contributes to the maintenance of the sick role (Fordyce, 1976). Pain behaviour is reinforced by others. When Pauline exhibits pain behaviour her family and health professionals pay her attention. It may also serve as a way to avoid an unpleasant task. This is known as avoidance behaviour. Patients are not to blame for their pain behaviour, as it is rarely consciously or manipulatively 'put on' but is a habit of which the pain sufferer is often unaware. Pain cannot be seen or recognised by others: behavioural changes may increase their attention.

Reinforcement

When Pauline exhibits pain behaviour her family try to support her by suggesting medication or massaging her back and talking. When she is sitting quietly, perhaps absorbed in reading, they are more likely to move to another room. She thus learns that showing pain is rewarded by contact with others.

Reinforcement is anything that rewards or results from a certain behaviour, thus encouraging the behaviour to be repeated. We all respond to praise by feeling good about ourselves and continuing the activity that was praised. For pain sufferers avoidance of exercise and rest may become reinforcing as it temporarily reduces the pain level. Rest may be appropriate for acute pain but not for chronic pain as it is unhelpful and maintains the 'sick' role. Everyone who has contact with pain patients is in the position to reinforce. Reinforcement can maintain pain behaviour after the initial injury has long since healed (Fordyce, 1976). Patients are rarely aware of this pattern of behaviour.

Contingency management

The aim of contingency management is to reduce pain behaviour and to encourage more helpful activity patterns. Simply, this means being specific about reinforcing things which are desirable to encourage. Thus the patient is reinforced, e.g. by praise when they try to walk or achieve a goal. Meanwhile complaints of pain and pain behaviour are not attended to; instead patients are encouraged to discuss issues in a problem solving way rather than moan and complain, which does little but drive others away. It is very important that this strategy is explained to patients, so they under-

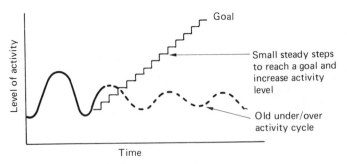

Figure 7.3 Pacing

stand the reasoning and learn to reinforce themselves for positive changes. The frequencies of reinforcement should be decreased towards the end of treatment as patients need to learn to reinforce themselves for their own achievements. Self attribution – crediting oneself for achievements and effort – is vital for the maintenance of progress; thus when patients thank the therapist for 'making them better' the therapist should remind them that the patients' own efforts caused the improvement.

Coping strategies

These are ways in which people cope with pain. Pauline copes by taking pills and resting. In her case more helpful and functional strategies could be used. Such strategies include relaxation, distraction and encouragement to change panicky thoughts into more realistic ones. Recognising and being pleased with achievements, however small, and the avoidance of 'catastrophising' – always expecting the worst to happen – is important. This is achieved by using other more helpful coping strategies. Thus the catastrophising thought 'I am going to die of the pain,' could be replaced with a more realistic one of, 'the pain is bad but I coped before and I need to plan how to help myself now'. In addition to helping patients acquire more realistic ways of thinking, the cognitive approach to therapy has also been shown to reduce feelings of depression and anxiety. There is not room to discuss this important subject in detail. The interested reader is advised to refer to the reading list.

Goal setting

To make changes, pain patients are encouraged to set their own goals. These must be relevant, realistic and achievable. Pauline would set very different goals compared with a 50-year-old ex-lorry driver. Paraplegic pain sufferers would set their own manageable goals, as no one is too disabled for this approach. Goal setting can be difficult for many patients who have given up so much. Support, education, and patience are required from the therapist.

Pacing (Figure 7.3)

This is a vital part of pain management as a way of breaking out of the under/overactivity cycle. Pacing means increasing the activity level by small steady steps at a rate set jointly by therapist and patient towards the longer term goal. Patients start from a level that is easily achievable, called a baseline. Patients increase daily by an agreed amount, and not according to the pain level. Conversely, they are *not* pushed to increase *beyond* their tolerance. Thus even when the pain is less severe, patients keep to the guide lines. Pacing also means breaking large tasks such as shopping and housework into smaller sections and activities, scheduling in breaks and relaxation. As with goal setting this is not an easy task; habits have to change.

Medication

There is much debate surrounding the role of medication in chronic pain. Medication must be taken on a time-contingent basis, i.e. by the clock, rather than when the pain is at a high level. If medication is always taken in response to pain it can encourage the overdoing of activities, thus in fact causing more pain in the long term. It is easier to reduce if drugs are taken in a planned way, rather than when desperate. Medication ceases to be so reinforcing, because it is taken by the clock whether in pain or not.

Alternative coping strategies can be learnt without patients becoming anxious when they think of taking less medication. Patients can be taught to relax for 10 minutes rather than take a pill. Most patients admit to feeling no extra pain once pill-free and can enjoy being rid of side effects. This method can also be used for all types of analgesics as well as benzodiazepines, sleeping pills and tranquillisers.

Education

Acute and chronic pain differ in many ways. Frequently health professionals and patients use their experience of acute pain as an inappropriate model. Both the patient and the staff involved have to be educated about the particular problems of chronic pain.

Important principles which should be taught include the following:

Increased pain does not mean that more damage is being done; any damage has long since healed and simple anatomy and physiology should be taught as a basis for more understanding on this subject.

Pain cannot be seen on an X-ray, or scan, but is a complicated process involving all parts of the body and brain.

More operations and invasive procedures are not always the answer and can cause further damage and pain.

Excessive rest or activity is unhelpful:

Patients have to come to terms with their pain and accept that a cure may not be possible.

Psychological ways to help cope with the pain do not mean that the pain is imaginary or psychosomatic. It is vital that patients believe that their pain is believed and accepted.

It is helpful if leaflets are given as well as verbal explanation.

The interdisciplinary team

An interdisciplinary team including nurses, physiotherapists, occupational therapists, psychologists and doctors is useful as many skills are needed for this approach.

Physiotherapists prescribe graded exercises to improve fitness levels, loosen scar tissue and teach patients about healthy muscles and joints.

Occupational therapists assess problems with activity levels, body mechanics, teach goal setting and look at work issues.

Psychologists teach new coping strategies such as changing unhelpful thoughts into more realistic ones by using cognitive therapy. They also teach relaxation and design contingency management programmes. Many psychologists are involved in the assessment of patients who may be appropriate for this type of approach.

Doctors have a vital role in reassuring the patient that this is the correct treatment and further invasive procedures are not appropriate. Medication changes and withdrawal are usually initiated by the medical team.

The nurse's role

Let us return to Pauline to illustrate how nurses can use the cognitive behavioural model.

Nursing input will depend on the environment in which Pauline is encountered. In Pauline's case this could be: a hospital ward, a pain clinic, in the community or in a specialised behavioural unit.

Wherever it be, the general approach taken should be broadly the same. Even if the whole approach cannot be embraced, nurses may be able to use elements in their practice. The overall goal should remain to help patients improve their functioning despite the pain.

Pauline's treatment

Pauline's GP suggested that Chris, a primary nurse with an interest in pain, might be able to work with her as things seemed to be getting worse.

Chris quickly became aware that the current nursing and medical interventions were helping few of Pauline's problems, despite frequent visits to hospital and the pain clinic. Chris believed that the cognitive behavioural approach would be the appropriate model of care.

Assessment

Before this approach was initiated, Chris confirmed that active treatment was no longer suitable, by looking through medical notes and discussion with other involved colleagues. To ensure that Pauline became a partner in the

WEEKLY ACTIVITY GOAL CHART

Name _____   Week _____

	MON How often/ much ✓	TUES How often/ much ✓	WED How often/ much ✓	THURS How often/ much ✓	FRI How often/ much ✓	SAT How often/ much ✓	SUN How often/ much ✓
Sitting base line = 10 minutes	10 mins /hour ✓✓✓✓	10 mins	12 mins	12 mins	13 mins	13 mins	14 mins
Walking base line = 9 minutes	9 mins /hour ✓✓✓✓	9 mins	10 mins	10 mins	11 mins	11 mins	12 mins
Typing base line = 5 minutes	5 mins /hour ✓✓✓	5 mins	6 mins	6 mins	7 mins	7 mins	8 mins
Relaxation session four times daily	10 mins ✓ 4 mins ✓ 15 mins ✓ 8 mins ✓						

Figure 7.4 Weekly activity goal chart

treatment, the rationale and aims of the cognitive behavioural approach were explained. Following discussion, Pauline began to understand that a cure was not possible but making some changes to her lifestyle could improve her quality of life.

Plan

With Chris's help Pauline set the following long term goals:

1. Return to some form of part-time work.
2. To go out socially once a week.
3. To entertain friends once a month.
4. To go clothes shopping with her daughters.
5. To play some form of sport weekly.

All these goals were achievable in the long term and activities that were important to Pauline. To help achieve these aims, several short term goals were identified; sitting, walking, and typing. These activities Pauline saw as her building blocks to the future. Difficulties with these meant difficulties with most activities.

Intervention

Traditional care plans may not be appropriate as patients need to have their own goal sheets and evaluation on which the therapist advises. Goals and plans are thus shared.

Pauline set baseline levels, i.e. levels that she was currently able to do on an activity goal sheet (Figure 7.4).

Progress was monitored using this sheet. Pauline decided that she wanted to increase these levels by 1 minute every other day. She learnt that she must keep to these levels even on 'good days'.

Learning to pace her activities throughout the day was vital. Using ironing as an example, she planned to keep the ironing board up all day, doing only two items at a time, and giving herself short rests throughout the day. Her old pattern meant ironing without stopping, then collapsing for several hours. She found pacing also helped prevent increased pain. When the pain level did increase Pauline learnt not to panic. With help from Chris she gradually learnt relaxation techniques, to use when becoming tense and panicky. Education about pain mechanisms increased her sense of control making her feel less 'abnormal' for having this continuing pain. Chris arranged contact with other chronic pain patients which allowed her to share experiences and feel less alone.

Pauline learnt to reinforce herself for her progress, sometimes by a rest or occasionally enjoying a chocolate bar. She learnt to feel pleased with even small changes. It was identified that in the past she was often very hard and critical on herself. There was discussion with her family about the kind of support she wanted. Pauline asked them to reinforce her by praise each time she achieved a goal, paced things or achieved something new. She reassured them that the programme was safe and no damage was being done. Together they worked on joint goals. Husband and wife decide to visit the local pub for just one drink as a step to improving their social life. Pauline's daughters agreed to go swimming weekly with her, which was something they would enjoy too.

The community physiotherapist taught some appropriate exercises involving stretch and general fitness. These, as with the goals, started from a baseline with small daily increases. Pauline was not pushed but just reinforced for any attempt at the exercises.

Pauline looked at work issues with the occupational therapist. Together they decided that full-time work was unrealistic for the time being. The occupational therapist worked closely with Chris to decide what activities were realistic. A voluntary job, which did not involve too much sitting or writing, for a couple of hours a week would be enjoyable. Body mechanics and ways of improving her posture were also discussed.

Medication use was an important issue, as it has been her primary way of coping. Pauline realised that if she paced her activities there would be less need for pills. Her nurse discussed with her the benefits of taking her medication 'by the clock', i.e. by a time contingency rather than pain contingency. Thus Pauline decided to take two coproxamol at meal times and set a goal of cutting out one pill every 5 days. Instead of taking some coproxamol she tried to use relaxation instead.

Sleep and diazepam use were a problem. Chris discussed the unwanted effects of diazepam and issues of tolerance and dependence. Pauline realised that a more sensible daytime routine would help her sleep, as she would not be overtired and full of aches and frustration. The use of relaxation would help reduce tension at night, together with a winding down time and avoidance of tea and coffee. Thus Pauline agreed to reduce her diazepam by 2 mg per week. She understood that possible withdrawal symptoms could be distressing but would end eventually. Relaxation helped too, as did a self-help leaflet.

The staff team working with Pauline all used this model, noticing changes, reinforcing Pauline for her achievements and working together, communicating regularly on her progress.

To ensure maintenance of the progress made once official therapeutic contact ceased, Pauline devised a plan for coping with set-backs and flare-ups in pain. Main elements involved cutting back on the number of exercises and activities by half for a few days then gradually building up again. Relaxation and scheduled rest periods were vital. Thus rather than fighting the pain during a flare-up by continuing at a high activity level which would inevitably lead to collapse and a hospital admission, Pauline would instead use a prearranged plan. Pauline discussed this plan with her family so they could work with her during a difficult time.

Progress and maintenance

Pauline continued with her goals after her official treatment had ended. Six months later Pauline was doing voluntary work. She could sit for 30 minutes, stand for 20 minutes, and type a whole page without stopping, a real achievement. She was swimming weekly and went out each Friday with Bill. Pauline was now in the habit of spreading out her activities throughout the day and found she had much more energy by evening. Her family told her she was a much nicer person to live with.

Diazepam had stopped completely, and her sleep was no worse. Pauline only took one coproxamol in the morning and one in the afternoon.

Evaluation

At times the pain still depressed Pauline and some days she did slow down and rest more, but she saw this as just a temporary setback of which she was in control as she had plans for coping with flare-ups of pain. She noticed that lying in bed made her more depressed, not more rested. She wished she saw more of her friends but accepted that renewing her social life took time. Overall she was pleased with herself; she accepted the pain would probably always be with her but was no longer afraid of the future. The cognitive behavioural approach enabled Pauline to increase her function and improve her quality of life despite the continuing pain. In Pauline's words 'I feel I now control my pain rather than It controlling me.'

Limitations to this approach

Some patients find there are too many re-inforcements for remaining in the sick role to improve their functions.

In some cases there may be long standing family problems or mental illness that block any possible changes. Nurses must be realistic in what they hope to achieve and realise that not all patients will respond to treatment. Pauline was able to make changes; success or failure depends not only on 'pain level' or 'pain toler-ance' as these are very subjective measure-ments and often vary depending on distress at the time. Patients often increase their function even with increased pain, by learning new skills to cope better.

Implementation

A nurse interested in using this approach must prepare the ground well.

Ward staff at all levels have to understand the model, as one staff member reinforcing pain behaviour could sabotage all other efforts. This is called intermittent reinforcement.

The ward routine needs to be flexible to allow self-medication, the setting of relevant goals, and involvement of the family (including week-end leave).

Some patients may find it confusing to be surrounded by acutely ill people whose pain is being controlled, and thus comply less willingly with the cognitive behavioural approach.

As many of the inter-disciplinary team as possible should be available. Physiotherapists and occupational therapists may well be part of an existing team, but psychologists may be more difficult to obtain. Nurses could find it useful to consult with a psychologist on specific behavioural problems if the latter is unable to have direct patient contract.

Specialised units

The development of pain management units with specialised staff has aimed to overcome the difficulties described above. Patients also benefit from the support and encouragement of fellow sufferers.

INPUT, the Inpatient Pain Management Centre at St Thomas' Hospital London, is a self contained unit treating chronic pain patients on both a 4-weekly inpatient and an 8-weekly outpatient course. Staff in the unit include a doctor, nurse, psychologists, physiotherapist, occupational therapist and administrator.

For the Inpatient Programme, five inpatients are admitted at 2-weekly intervals. Patients have their own rooms, and are self caring. There are no staff at night and patients make their own meals. There is a full timetable of physiotherapy, goal setting, education and relaxation sessions, all of which are undertaken in a group environment. Family involvement is encouraged. An inpatient programme needs its own unit, staff and facilities with an informal and unclinical atmosphere where patients can be self caring.

The outpatient course is 3 hours each week with similar content. A key worker system is used to ensure continuity each week. A key worker can be an occupational therapist, nurse or psychologist.

It is not yet clear from research if one method has more advantages than another. Obviously an inpatient course is more intensive and com-prehensive but with an outpatient course patients gain more experience of achieving their goals, problem solving and reducing their medication in the home setting. While the inpatients do go home at weekends, some find it difficult to maintain their progress at home. Outpatient courses are cheaper to run, need fewer staff hours and require one room rather than a special ward or unit. Similar pro-grammes are run in America and Australia and a few exist in Britain and Europe. In the USA some Pain Management Centres encompass all the areas of pain control, from nerve blocks to behavioural therapy. This has the advantage of staff gaining experience in all areas of pain treatment and patients having access to all forms of treatment. It must be hoped that such centres will be developed in Britain and Europe.

Research

Predicting which patients will do well is at present unreliable. Sometimes the most sur-prising people make great gains, while more apparently promising patients find it difficult to make changes.

An increasing body of research is evaluating

the effectiveness of this treatment of pain and the sort of patients whom it helps (Linton, 1982; Keefe *et al.*, 1986). Most studies find that the cognitive behavioural approach does significantly improve patient functioning but as yet there is little written specifically on the nurse's role.

Summary

Nurses have much contact with chronic pain patients. Listed below are some key points on this developing role of nurses.

1. Believe that the pain is real, not just psychological or exaggerated.
2. Assess whether the patient presents with the chronic pain syndrome.
3. Look at patients' activity level and identify the problems.
4. Teach pacing and goal setting.
5. Assess education needs and provide necessary resources.
6. Encourage and plan drug reduction if appropriate.
7. Reinforce all attempts at improvements and achievement of goals.
8. Encourage patients to attribute all gains to their own efforts.
9. Work with patients' families so they can provide the right type of support.
10. Work as part of an interdisciplinary team.
11. Know your own limitations – refer on if necessary or work with other appropriate professionals.
12. Evaluate all of these interventions to increase the body of knowledge in this developing area.

Conclusion

There are many challenges ahead for nurses who wish to use this new approach. Behavioural interventions are a new dimension in the care of patients who have in the past been told either to put up with the pain or continue a never ending and often expensive search for the elusive cure. Many Pain Clinics are now incorporating behavioural management into their service. Nurses who work with chronic pain patients now have an opportunity, perhaps a duty, to improve their care of this client group by using this approach in their practice.

Acknowledgements

I would like to thank my colleagues at St Thomas' Pain Management Centre, especially Dr Phil Richardson, for their help and advice with this chapter.

References

Fordyce, W. E. (1976) *Behavioural Methods for Chronic Pain and Illness*. Mosby, St Louis

Keefe, F. T., Gil, K. M. and Rose, S. C. (1986) Behavioural approaches in the multidisciplinary management of chronic pain: programmes and issues. *Clinical Psychology Rev*, **6**, 87–113

Linton, S. J. (1982) A critical review of behavioural treatments of chronic benign pain other than headache. *British Journal of Clinical Psychology*, **21**, 321–337

McCaffrey, M. (1979) *Nursing Management of the Patient with Pain*. JB Lippincott Co., Philadelphia

Useful reading

Blackburn, I. M. and Davison, K. (1990) *Cognitive Therapy for Depression and Anxiety*. Blackwell, Oxford

Broom, A. and Jellicoe, H. (1987) *Living With Your Pain, A Self Help Guide*. BPS Methuen, London

Loeser, J. D. and Egan, K. J. (1989) *Managing the Chronic Pain Patient, Theory and Practise at the University of Washington Pain Centre*. Raven Press, New York

Phillips, H. C. (1988) *The Psychological Management of Chronic Pain*. Springer, New York

Roland, M. and Jenner, J. R. (eds) (1989) *Back Pain, New Approaches to Pain*. Manchester University Press, New York

Snelling, J. (1990) The role and the family in relation to chronic pain, a review of the literature. *Journal of Advanced Nursing*, **15**, 771–776

Walker, J. (1987) Chronic pain. *Journal of District Nursing*, **June**, 6–8

8

Care of the dying

Christine Pearce

Introduction

If nurses are to understand their role in the management of cancer pain it is helpful to look first at care of the dying in broad terms.

Individuals within society can be said to adopt roles according to their situation. For example, a person will adopt a role in the family, another role in the workplace, a third role with friends and so on. These roles can be described as a collection of expectations which involve both rights and duties.

The *sick role* was first described by Parsons (1951), as one in which the individual has a right to be exempt from the responsibilities of their usual role, and a right to be cared for.

The duties of the sick role are twofold. Because society regards illness as an undesirable state, the patient must wish to get well. The person who lacks this desire is not favourably regarded by their fellows.

A second duty is the obligation to obtain help, aimed at the restoration of health, and to cooperate with prescribed treatment.

As with other social roles, the sick role determines how the person responds to their situation.

In 1977 Noyes and Clancy described another aspect of social behaviour that they termed the *dying role*.

The social role of the dying person, though initially similar to that of the sick role, differs in one important respect; while the sick role terminates in the restoration of health, the other ends in death.

As a person enters the dying role, it is important for them to retain the desire to live, since by 'giving up' too readily it may be thought that they are rejecting both loved ones and social obligations.

Ideally, the person may relinquish unrealistic hopes of recovery, but retain the 'will to live'. The relevance of such a theory is founded on observations which suggest that this optimum motivational state will allow the patient to benefit most from care offered, thereby achieving the best quality of life for the time they have left. It is to help the patient achieve this ideal state that the nurse must direct care.

The hospice movement

The concept of helping a person adjust emotionally to death whilst retaining hope, has long been at the heart of those providing terminal care. Historically the needs of the dying have been met either in their own homes, or in hospices which until recent years would most commonly have been run by religious orders.

Over time the Hospice Movement has developed considerable expertise in care of the dying, and thanks to the pioneering work of Dame Cicely Saunders, the hospice philosophy is now widely recognised and has spread into care given by other health care professionals (Saunders, *et al.*, 1981).

Cicely Saunders' aim was to create an environment in which patients and their families would be helped and supported, in adjusting emotionally and spiritually to approaching death.

Pain and other distressing symptoms were assessed and treated more scientifically than before, and new knowledge was disseminated to professional and non-professional carers alike.

In the last 15–20 years, there has been a dramatic increase in the success of health care professionals specialising in terminal care, to control pain and distressing symptoms. This knowledge and expertise can be applied and adapted to help all dying patients.

Current options for terminal care tend to fall into three categories: 1) home care, 2) hospice care and 3) hospital care. For most people with terminal illness, their preferred choice of place in which to die remains their own home (Parkes, 1985).

The current emphasis on community care can help patients in this respect, as services for the terminally ill have developed quite dramatically over the last 13 years (see Table 8.1).

Table 8.1 Development of services for care of the dying patient

Service	1981	1993
In-patient units	58	193
Bed number	1297	2993
Home care teams	32	400
Hospital support teams	8	216
	1989	1991
Day care centres	65	200

(St Christopher's Hospice Information Service, 1993)

Community care

In caring for the dying patient at home, the key person to the quality of care given is the district nurse.

The district nurse works a little like the conductor of an orchestra who, by knowing the musical score intimately, will draw into play the appropriate instruments, at the correct time, in order to achieve the best and most sensitive interpretation of the composer's work.

Like the conductor, the district nurse must know well the available services and expertise, and be able to utilise these resources at the appropriate time according to the patients' and families' wishes.

With the development of community care through improved funding, specialised expertise is available for the district nurse to make use of.

Home Care Teams comprise a number of health care professionals, specialising in care of the dying. Ideally the team will have nursing staff, usually Macmillan nurses, a doctor, a social worker, physiotherapist and in some areas a psychologist, a chaplain and occupational therapist. The expertise of the home care team can be used by the district nurse to augment the quality of care already given in the patients' home.

Home care teams can not only help the district nurse to care for the patient, but can also provide valuable support for the family during the patients' illness, and after the patients' death in the form of bereavement counselling.

The district nurse can also benefit professionally by working closely with the home care team.

Hospice and continuing care units (in-patient units)

The majority of hospice and continuing care units offer services which can be classified as: pain and symptom control, rehabilitation, respite care and continuing/terminal care.

Pain and symptom control techniques may range from the simplest of complementary approaches such as massage and relaxation, to highly specialised orthodox medical interventions like neural blockade and the implantation of drug delivery systems (Cherry and Gourlay, 1987).

Rehabilitation may be offered on an in-patient basis or as an outpatient visiting Day Care Units for treatment.

Rehabilitation is seen as a particularly valuable service; the aims being to assist the patient to return home for as long as is possible, and to support the carers with resources and advice. Physiotherapy and occupational therapy will help the patient regain strength and confidence and facilitate necessary adjustments to the patients' living accommodation so that their return home has the minimum of problems.

Day care services offer in many cases both in-patient and out-patient company, activities for those who wish, warmth, food, help with bathing, hair care and chiropody services as well as specialist nursing and medical help.

Respite care. Many patients with terminal illness are cared for at home by relatives and friends. This may become increasingly difficult as the illness progresses.

Hospices and many continuing care units can

offer the family respite from the weight of such care by admitting the patient for a period of time. This facility is very often as much of a relief to the patient as it is to the family. Respite care can assist the family to recharge their batteries and so continue the care at home for as long as possible.

Continuing terminal care. Although the majority of patients report that they wish to be cared for and die at home, for various reasons a significant proportion will be admitted to hospital or hospice. The patient may become so dependent on nursing care that neither the family nor community services can manage. The family may feel that when death is imminent, they are unable to cope as anticipated. A patient may express the wish to die in a hospice or hospital so as to spare the family the distress of the death at home.

The hospice is seen as a part of the community and if the patient is unable to remain at home to die then admission to a hospice can be offered.

Support for the relatives is available and experienced staff can provide comfort and understanding at this distressing time. After the patient's death, bereavement services are offered and Befrienders (trained volunteers) can visit the relative to offer emotional as well as practical support.

Hospice staff liaise closely with the primary care team, home care teams and hospital staff in order that the best possible care can be given.

Hospital based care for the dying

For those who work in the hospital setting there are a number of factors which make the provision of quality care for the terminally ill difficult to achieve.

Hospitals in the main are geared to the provision of acute and curative care, and demands on the service make it difficult to offer the type and range of care provided by hospice and continuing care units.

Curricula for medical and nurse education dedicate comparatively little time to topics related to care of the dying, so that specific communication skills and pain and symptom control techniques in terminal care are only briefly touched on in many cases.

The ranges of the complementary approaches to pain and symptom control used in most hospital settings is often quite limited, sometimes due to a failure to recognise the contribution such techniques have to offer, sometimes perhaps through lack of knowledge.

Staff skill mix may be inadequate in some clinical areas when caring for the specific needs of the dying patient and the family. The pace of work within the hospital setting is not generally conducive to rest and quiet for patients and their families facing death, and facilities are rarely available for relatives to stay or participate in care. When staff make time to spend with relatives, that time can be often punctuated by frequent interruptions.

Terminally ill patients in hospital report a number of problems which can be seen to stem from the difficulties previously identified.

Some patients report difficulties in obtaining information and the time to discuss concerns with medical and nursing staff, particularly when seeking information about prognosis. The patient's perception of whether staff believe the amount of pain they experience is often a negative one, and their pain control can be affected by these feelings.

Some of the difficulties are almost impossible to overcome without considerable changes to the hospital system. Many, however, can be considerably improved with better education at an early stage of training.

Hospices and continuing care units are not necessarily better than hospitals at giving appropriate care for the terminally ill, but they are different in emphasis, atmosphere, expertise and approach. Most are comparatively small so are privileged in being able to concentrate on those aspects that are of greatest concern to the patient and family.

There are of course many different illnesses from which an individual may die. Cancer, though by no means necessarily the worst of these illnesses, is, however, one of the most common. One person in three will be diagnosed as having cancer.

The care and attention a patient with cancer receives from the moment of diagnosis will affect the way in which that person copes with the illness and will similarly affect those close to the patient. The nurse will be the person most in touch with the patient at all stages throughout their illness, so that the nurse's role in caring for the patient with cancer is of fundamental importance.

The public perception of cancer

An individual's perception of cancer tends to be based on information gained from the media, often in the form of newspaper reports and magazine features; the recollections of friends or relatives, and personal experience.

In the first instance media reporting is rarely complete and can sometimes be misleading; in the second instance one individual's experience cannot be seen as a predictor for another's.

This combined effect can be a profoundly negative one, leading people to assume that cancer inevitably means unbearable pain and suffering, and ultimately an undignified death.

For some individuals the belief remains that cancer is in some way a punishment for what they may consider to be their inadequate lifestyle, and that suffering is the penalty they must pay.

This negative view of cancer clearly has implications for both patient and carers alike.

Research indicates that cancer patients who have a positive outlook and take an active role in their own care live longer than those who do not (Weisman, 1977).

Morris *et al.* (1986) observed that denial of cancer appears to have similar effects to an actively positive outlook.

The patients who suffer most would appear to be those who 'give up' and see pain and distress as unavoidable. These individuals present with difficult physical and emotional problems, and die soonest.

Patients' concerns post-diagnosis

The question often asked is 'why is cancer so special?' An attempt to answer this question might begin with a look at the extent of the problem.

The statistics tell us that one in three individuals will have cancer at some point, and that one person in five will die from cancer (Marie Curie Memorial Foundation, 1990).

Driever and McCorkle (1984) set out to identify what patients with different types of illness (lung cancer or myocardial infarction) reported as concerns at 3 months and 6 months after diagnosis.

The study identified four categories of patient concern:

- *Patient status*: an overall description of the subject's current state, e.g. degree of incapacitation, and progress in resumption of 'normal activities'.
- *Patient activities*: the kind and quality of pre-illness activities the subject was resuming relative to the number and severity of disease symptoms experienced.
- *Patient symptoms*: the number and severity of symptoms related to activities of daily living that the subject reported.
- *Patient attitude*: the kind and degree of the subjects' outlook on their experience with their disease and its effects on their activities of daily living and expectations for their future.

Generally, both lung cancer and myocardial infarction patients indicated a similar pattern of concerns in all four categories. Despite this similarity, lung cancer patients reported significant differences in severity for patient status and symptom concern, particularly at 6 months postdiagnosis. The conclusions were that myocardial patients were reportedly doing better, engaging in more 'normal activities' having minimal symptoms and having a 'positive outlook' as compared to persons with lung cancer.

It is not necessary, therefore, to assign rank to illness in order to provide quality of care. The imperative is to understand and respond to the patient's experience of their illness, whatever that may be.

Another way of investigating patients' concerns regarding their cancer is to look at the life cycle (Erikson, 1983) (Figure 8.1).

Patient's concerns will be influenced by their point in the life cycle.

The diagnosis of cancer at different points in this life cycle will present the individuals concerned with different problems. For example, the mother with young children may worry primarily about who is to care for them after her death.

There may be conflicts of interest between grandparents, as to who should be their guardians. There may be worry about income loss, if the father has been absent from his work. All of these fears and anxieties will influence the patient's pain.

A nurse who has an understanding of this concept is in a position to anticipate problems a patient may experience, and offer help before the problem becomes overwhelming. Undoubt-

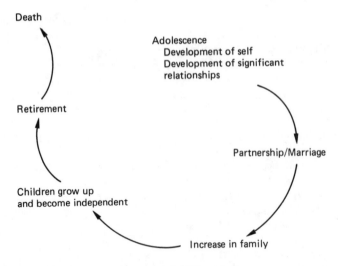

Death

Adolescence
Development of self
Development of significant
relationships

Retirement

Partnership/Marriage

Children grow up
and become independent

Increase in family

Figure 8.1 The life cycle

edly the most consistent fear that cancer patients report following diagnosis is the fear of dying and in particular fear of dying in pain (Hauck, 1986). Cancer, however, is not synonymous with pain. Approximately two-thirds of patients experience pain, which means that one-third of patients do not (Twycross and Lack, 1990).

Pain may be the presenting symptom, or it may not present until diagnostic or therapeutic procedures are commenced or at a late stage in the course of the illness.

Physical pain

Pain can be defined as 'an unpleasant sensory and emotional experience associated with actual or potential tissue damage, or described in terms of such damage', (Merskey, 1979).

Pain in cancer patients may be:
1. Caused by cancer, e.g. metastatic bone pain, nerve compression, soft tissue infiltration, visceral involvement, muscle spasm, lymphoedema, raised intracranial pressure and myopathy.
2. Related to treatment, e.g. postoperative pain, postoperative complications and post-radiation fibrosis.
3. Associated pain, e.g. constipation, decubitus ulcer and post-herpetic neuralgia.
4. Unrelated pain, e.g. musculoskeletal and migraine.

These different types of pain require careful diagnosis, since they may demand quite different types of treatment. Often cancer patients report multiple pains.

Pain, however, is not simply a physical response to tissue damage. Dame Cicely Saunders (1989) describes a concept of 'total pain' (Figure 8.2) in relation to terminal illness. This concept is based on observations that an individual's experience of pain is a combination of emotional, spiritual and social pain as well as physical pain. These factors combine to augment the experience of pain. The more aspects of the pain experience which are involved, the more complex is the pain problem.

Social factors may involve problems such as the change of role within the family. This may be due to an inability to perform customary activities around the home.

Leisure activities may be impaired or even curtailed, and the circle of friends may diminish.

Touch, both in the broad social context and in relationships with a partner, may alter. A partner may reduce or completely withdraw from physical contact, for fear of causing hurt or harm. The patient's perception of their own altered body image, as in breast cancer, may cause great distress and can leave the cancer patient feeling isolated and alone.

Spiritual questions such as 'Why has God let this happen to me?' are often expressed.

Concept of total pain

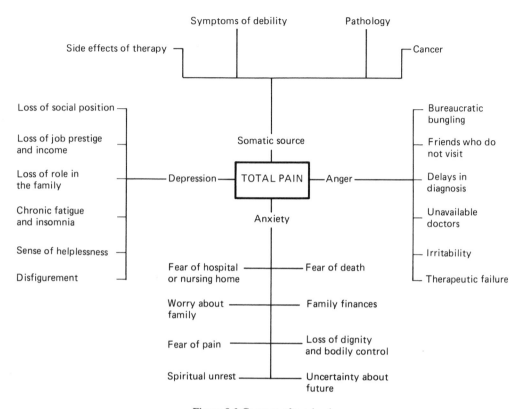

Figure 8.2 Concept of total pain

The individual may seriously doubt the existence of a God whom they consider to be so cruel; or feel that they are being punished in some way.

Emotional pain can occur due to distress felt by patients with terminal illness, when they consider leaving loved ones, or perhaps lost opportunities, 'If only I had . . .'.

These problems are only part of a highly complex situation, and can bring about anxiety, anger or depression, all of which make pain more difficult to tolerate (see Figure 8.1).

It may not be possible to alleviate all the problems identified in the total pain concept, but there are many areas where considerable help can be given.

Fear of death is a very real fear for many cancer patients, but when encouraged to express these fears in more detail, patients tend to talk more of fear related to the manner of their dying.

This fear is linked to the sense of loss expressed by patients; loss of physical as well as emotional control.

The nurse's role in the management of cancer pain

In order for pain to be controlled, patients must be able and willing to communicate their pain to health care professionals. Some individuals find this more difficult than others. If the nurse is to help patients communicate their needs, a basic understanding of the processes that inhibit expression of pain is important.

In Western culture particularly, great value is placed on being seen to be strong. In literature, heroes are classically described as individuals who can tolerate extreme pain without complaint.

Children are generally discouraged from expressing pain freely, and gender variations are pronounced, 'boys don't cry'. The ill patient in hospital may be reluctant to express pain for fear of the consequences, a prolonged stay in hospital for example, or unpleasant treatment.

They may not feel able to 'bother' busy medical and nursing staff; or to 'worry' family or friends with their complaints of pain.

Given this background of learned responses, it is not surprising that many people need to be 'given permission' to express their pain. The kind of relationship the nurse has with the patient will influence the quality of communication. When trust between nurse and patient has been established, pain assessment can begin.

Depending on the severity of the pain, this assessment can be brief and specific; requiring only such information as to facilitate prompt pain relief; or considerably more detailed as would be the case for a patient with pain of a more chronic nature.

The nurse can relieve some of the fear by encouraging the patient to talk about their concerns, and by assuring the patient that every effort will be made to provide comfort and support throughout their illness.

In many instances, while waiting for the doctor, the nurse will have an opportunity to perform simple nursing procedures. Helping the patient to find the most comfortable position, for example, will promote comfort, and may alleviate some of the patient's initial anxiety and therefore some of the pain. Details of the pain assessment must be passed on to the doctor promptly and as clearly as possible; and the administration of prescribed drugs carried out immediately. The timing of the evaluation of effect will depend on the type of drug or treatment prescribed and requires that the nurse knows enough about the treatment to time the evaluation correctly. Too soon, and the treatment has not had sufficient time to work; to late and the effect may have disappeared. A professional responsibility of every nurse is to keep informed about treatments being offered. A detailed understanding of how drugs or other interventions (e.g. nerve blocks) work; and potential side effects and how to recognise them is essential.

With so many drugs in use, and new drugs coming on to the market all the time, this is not an easy task. There are, however, a smaller number of drugs and treatments that are constantly used, and the nurse can concentrate her energies on learning those in detail.

Knowledge of these treatment interventions will need to be continually updated in the light of advances in pain relief techniques.

This understanding is fundamental to the nurse's role in patient teaching, for if an individual is to benefit from treatment, they must first comply with that treatment (Sarneckey and Sarneckey, 1984). To comply, the patient must understand what is expected of them.

The nurse's role in this respect is to give patients as much information as they need, in a form they can understand. This may be information about drugs and how to take them, about preparation required for treatment to begin, or details of how patients can help themselves during treatment. To share this information with the patient is to give back a degree of control, therefore enabling the patient to get the maximum benefit from treatment.

This information may also be shared with other health care professionals involved in the patient's care, and the patient's relatives as appropriate.

In summary then, the nurse's role in pain management can be seen as follows:

1. To encourage patients to express their pain.
2. To accurately assess the patient's pain.
3. To perform simple nursing actions aimed at reducing anxiety and promoting comfort.
4. To report promptly the results of pain assessment to the patient's doctor.
5. To safely administer drugs prescribed by the patient's doctor.
6. To evaluate accurately the effect of drugs or other treatment intervention.
7. To provide the patient with such information as to enable informed consent and compliance.
8. To maintain and update own knowledge and that of other health care professionals in current pain relief treatments and techniques.

Taking the last point first, it is appropriate to review the current options available to patients for the control of cancer pain.

As can be seen in Table 8.2, when cancer pain is first reported, the clinician is presented with a wide range of treatment possibilities.

The initial therapy decisions will be based on the stage of the cancer and the patient's general fitness as well as their desires for treatment.

Table 8.2. The treatment of cancer pain

	Pain Initial therapy	
Symptomatic	C O	Anticancer
	N	curative palliative
	T	
Oral analgesics	I	Radiotherapy
Co-Analgesics	N	Chemotherapy
Local analgesic blocks	U	Surgery
Physical therapy	I	Hormone therapy
Massage, relaxation,	N	
hypnotherapy	G	Pain persists
	C	Parenteral opioid
	A	+/− adjuvants,
	R	+/− non-opioids
	E	
		Pain persists Interrupt pain pathway +/− adjustment of drugs

Therapy will be offered curatively, or for symptom control alone if the cancer is too far advanced for cure.

Pharmacological intervention for pain control has been shaped by guidelines from the World Health Organisation (WHO) and its panel of experts. WHO states that analgesics should be prescribed very specifically, and describes a concept called the analgesic ladder (Figure 8.3). In this approach the choice of drug used is based on analgesic response, thereby tailoring the analgesic to the patient's needs.

If pain fails to respond to a non-opioid, then a weak opioid may be effective; if a weak opioid fails then a strong opioid is indicated.

Drugs used in such a way must be prescribed and given regularly, and titrated in such a way as to prevent the pain from returning. 'Traffic' on the ladder need not necessarily be one-way. If the patient reports overwhelming pain, it may be appropriate to start at the second or even third step. Once pain is under control the patients' requirements for analgesia will in most cases fall and the drug regime can be revised.

Co-analgesics are drugs other than analgesics but which also relieve pain. These drugs may include corticosteroids, antispasmodics and antibiotics, and can be effective with or without concurrent analgesics.

Psychotropic drugs have a place in the control of cancer pain. Antidepressants such as amitriptyline can be helpful in nerve destruction pain, and anticonvulsants like sodium valproate can be used to control the stabbing pain that sometimes accompanies nerve compression.

Local analgesic blocks can be another useful form of co-analgesia and physical therapies such as physiotherapy, massage, aromatherapy, relaxation techniques and in some instances hypnotherapy can be most beneficial at any point in the patients' illness.

Treatment of cancer pain

Anticancer therapy can be used as previously stated with cure as its goal, but should cure be unrealistic, then anticancer therapy in the form of radiotherapy, chemotherapy, hormone therapy and surgery may be highly effective in pain control. The mode of action in this case is most commonly effected by reducing the bulk of the tumour, and thus relieving the pressure on adjacent structures and organs.

Should pain continue, then it may be appropriate to consider parenteral opioids. Normally a test dose is administered, which, if effective can then be given continuously via a syringe driver for example, or in an increasing number of cases via an epidural or intrathecal drug

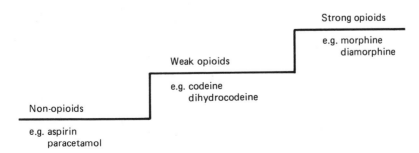

Figure 8.3 The analgesic ladder

delivery system, a drug reservoir which can be implanted under the skin to enable the patient to be cared for at home.

The interruption of the pain pathway, only appropriate for a comparatively small number of patients, can be of use, and in some cases a single intervention may be all that is required. Whatever treatment modality is chosen, the basic principles of pain control must be followed if treatment is to be truly effective.

Those principles are:

- Ask questions and observe the patient, do not wait for reports of pain before acting.
- Accurately diagnose the cause of pain so that the correct drug or intervention can be used.
- Use regular analgesics in doses titrated to each individual so that the return of pain is prevented.
- Set realistic goals. Perhaps an initial goal might be a pain-free night.
- Evaluate the effectiveness of treatment and review options often.
- Acknowledge that treatment interventions are only a part of the overall management and that empathy and understanding, diversion through activities and mood elevation are equally essential components of good care.

Pain management skills development

Having identified an outline of the nurse's role in pain management, it is important to identify the specific skills a nurse must develop in order to fulfil this role. Taking the first point of contact with the patient, and the establishment of a therapeutic nurse/patient relationship, it is necessary for the nurse to employ good communication skills, particularly listening skills.

Listening skills

Effective listening involves a range activities. To begin with it is necessary to *attend* to what the patient is saying. Ideally this can best be done sitting, rather than standing by the patient; this facilitates comfortable eye contact at the patient's own level. Distractions should be kept to a minimum, and time set aside for listening. The nurse must appear to have plenty of time so that the patient does not feel rushed.

These ideals may of course be difficult to achieve in a busy clinical area, but efforts should be made to get as near to them as is practicable.

Questioning technique

Appropriate questioning technique is crucial for accurate assessment of the patient's pain.

The type of questioning technique will depend upon the information required. Open questions, e.g. 'Tell me about your pain', will allow patients to talk freely, while closed questions, e.g. 'What medication are you taking now?' will help patients focus on quite specific details.

The combined skills of listening and questioning will help the nurse, if required, to act as the patient's advocate, conveying the patient's wishes to other health care professionals.

Information sharing

The patient who is diagnosed as having a terminal illness faces an uncertain future in which contact with health care professionals will dominate.

Regardless of whether the treatment to be offered is aimed at cure, or palliation, the relationship established between nurse and patient is vital at all stages to the patient's wellbeing. Following the diagnosis of cancer, there are many bewildering facts for the patient to take in, many of which may take some time to assimilate. There will be difficult decisions to make about treatment, and painful considerations about the future. In order to make these decisions, the patient needs as much information as is available, time to consider all the options, informed staff to discuss their concerns with, and above all the opportunity to ask questions.

For trust to exist between patient and nurse, the nurse needs to assess, acknowledge and accept the patient's feelings. The nurse must understand that pain is an entirely subjective experience, and that the patient must be listened to and assessed on that basis. 'Pain is what the patient says it is and exists when the patient says it does' (McCaffery, 1972). For the patient in pain, trust may begin when the patient feels that their pain is believed.

The negative effect that anxiety has on an

individual's experience of acute pain is well described (Hayward, 1975); information sharing can relieve much unnecessary anxiety. Clear unambiguous explanations from nursing and medical staff will afford the patient opportunities to understand what is happening to them.

Information sharing can also be achieved in the form of printed information booklets, of which there are many available, (see the Resource section), or printed information which can be produced locally, e.g. ward information leaflets etc. The patient who is well informed is in the best position to make decisions about their future.

Should the fully informed patient decide against the doctor's recommendations, this choice should be respected.

Observation skills

To add to the overall profile of the patient's pain, observation skills will be required, such as noting the patient's posture, and activities, interaction with family members or other patients.

Theoretical background

It is essential for the nurse to have knowledge of appropriate assessment instruments, and their application in the clinical area. A great deal of information on pain can be found in nursing journals and textbooks as well as psychological and medical journals.

With so much information available, it would be impractical for the nurse to try and find it all.

Librarians and information scientists can be most helpful in this respect, by carrying out literature searches. The librarian will need to know what the nurse is looking for in as much detail as possible, and be given plenty of time in which to carry out the search (Pollock, 1984). Other sources of information may be local Pain Interest Groups, or Research Interest Groups (see Resource section).

Nursing measures in cancer pain management

There are particular nursing activities that can bring great comfort for the patient with cancer pain.

Helping the patient to find a comfortable position has already been mentioned; other procedures can include the elevation of a painful limb, the application of a heat pad or ice pack if appropriate (compression bandaging can be of great benefit to the patient with lymphoedema: Badger and Twycross, 1988) and gentle massage, or relaxation techniques when employed, can in some cases achieve a reduction in the dose of drug required for pain relief.

Patient control

One of the overriding feelings reported by cancer patients is one of loss of control over their destiny. This sense of helplessness is as demoralising as it is frustrating.

In terms of pain management, it is both desirable and possible to give back control to the patient. This can be done in a number of ways.

To begin with, where possible the patient should be given the opportunity to assess their own pain, and document it. The use of pain assessment charts described later in this chapter is a practical way of achieving this. By having the patient involved in this way, not only is a degree of patient control restored, but the patient will see that their own experience is being respected. If the patient is receiving medication for the relief of pain, it is more likely to be effective if the patient is taught how to self-medicate, and where possible, allowed to do so.

The idea that patients will take more medication than they need is now seen to be erroneous.

In studies carried out on patient controlled analgesia systems, patients with acute pain were reported to have taken less of the prescribed medication than those patients given the medication by nursing staff, while at the same time achieving an equally good level of pain control as those patients being medicated by the nurses (Hill *et al.*, 1986).

Incidence of drug addiction in cancer patients is exceedingly rare. Cancer patients who have been taught about their medication, and are given the freedom to use that information appropriately, are observed to achieve high levels of pain control. With the correct type of support this is possible for the majority of cancer patients.

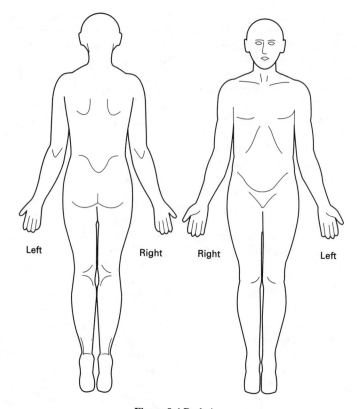

Figure 8.4 Body image

Pain assessment skills

It is important to remember that not all patients who have cancer experience pain. About one-third of cancer patients do not experience pain.

Of the cancer patients who do report pain, a significant proportion of that pain may be due to problems other than the cancer; to the side effects of treatment for example, to generalised debility, or to a concurrent disorder such as arthritis (Twycross and Lack, 1990).

Current treatments for pain are quite specific, so it is vital that the cause of the pain is identified and appropriate treatment offered.

If the nurse is to accurately assess the patient's pain, in addition to observations of the patient and their interaction with other people, a series of questions will need to be asked.

To obtain a comprehensive picture of pain experienced by the cancer patient, a number of areas of need to be investigated:

- Site(s)
- Intensity
- Frequency
- Feelings about medication/treatment
- Duration
- Character of pain
- Alleviating factors
- Aggravating factors
- Past/current medication or treatment
- Efficacy of medication or treatment
- Effects of pain on sleep pattern
- Effects of pain on desired activities
- Expression of pain to others
- Desires for pain relief
- Feelings about pain now

Perhaps the most obvious first question relates to the site of the patient's pain: 'Where are you hurting?' or 'Where is the pain?'

One way of recording the pain site is to use a body image chart, on which the patient is asked to shade in the area(s) that are affected. When there is more than one pain site, the patient is asked to label the sites A, B, C, D and so on (see Figure 8.4)

The patient will be looking at a mirror image of themselves; the body image should be orientated left and right (as above), in order to avoid confusion.

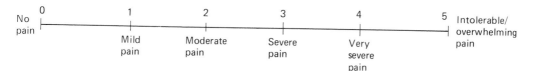

Figure 8.5

PAIN ASSESSMENT CHART

KEY TO PAIN INTENSITY

CONTINUATION NO: _____

0 = no pain
1 = mild pain
2 = moderate pain
3 = severe pain

4 = very severe pain
5 = intolerable/overwhelming pain

s = sleeping

DATE	TIMES	PAIN SITES								ANALGESIA NAME, ROUTE & DOSE	PATIENT ACTIVITY AND COMMENTS
		A	B	C	D	E	F	G	H		
10/11/93	08¹⁰	7								Morphine elixir 5 mg orally	Patient distressed by this pain. Tired and tearful.
"	08¹⁰		3							Flurbiprofen 2 tabs	
"	09⁰⁰	5								Morphine elixir 5 mg orally	Patient reports some relief but is still distressed.
"	10⁰⁰	1									Patient reports this is the best she has felt in four days.
"	12³⁰	0									Patient reports that site B is now pain free.

Figure 8.6 Example of a completed pain chart

Having established where the patient is hurting, the next step is to find out how bad the pain is (pain intensity). There are a number of assessment tools that are available for this purpose.

Numerical assessment

Patients can be asked to assign a number between 0 to 10 to the pain they are feeling, 0 being no pain, and 10 being excruciating pain.

Verbal descriptors

The nurse can ask patients to use words to describe pain intensity. The words most commonly used are: No pain, just noticeable, weak, mild, moderate, strong, severe, excruciating (Tursky 8-word randomised score; Tursky, 1976).

Patients are asked to choose the word that best describes the pain they are feeling at that moment. The words can be set out on a chart alone, or incorporated in a scale (Figure 8.5) (Sharp, 1986).

Another way of measuring pain intensity is to use a visual analogue scale (VAS) (see Figure 2.2, p. 8). The patient is asked to make a mark on the line, at a point which represents how bad the pain is at that moment. The line is 10 cm long, so by measuring the position of the patient's mark on the line, pain intensity can be recorded on a pain chart (Figure 8.6).

By taking a series of measurements as often as is appropriate, the pattern of the patient's pain can be seen quite clearly. This record of pain can play a useful role in helping nursing and medical staff to make decisions about which treatment to offer.

A proportion of cancer patients who report pain may report two or more pain sites. Where more than one pain is reported, it may help to identify which the patient considers to be the worst. This may not always be the one described as being the most intense.

The hypothetical question 'If only one of your pains could be relieved, which one would you choose?', can allow the patient to consider which pain has the more profound affect on their life.

This information can help the nurse to set individual nursing priorities.

There is much academic discussion about the realiability and validity of visual analogue scales in pain assessment (Scott and Huskisson, 1976).

Some researchers report that they are better with the line in the vertical plane, as Hayward did in his study of postoperative pain (Hayward, 1973), while other researchers suggest that there is little significant difference between horizontal or vertical scales.

From the nursing viewpoint, the important factors to consider when introducing any assessment tool are:

● Does the patient find it easy to use?
● How much time does it take for the patient to self-assess?
● Will the use of the tool significantly increase the patient's chances of achieving pain control?

There is evidence that after only a brief teaching period, that is less than 2 minutes, patients have little difficulty in using the visual analogue scale, and that the time taken to self-assess is approximately 20 seconds.

The impact of VAS assessment on pain control is largely dependent on its correct introduction to the clinical area, and on the nursing and medical staff taking it into account when deciding on treatment options. Those clinicians and nurses who use the VAS regularly in pain assessment report that it is a sensitive and useful instrument (Scott and Huskisson, 1976).

The character of pain

To gain an impression of the character of reported pain, the nurse can ask the patient 'Can you tell me what the pain is like?' or 'Can you describe your pain?'

Words patients choose to describe pain, e.g. burning, aching, dull or sharp, fearful or gruel-ling, help to give some depth of understanding to the pain problem.

A pain questionnaire developed at McGill University (Melzack, 1975) from earlier work, demonstrated high agreement among patients, students and physicians on the meaning attached to pain adjectives.

The McGill pain questionnaire groups pain descriptors into three main categories reflecting the underlying dimensions of pain:

● Sensory words which describe pain in terms of time, space, pressure, heat and other properties.
● Affective words which describe the pain in terms of tension, fear and autonomic properties.
● Evaluation words which describe the intensity of the total pain experience.

Since its introduction, the McGill Pain Questionnaire has become respected in both clinical evaluations and treatment trials, in addition to experimental pain models in volunteers. Although the need for regular use of the McGill pain questionnaire in nursing assessment is unlikely, knowledge of the theory and its relevance to pain diagnosis can assist the nurse in understanding the assessment findings more fully.

Frequency and duration of pain

In order to establish the extent of a pain problem in terms of time, the nurse needs to ask 'How often does the pain occur?' and 'How long does the pain last each time?' Patients may report a constant background pain with severe short-lived exacerbations, indicating a pain that is intermittent in nature.

If a patient reports pain that occurs three or four times each day, and lasts about an hour and a half each time, it can be seen that the patient is experiencing unrelieved pain for a total of around 6 hours out of every 24. A further question, 'When does the pain occur?' may reveal that the pain tends to occur at particular times in the day or night, e.g. during working hours, or in the latter part of the night.

Clearly if the patient is experiencing 6 hours pain during each working day, the effects on concentration, and ability to perform working tasks, may be profound.

The discovery of when the patients' pain occurs can lead to the questions, 'What makes the pain better?', and 'What makes the pain worse?'

The patient with an oesophageal cancer may report pain or discomfort when eating certain foods, in which case the nurse can offer dietary advice such as reducing the intake of spicy food and avoiding liquids that are very hot or very cold. Bright light may provoke headache for the patient with a cerebral tumour; if so the nurse can offer gentle lighting in the patient's room or bed area.

Cold may bring a facial pain in the patient who has trigeminal nerve damage, so the nurse can advise about the triggers to avoid, such as draughts, and hot or cold drinks.

Identification of trigger factors that aggravate or alleviate pain will give the nurse an opportunity to understand what type of pain the patient is reporting and plan the care accordingly.

The effects of pain on desired activities

For the nurse to truly understand the effect of pain on both the patient and family, it is necessary to discover the effects of pain on aspects of the patient's life.

Response to the question, 'What does your pain stop you from doing, that you *want* to do?', will give the nurse an insight into some of the patient's values, and the influence of pain and quality of life at that time.

The young mother who cannot cuddle her child because of pain may suffer more than if the pain was only stopping her from doing household chores such as ironing. Add to this the meaning of pain related to cancer, and the pain itself becomes less tolerable.

In consequence, pain may be more difficult to control. If the nurse can identify the activities the patient wishes to regain, the resources and treatment may be appropriately concentrated to maximum effect.

Effects of pain on sleep

Questions related to the effect of pain on sleep can yield valuable information about the type of pain the patient may be reporting, and the effect of current treatment. It is important when asking about pain related to sleep that the nurse establishes pain as the problem, and not other factors that may interfere with sleep, such as room temperature, noise, etc., especially in the hospital environment. Two questions are particularly helpful in this respect; 'Does pain *stop* you from getting to sleep?' and 'Does pain *wake* you after you have fallen asleep?'

If pain stops the patient from getting to sleep, it may be that the medication needs reviewing, or that the hours of darkness increase patient's feelings of isolation, and fears of dying. In this case the nurse may be able to make time to spend with the patient, listening to them if they wish to express their fears, or offering massage to help them relax. If the pain wakes a patient from sleep, perhaps the medication is not lasting through the night, or perhaps pain is occurring on movement during sleep. In both cases the doctor may wish to revise the drugs being prescribed.

If the pain is related to movement, the nurse may be able to identify ways of providing better support, or comfort for the patient when lying in bed.

It is possible that a simple activity is missing from the patient's bed-time routine, a warm, relaxing bath before bed, or a nightcap.

The nurse can help the patient by facilitating as near a normal bed-time routine as is practicable.

If pain is allowed to interfere with sleep for long, the patient will arise in the morning feeling tired or exhausted. The resulting fatigue will further exacerbate the pain.

Past or current medication/treatment

Details concerning the treatment or medication are essential. The nurse will need to know precisely what medication the patient is currently taking, and if it is being taken exactly as prescribed.

A patient who is frightened of strong drugs such as morphine may be reluctant to refuse the prescription from the doctor, but may not necessarily be taking them as advised.

Such non-compliance as this may stem from a fear of becoming addicted to strong drugs, or it may relate to worries about becoming drowsy. Cancer patients may fear that if they take morphine early in their illness, it will not work if they need it later on. They may perhaps feel that taking strong drugs will hasten their death.

These concerns are sometimes held not just by patients, but by health care professionals themselves, and relate to myths that have grown up around morphine and similar drugs.

The myths are a) that morphine means the likelihood of addiction, b) that tolerance (the need to continually increase the morphine dose to achieve the same analgesic effect) frequently occurs, and c) that morphine will hasten death. Patients and staff alike must understand that these myths do not stand up to close scrutiny.

Addiction to morphine in patients who have pain is an extremely rare occurrence; as is tolerance (Twycross and Lack, 1990). By relieving pain, morphine far from hastening death will reverse the vasoconstriction, muscle tension and anxiety that accompanies pain, thus allowing the patient to feel more comfortable and relaxed.

Drowsiness is a common experience for the cancer patient who is beginning on morphine, but lasts for a few days only if morphine is prescribed appropriately.

It is important to establish early on what patients' fears are related to strong medication, since if these fears lead to non-compliance they may result in patients being prescribed drug doses less than or in excess of their needs, which in turn could lead to unacceptable side effects and even less compliance than previously.

Another aspect of treatment/medication that must be investigated is the effect: 'How good was the medicine at relieving your pain?' 'How much of the pain did the treatment take away?'

To complete information related to treatment, it is necessary to ask the patient 'How do you feel about the treatment?'. This will give the patient an opportunity to express their concerns and clarify their thoughts regarding future treatment options.

Some side effects of treatment may be so distressing to the individual that they would prefer to choose another option if one is available, or even go without treatment at all. An important part of the nursing assessment of pain is to find out to whom the patient has communicated their pain. Response to the question, 'Who have you told about your pain?', will help in the prediction of potential problems. If the patient does not express the pain to a relative for example, it is possible that the relative will have unrealistic expectations of the patient. This can lead to difficulties within the family as a whole.

If the patient does not express the pain to their doctor, then appropriate treatment cannot be prescribed, and pain may persist unnecessarily.

The patients' goal for pain relief, 'How much pain do you want to be rid of?,' needs to be established early on in the treatment process, and reviewed as the patient's situation alters.

If for example the appropriate drug to treat the pain results in unacceptable side effects, the patient may prefer to have less of the drug and tolerate a little pain. This kind of compromise can only be made by returning a degree of control to the patient, and respecting their wishes.

These pain assessment activities can be used to provide a firm basis for the planning of nursing interventions, and will also assist the medical staff in diagnosing the cause of the pain.

In the community, similar assessment methods can be adapted to suit the home care setting (Raiman, 1986).

When a patient reports pain, the community nurse can introduce the pain diary and explain its use. After checking that the patient has understood how to record their pain, the nurse can plan when to see the patient again. On the nurse's next visit the information recorded by the patient in the pain diary can form the basis of a more detailed pain assessment. Used in this way the pain diary is a very valuable method of communicating the patient's pain to the general practitioner, and over a period of time provides a comprehensive history of the patient's pain experience.

Introduction of pain assessment methods to the clinical area

If the introduction of pain assessment methods to the clinical area is to be successful, both nursing and medical staff should be involved in the process from the very beginning. The nursing staff must be taught the skills necessary for them to understand and use assessment instruments effectively, and the medical staff will need to recognise the value of assessment in their management of the patient's pain.

The first task of the nurse is to ascertain what problems, if any, exist with the current pain assessment techniques. This can be achieved by carefully observing pain problems within the clinical area and discussing the possible causes of these problems with team members. This may be a relatively simple procedure, following the same problem-solving steps, familiar to nurses in their everyday planning of care.

When the problems of pain assessment have been investigated, the nurse can clearly identify necessary aims and objectives for the project. These objectives will be instrumental at a later date, in the evaluation of outcomes.

If the introduction of a pain measure is seen to be appropriate, the nurse can choose from measures already in use, or perhaps design a measure specific to the needs of the patients within the clinical area. If the pain measure is a new design it must then be tested by a number of patients and the findings discussed (Gracely, 1990). Necessary modifications can be made at this point before the measure is tested over a longer period.

When the pain measure has been in use for a period of time, the nurses can evaluate its effects on pain management, and communicate their findings to other nurses.

Introduction of new nursing measures

Massage

The precise mechanism by which massage relieves pain although much debated, has been subjected to limited experimentation.

The work that has been carried out so far suggests effects in four main areas.

1. Effects on the circulation

The erythema that follows massage is attributed to an increase in blood flow. A number of individuals have reported a measured increase in circulation from various massage techniques (Skull, 1945; Wakim et al., 1949, 1980). Extrapolation from these observations suggest that massage thereby removes waste products and promotes healing.

2. Effects on lymph flow

As early as 1894, the effects of muscle contraction on lymph flow was demonstrated, and it is suggested that massage can have a primary effect on lymph flow. Massage for lymphoedema, however, must be gentle: light strokes applied to the skin surface, not sufficient to increase blood flow. Elkins et al. (1955) and Wakim (1955) demonstrated that massage and compression of an oedematous extremity can increase lymph flow and reduce oedema. Compression bandaging and massage is now com-

monly used to great effect in many hospices and continuing care units.

3. Effects on muscle spasm

One of the primary aims of many massage techniques is the relief of muscle spasm. Cyriax (1971, 1975) has suggested that deep massage can separate adhesions and restore movement between individual muscle fibres. Wakim (1980) describes the effects of massage as relieving muscle fatigue by improvements made in the circulation and the removal of waste products.

4. Effects on endogenous beta-endorphin production

Beta-endorphin is a naturally produced peptide known to modulate pain. It is felt that massage can raise an individual's pain threshold, possibly by stimulating the release of beta-endorphins into the circulation. For the person with cancer, touch may have become markedly reduced, for reasons stated earlier. The value of massage techniques in the care of the dying patient is seen in pain control, the management of lymphoedema and also in communication. Hospice staff report that patients will often talk more freely about fears and concerns during or after massage.

Although hospice and continuing care units have developed these techniques, the skills remain largely underused in the hospital setting, lack of knowledge being perhaps the main reason. For the nurse to employ massage skills in the relief of cancer pain, an understanding of the range of massage techniques and their appropriate application is essential.

Massage is described as the touching or application of forces to the soft tissues, usually muscles, tendons or ligaments, without causing movement or a change in the position of a joint (Wall and Melzack 1990).

There are a number of different massage techniques and each one is performed with a specific aim in mind. The techniques most commonly used are:

Stroking or effleurage

This technique requires the nurse to make light movement of the hands over the skin, in a slow and rhythmic fashion. The hands are in constant contact with the skin and follow exactly the contours of the area being massaged.

Effleurage may be very gentle or applied with more definition to deeper tissues. Light effleurage is soothing and designed to be non-painful. Deeper effleurage can be mildly uncomfortable and is always applied in the direction of venous flow for maximum benefit.

Kneading and petrissage

For this technique the nurse will need to grasp, lift, knead or push the tissues being massaged.

The skin should move with the hands over the underlying tissues. The technique differs from effleurage in this respect. These techniques are more commonly applied to muscles which can be gripped and kneaded, moving from area to area.

Connective tissue massage

For this the nurse will need to use deeper stroking movements, aimed specifically at freeing subcutaneous and connective tissue adhesions. This results in a sensation of warmth and hyperaemia of the skin.

Friction and deep massage

The goal of this technique is to loosen scar tissue or adhesions between deeper structures, such as tendons, ligaments, muscles. These procedures are thought to assist in the absorption of localised effusion (Cyriax 1971; Wood 1974).

Several sessions may be required to obtain maximum benefit, followed by gentle exercise to promote mobility.

Tapotement percussion or clapping

This method employs a series of gentle taps or blows to specific areas.

Tapping is performed using only the tips of the fingers. The ulnar border of the hand may be used or the flat or concave palm.

These percussive movements are usually used in postural drainage of the lungs, or to promote muscle contraction and relaxation and therefore increased circulation.

Shaking and vibration

This method of massage requires the nurse to use either coarse or fine vibratory movements on a part of the patient's body.

This technique is used almost exclusively for postural drainage of the lungs.

For an individual experiencing cancer pain, the two most commonly used massage techniques are stroking or effleurage, and kneading and petrissage. To perform any of these techniques the nurse must receive specific training, and time to practise before using the skills with a patient.

Some general guidelines to follow when performing massage are:

1. The room must be warm; a recommended minimum room temperature is 70°F (21°C).

   Use blankets to cover the areas not being massaged.
2. A firm surface for the patient to lie on is preferable, although massage can be performed with the patient sitting in a comfortable chair.
3. Use a light vegetable oil to lubricate the hands, to prevent friction. Sunflower, grapeseed or olive oil are amongst the best.
4. Pour oil onto the hands (never directly onto the patient's skin) to warm it, before commencing the massage, and use sparingly or the massage will be difficult to perform.
5. Try to keep contact with the patient at all times, lifting one hand at a time when moving from one area to another. Feedback from the patient on the pressure and speed of the strokes is essential if the massage is to be of benefit.
6. Do not massage an area where pain is present.

   Avoid areas that are bruised or inflamed or where there are sensitive veins or tissues.
7. A massage is often particularly beneficial if given after the patient's bath or shower.

Nurses experienced in massage techniques report that for the patient with advanced cancer, massage is best confined to those areas of the body that are most accessible with comfort, e.g. hand and arm, foot and calf, and neck and shoulders. These areas can be massaged with minimum disruption to the patient's position and still provide enormous comfort and pain relief.

Massage is often of particular value at night. If the patient has woken anxious or frightened; the comfort and support that such a procedure provides is often instrumental in encouraging the patient to talk more freely about what worries them. The time given to massage tends to be up to 20 minutes, but the patient must be allowed to communicate their wishes, and shorten or lengthen the session accordingly.

Relaxation training

Simple relaxation techniques can be learned by the nurse and taught to the patient, and when used as a regular part of each day can be helpful in managing pain.

The first step is to encourage the patient to become conscious of tension when it occurs. This will help the patient to concentrate their efforts on reversing its effects.

There are very many different relaxation methods. Two are of particular value to teach cancer patients and are quick and easy to learn (Moyes T, Relaxation training: a manual for therapists, 1984).

The 10 to 1 count

This is possibly the most widely used method and involves counting backwards from 10 to 1.

The patient is asked to visualise each number in turn, consciously releasing more tension with each visualisation, and relaxing more deeply with each exhaled breath.

This exercise can be combined with another in which the patient is encouraged to concentrate on each of the major muscle groups (starting with the muscles in the feet), with each descending number. The patient is asked to tense and relax each muscle group in turn.

When a patient has mastered this technique it may be possible to achieve the same relaxation in the count of five.

2. Clock-watching

In this exercise the patient is taught to imagine the face of a clock, with one hand moving anti-clockwise from 12 (the starting point). As the hand moves backwards around the clock face from 12 to 1, relaxation should become progressively deeper, so that by the time it reaches 12 again relaxation should be as deep as possible.

Both these exercises can be used by patients who are mobile or confined to bed; they can be used individually or as part of a group exercise.

Relaxation tapes are now produced commercially and can be of benefit to a patient when first attempting to learn relaxation skills. Alternatively, the patient might play a tape of their favourite music to help them relax.

Establishment of these massage and relaxation techniques as part of a daily routine can be of great value in managing cancer pain, and should be included in care planning from the first point of contact with the patient.

Patient education

The importance of sharing information with the cancer patient has been introduced at the beginning of this chapter. A range of activities can be involved in this process, and where appropriate should include the family as much as the patient. The primary aspects of patient education are:

- Information-sharing aimed at helping the patient understand the illness.
- Information-sharing aimed at helping the patient understand treatments.
- Information-sharing that will enable the patient to help himself.
- Information-sharing that will help the family to support the patient.

Understanding the illness

Historically there appears to have been a reluctance on the part of some health care professionals to give patients information about their illness in such a way as to be understood.

The use of clinical terms such as malignancy or neoplasm, used without explanation or clarification, can lead to considerable misconceptions and lead to either heightened anxiety or unrealistic expectations.

In studies of dying patients, around 90% of the patients who had been told about their illness believed it had been advantageous to know (Owens and Naylor, 1989).

The nurse's responsibilities in this respect are to make information available to patients, and to provide opportunities for the patient to seek further information as and when desired.

In this situation the nurse can facilitate patients' understanding by using some relatively simple communication skills.

Reflecting

If a cancer patient asks a question concerning their prognosis, 'Am I going to die, nurse?', or 'I'm not going to get better am I, nurse?' rather than giving an immediate answer, it is often more helpful to reflect the question 'Do *you* think you are going to die?' or perhaps 'What do *you* think is happening?'. In this way the patient is given the opportunity to explore their own thoughts and feelings in their own time.

In the majority of cases the patient has already considered the problem and is seeking only confirmation.

By reflecting the question, the nurse is less likely to cause unnecessary distress, in the patient who is as yet not ready to take in such news.

Research suggests that to deny patients information about their illness and prognosis can in many cases increase distress, and deprive them of opportunities to say their good-byes, finish tasks, or 'put their house in order'.

Understanding of treatment

As stated earlier, information-sharing related to treatment is of primary importance in patient compliance.

Information booklets are of benefit, particularly if used in combination with further consultation and discussion with nursing and medical staff.

There are also organisations such as BACUP that provide an extensive information and support service (see Resource section).

Another possible source of information and support can come from patients who have successfully undergone treatment, and are willing to talk about it to patients being offered the same treatment.

Self-help information

The ways in which patients can help themselves during treatment and medication have already been covered, as has massage and relaxation training.

The patient can be also be advised about contact with local self-help groups; these can be a rich source of assistance and support for patient and relative alike.

Information and training for relatives

Where possible the skills such as those of massage and relaxation can be passed on to friends or relatives who are the main carers.

This can be of special value in the home-care situation, and provides the relative with a very practical and positive way of helping in the provision of pain relief and comfort.

The following case histories may help to illustrate how some of the nursing management activities described in this chapter can contribute to the relief of cancer pain. One case history is taken from the hospital setting, one from a hospice, and one from a home-care situation.

Case history 1

Mr X, a retired teacher was about to receive surgery to remove a tumour in his oesophagus. Mr X had insisted from the outset that he should be told all about the diagnosis and treatment, but he also admitted that previous experience of surgery had made him extremely fearful of pain, to the extent that he was considering refusing the operation.

The nurse arranged for him to see the doctor again to discuss Mr X's worries, and for the doctor to explain in more detail what the operation would mean. The nurse then introduced Mr X to pain assessment charts used as part of the nursing care, and offered him the opportunity to learn how to self-assess.

It was explained to Mr X that he could then use the assessment charts to help him communicate his pain to the staff after his operation.

Mr X was grateful to be involved in this way and reported that he felt it had given him much more control over his own pain and confidence in the staff during the postoperative period.

Case history 2

Mrs Y, a 71-year-old retired cleaner, was admitted to the hospice with gross lymphoedema of her left arm secondary to breast cancer. The lymphoedema had gradually been worsening over the last 8 months, despite treatment with a compression sleeve, light massage, and skin care. Mrs Y was admitted to the hospice unable to lift her arm more than an inch or so away from her side, and in extreme pain from the lymphoedema.

The physiotherapist planned and implemented compression bandaging and gentle massage and exercises as part of the care plan, and with nursing staff continued the process over the next 17 days.

The effects were marked, with pain relief and restoration of function achieved to a high degree.

Mrs Y was discharged home able once more to care for herself.

Case history 3

Mrs G, a young mother with ovarian cancer, being cared for at home, was thought by her relatives to have accepted the news of her illness and prognosis, and was coping 'admirably' with her deteriorating health.

Mrs G had two children; a boy of 5 and a girl of $2\frac{1}{2}$ years old.

The district nurse visiting Mrs G noticed that she appeared to be requiring more and more medication to control her pain, and so encouraged Mrs G to keep a pain diary for a week. Details of her sleep pattern indicated that Mrs G was getting less than 2 hours sleep each night.

On further investigation it appeared that this had been the pattern for the last 6 weeks. This was making Mrs G irritable with the children, whom she now could barely tolerate in the same room with her.

This was a source of great distress to the whole family, and Mrs G felt that her children's abiding memory of her would be very negative and hurtful to them as they grew up.

After sharing Mrs G's pain diary information with the general practitioner, the district nurse taught Mrs G some basic relaxation skills, and supplied her with a relaxation tape to help her establish the technique as part of her pre-sleep routine.

Over the next 9 days Mrs G's hours of sleep rose to between 5 and 6 hours each night. Her improved sleep pattern helped in relieving depression that had impoverished her quality of life.

Mrs G reported that her pain was less severe and her analgesic medication was modified accordingly. Without the side effects of her medication, she found that her concentration improved and that she was able to enjoy the company of her children again.

The same relaxation skills were taught to Mrs G's husband and mother, who were the main carers; and these helped them to continue caring for Mrs G at home, until her death some 2 months later.

In all these cases the nursing management of the patients' pain involved the application of many of the core points described in this chapter:

Establishment of trust
Assessment
Review
Patient control and education
Family involvement
Advocacy

These skills are not all easy to accomplish, but with the cooperation and support of colleagues, they can be effectively utilised to provide optimum pain control for the patient with cancer.

References

Badger, C. and Twycross, R. G. (1988) *Management of Lymphoedema*. Sir Michael Sobell House, Churchill Hospital, Oxford, OX3 74J

Cherry, D. A. and Gourlay, G. (1987) The spinal administration of opioids in the treatment of acute and chronic pain: bolus doses, continuous infusion, intraventricular administration and implanted drug delivery systems. *Palliative Medicine*, **1**, 89–106

Cyriax, J. (1971) *Textbook of Orthopedic Medicine*, Vol 2, 8th edn. Bailliere Tindall, London

Cyriax, R. (1975) *Textbook of Orthopedic Medicine. Diagnosis of Soft Tissue Lesions*. Vol. 1, 6th edn, Balliere Tindall, London

Driever, M. J. and McCorkle, R. (1984) patient concerns at 3 and 6 months postdiagnosis. *Cancer Nursing*, **June**: 235–242

Elkins, E. C., Herrick, J. F., Grindlay, J. H. *et al.* (1955)Effect of various procedures on the flow of lymph. *Archives of Physical Medicine*, **34**, 31

Erikson, E. H. (1985) *Life Cycle Completed*. Norton,

Gracely, R. H. (1979) Psychophysical assessment of human pain. *Advances in Pain Research and Therapy 3*. Raven, New York, pp. 805–824

Gracely, R. H. (1990) Pain language and ideal pain assessment. In: *Textbook of Pain*, 2nd edn (eds Melzack and Wall), Churchill Livingstone

Hauck, S. L. (1986) Pain: Problem for the person with cancer. *Cancer Nursing*, **9(2)**, 66–76

Hayward, J. (1975) *Information – A Prescription against Pain*. Royal College of Nursing, London

Hill, H. F., Saeger, L. C. and Chapman, C. R. (1986) *Patient Controlled Analgesia, in Cancer Patients Following Bone Marrow Transplantation:*

a Pilot Study. Unpublished manuscript, Fred Hutchinson. Cancer Research Centre, Seattle, Washington

Kalso, E. and Vainio, A. (1990) Morphine and oxycodone hydrochloride in the management of cancer pain. *Clinical Pharmacology and Therapeutics*, **47(5)**, 639–646

Marie Curie Memorial Foundation (1990) *Annual Report*

McCaffery, M. (1972) *Nursing Management of the Patient with Pain.* Lippincott, Philadelphia

Melzack, R. (1975) The McGill Pain Questionnarie: major properties and scoring methods. *Pain*, **1**, 277–299

Merskey, H. (1974) Pain terms: a list with definitions and notes on useage. Recommended by the IASP Subcommittees on Taxonomy. *Pain*, **6**, 249–252

Morris, J. N., Suissa, S., Sherwood, S. *et al.* (1986) Last days: a study of the quality of life of terminally ill cancer patients. *Journal of Chronic Disease*, **39(1)**, 47–62

Moyes, T. (1984) *Relaxation Training: A Manual for Therapists.* Sub-Debt Clinical Pyschology, The Whelan Building, Liverpool University

Noyes, R. Jr and Clancy, J. (1983) The dying role: its relevance to improved patient care. In: *Hospice Care, Principles and Practice.* Eds C. A. Corr, and D. M. Corr, Faber, pp. 12–21

Owens, R. G. and Naylor, F. (1989) *Living While Dying.* Thompsons Publishing Group

Parkes, C. M. (1985) The dying patient. Terminal care: home, hospital or hospice. *Lancet*, Vol. 1, 155–157

Parsons, T. (1951) *The Social System.* The Free Press, New York

Pollock, Ms (1984) Six Steps to a Successful Literature Search. *Nursing Times*, **October 31**: 40–43

Raiman, J. (1986) Monitoring pain at home. *Journal of District Nursing*, **May 1986**, 4–6

Sarneckey, M. T. and Sarneckey, G. J. (1984) Better patient compliance through effective instructional planning. *Military Medicine*, **149**, 221–224

Saunders, C. (1989) The management of terminal malignant disease, 2nd Edn. Edward Arnold, London

Saunders, C., Summers, D. H. and Teller, N. (1981) *Hospice: The Living Idea.* Edward Arnold, London

Scott, J. and Huskisson, E. C. (1976) Graphic representation of pain. *Pain*, **2**, 175–194

Sharp, S. (1986) Use of the London Hospital pain observation chart. *Nursing*, **11**, 415–423

Skull, C. W. (1945) Massage – physiological basis. *Archives of Physical Medicine*, **261**, 159

St Christopher's Hospice Information Service (1991) *Development of Services for Care of the Dying.* St Christopher's Hospice, 51–59 Lawrie Park Road, Sydenham, London SE26 6DZ

Starling, E. H. (1894) The influence of mechanical factors on lymph production. *Journal of Physiology*, **16**, 224

Twycross, R. G. and Lack, S. A. (1990) *Therapeutics in Terminal Cancer.* Churchill Livingstone,

Turskey, B. The development of a pain profile: a psychophysical approach. In: *Pain, a New Perspective in Therapy and Research* (eds M. Weisenberg and B. Turskey), Penguin Press, New York, p. 171

Wakim, K. G. (1949) The effects of massage on the circulation in normal and paralysed extremities. *Archives of Physical Medicine*, **30**, 133

Wakim, K. G. (1955) Influence on centripetal rhythmic compression on localized edema off an extremity. *Archives of Physical Medicine*, **36**, 98

Wakim, K. G. (1980) Physiologic effects of massage. In: Manipulation, Massage and Traction, 2nd edn (ed. J. B. Rogoff), Williams and Wilkins, Baltimore

Wall, P. D. and Melzack R. (1990) *Textbook of Pain*, 2nd edn. Churchill Livingstone, pp. 206–217

Weisman, A. (1977) *Coping and Vulnerability in Cancer Patients.* Project Omega, Harvard Medical School

Wood, E. C. (1974) *Beard's Massage Principles and Techniques.* W B Saunders, Philadelphia

Resources

The British Association of Cancer United Patients (BACUP)
121/123 Charterhouse Street,
London EC1M 6AA
Tel: 071–608–1661 Outside London 0800–181199
Cancer Link (Provides support and information about cancer)
17 Britannia Street,
London WC1X 9JN
Tel: 071–833–2451
The Marie Curie Memorial Foundation (Provides cancer care through in-patient units and home care nursing, and education services for professional carers)
28 Belgrave Square,
London SW1X 8QG
Tel: 071–235–3325
        071–435–4305
Cancer Research MacMillan Fund (Provides pain and symptom control advice, counselling services, and education for professional carers)
Anchor House,
15/19 Britten Street,
London SW3 3TZ
Tel: 071–351–7811

Educational courses for qualified nurses

English National Board for Nursing and Midwifery
Resource and Careers Services,
Woodseats House,
764a Chesterfield Road,
Sheffield S8 0SE
Tel: 0742–551064/65
Course: 931
The Continuing Care of the Dying Patient and the family
This course is aimed at giving the participants an appreciation and awareness of the clinical, pastoral and psycho-social aspects of the continuing care of the dying patient and the family.

There are currently 45 institutions approved to run the course.
Course: 285

Specialist Course in the Continuing Care of the Dying Patient and Family for nurses on part 1 of the Professional Register (RGN).
This course is for nurses with some experience in care of the dying patient and the family, and involves in-depth study of communication and bereavement counselling, symptom control, management of the service and principles of education.

There are currently 9 institutions approved to run the course.

Medical advice on cancer pain management can be obtained from:
The Pain Society,
9, Bedford Square,
London WC1B 3RA.

9

Pain in the elderly

Jan Walker

Introduction

The number of very elderly people in Britain is increasing rapidly at the present time. It is estimated that people over the age of 75 will comprise 45% of the retired population by the year 2000 (Rossiter and Wicks, 1982). The prevalence of painful and disabling conditions increases with age and arthritis is the most common cause of pain in the elderly. Masi and Medsger (1979) reported that as many as 85% of those aged over 75 suffer from significant degenerative joint disease. They also estimated that rheumatoid arthritis is present in 10% of those aged over 65.

A recent study of elderly people living in the community forms the basis for much of this chapter (Walker, 1989). Results indicated that 80% of elderly patients visited by district nurses in a south coast retirement area suffered from some degree of persistent pain. Seventy per cent of these were found to suffer from some type of arthritic pain which most commonly affected hips and knees. Other problems affecting the lower limbs included bunions, corns, ingrowing toenails, gout, old fractures, venous and diabetic ulcers, and peripheral vascular disease. It can therefore be seen that a large proportion of chronic painful disorders in the elderly directly restrict mobility and activity.

Other causes of chronic or persistent pain in the elderly include ischaemic heart disease, stroke, gastrointestinal disorders (including hiatus hernia, indigestion, gastric ulceration, constipation, haemorrhoids and diverticulitis), chronic respiratory disease, neurogenic pain (including neuralgias and neuropathies), back pain, and pressure sores. These are nearly all longstanding conditions involving either continuous or intermittent pain.

Many elderly people suffer from multiple pain problems. Out of the sample of 190 elderly people interviewed in relation to pain, 80% reported severe to excruciating pain, mostly on a regular basis. Sixteen per cent were never free of less than moderate pain (Walker, 1989).

The majority of older people appear to accept pain and cope well in spite of it. However, pain is often overlooked in nursing assessments (Walker and Campbell, 1989) and may not be recognised unless the patient complains about it. The failure of medical treatments to alleviate pain in this situation generates feelings of helplessness and frustration among medical and nursing staff. The more the patient complains, the more likely it is that the nurse will consider that he or she is exaggerating in order to gain attention (Walker et al., 1990).

The effective management of pain in the elderly depends upon adequate assessment. The assessment of pain and disability is the first stage in this process. Other factors are considered later.

Pain assessment in the elderly

Pain intensity

Chronic pain intensity can only be assessed by self-report. The most common measurement tools are the visual analogue scale (VAS), the numerical rating scale (on a 10 or 5 point scale) and the verbal rating scale. The literature suggests that failure to complete the VAS increases with age (Kremer et al., 1981). Walker (1989) found that the majority of those aged over 75 could not cope with either visual analogue or numerical rating scales. However Raiman's 6 point verbal rating scale (Raiman, 1986), shown in Figure 9.1, was readily received and

0	No pain
1	Just noticeable
2	Moderate
3	Severe
4	Very severe
5	Excruciating

Figure 9.1 Verbal rating scale (Raiman, 1986)

used by all patients regardless of age. Although this scale is less sensitive than the VAS, it provides a reliable measure of intensity for clinical nursing purposes.

It is of little value to complete any pain intensity rating scale with reference only to a single moment in time. However the rating scale can be most useful in conjunction with the questions:

'How bad is your pain when it is at its worst?' and

'How bad is your pain when it is least troublesome?'

The first question allows nurse and patient to identify how often the pain has been really bad and under what circumstances. The answers will help to isolate potential trigger factors for which avoiding action or treatment may be planned. The answer to the second question indicates if the patient is ever completely free of pain, or if the pain is substantially reduced at times. This enables both nurse and patient to identify the factors or circumstances which help to alleviate the pain and plan to extend or increase these.

These two questions may be used on a daily, weekly or even a one-off basis, in hospital or at home. Answers provide information from which to plan useful intervention strategies. It avoids problems associated with frequent monitoring of pain which focus the patient's mind on the thing he most wishes to forget.

For many elderly arthritis patients, the process of getting out of bed, washing and dressing in the morning causes excruciating pain. They may be unable to take analgesics first because of the imperative of getting to the toilet, therefore planning a strategy to avoid pain is diffi-

cult. However, patients may be encouraged to make strategic use of analgesics throughout the day in order to enable them to participate in activities and which will enhance their quality of life.

Pain location

It is important to know the location of the patient's pain, particularly since many of them will identify multiple sites. Body charts are commonly used for this purpose. However, many elderly people find it difficult to complete these themselves and frequently ask the nurse to mark the chart while they point to locations on their own body. Knowing the location of pain helps with diagnosis and with planning management priorities and strategies.

Pain-related disability

It is important to find out if pain prevents people from doing what they want to do. An activities of living checklist is helpful. A simple one might include dressing/undressing, washing/bathing, cooking, cleaning and general mobility. However, the list should be adapted according to the patient's circumstances. Bathing is not a problem for the patient who is content to have a shower, nor is cooking a problem for the patient who is happy to have meals provided.

The question 'Does pain stop you from doing what you want to do?' may identify activities such as gardening, shopping or knitting as a particular problem. This will help to establish the patient's priorities in terms of situations in which pain control measures or aids are required.

Pain quality

In addition to measuring the intensity, location and effect of pain it is useful to consider what it feels like to the patient. The McGill Pain Questionnaire (MPQ, Melzack, 1975) was designed with this in mind and contains lists of verbal pain descriptors. The full version looks intimidating. However, it takes only 5 minutes to complete with elderly patients. Arthritis pain is commonly described as gnawing, aching, stabbing and shooting. Venous ulcers are often described as aching, burning, stinging and itchy. People seem to feel relieved at being able to provide an accurate description of their pain. The main utility of this tool, in my opinion, is that it enables patients to feel secure in the knowledge that the nurse understands what they are feeling.

The MPQ includes two particularly useful dimensions – the affective and evaluative scales. Patients who describe their pain as 'miserable, intense or unbearable' (evaluative scale) are generally those who report that their pain is not under control. Patients who report that their pain is 'fearful or frightful, punishing, cruel or vicious' (affective scale), are generally not coping well and require help. These scales offer a useful indication of patients' attitudes towards pain.

Pain control and coping

A question which directly addresses the patient's ability to cope with pain is:

'Do you feel in control of your pain?'

Patients who answer 'yes' or 'on the whole' are generally coping well whatever their level of pain intensity. Patients who answer 'not really' or 'not at all' are having most difficulty in coping with pain. Such negative answers appear to reflect a lack of pain coping strategies.

Coping is reflected in the patient's mood state. Patients who appear anxious (worried, tense, uncertain, frightened), depressed (helpless, hopeless, worthless, guilty) or hostile (bitter, resentful, angry, irritable) are failing to cope with the problems they have, whether or not they are related to pain (Walker, 1989). Patients who are coping well with their lives generally report feeling calm, contented and optimistic. An assessment of the patient's mood state, based upon their use of these descriptors, is a valuable indicator of their quality of life which should be included in all assessments of patients with chronic conditions.

Additional factors which influence coping and quality of life are considered later in this chapter.

The nursing management of specific types of pain in the elderly

A starting point for the treatment of pain in the elderly is to ensure that the patient is receiving medical treatment which is appropriate for the cause of the pain. However, this chapter will focus upon issues in nursing rather than medical management. Three of the most common types of pain in the elderly are focussed upon below. They are arthritis, leg ulcers and neurogenic pain.

Arthritis

Osteoarthritis and rheumatoid arthritis are distinct diseases. However, in reality it is often difficult to distinguish between them in elderly patients. Indeed, patients may have both. Severe joint pain commonly accompanies both types of arthritis and may be difficult to relieve. Joint surgery may effectively relieve pain in hips and knees for those who are considered fit enough. Sadly this is often preceded by a long wait for out-patient appointments and surgery. During this time the pain increases and mobility becomes more difficult. Patients frequently worry because of lack of feedback about the result of tests or X-rays. They derive considerable benefit from having a little time to explain how they feel, receive information about what is wrong, what to expect, and what they can do to help themselves.

All types of arthritis can be exceedingly painful. The majority of patients with different types of pain problem identify arthritis pain as the worst. Arthritis is responsive to non-steroidal anti-inflammatory drugs (NSAIDs) and these often provide good relief from pain in the short term. However, there is a high incidence of adverse reactions, including gastric ulceration and haemorrhage, which cautions against continuous long term use. Many elderly people fail to discern benefits from these drugs after prolonged regular use, yet continue to take them if prescribed by their doctor. It is imperative to monitor the effects and efficacy of such drugs and to keep the doctor informed of the results. A periodic break from the drug might serve to reduce side effects and demonstrate the level of efficacy to the patient. Patients should be advised of the possible side effects of all drugs so that they can recognise early warning signs and stop taking them. Written information for elderly patients on the use of their drugs is helpful for them and for their carers.

The aim of analgesia for patients with acute or malignant pain is to maintain the patient in a pain-free state for as long as is necessary. With arthritis patients this aim is rarely attainable and improved quality of life may be a more realistic goal. Patients are commonly given paracetamol with variable (often minimal) effect, or codeine combination analgesics which provide good relief in the short term but which may cause painful constipation. Many patients prefer to put up with the arthritis pain than endure such undesirable effects.

Patients should be encouraged to develop their own pain-relieving strategies. These may include the use of hot water bottles, warm clothing, heat lamps, rubbing in topical ointments, gentle exercises and special diets. They do not always appear to have medical validity but enhance a sense of personal control over the pain. When these strategies are combined with strategic intermittent use of analgesics, many elderly patients manage to keep their arthritis pain tolerably well under control.

Leg ulcers

Leg ulcers, whether venous or arterial, are common in the elderly and can be extremely painful. One patient commented that she 'nearly went mad with the pain'. Walking is often very painful so patients tend to keep still, which does little to enhance the circulation. If patients also have arthritis this only makes matters worse as they stiffen up. However, as one lady said, 'I can't tackle the arthritis until the ulcer is better'. Regular movement and passive foot exercises must be encouraged for all patients.

There are a variety of different ways of treating leg ulcers which are beyond the remit of this chapter. The delivery of care is also important. Patients who require regular leg dressings frequently complain about changes in nursing staff and treatments. One patient counted 27 nurses over a 5 year period and asked quite reasonably 'how can they tell if it has progressed?'. It may be helpful to keep a chart of the size of the ulcer with descriptive comments, together with an assessment of pain intensity and quality which is completed on a regular basis. If this is left in the home for patients to examine and comment upon, it will increase their sense of control over what can be a very lengthy treatment. It will also demonstrate progress.

Another issue relating to leg ulcers is the frequently heard observation that patients remove their bandages or stick knitting needles down them just as the wound is on the point of healing. It is a common assumption that patients fear they will lose the regular attention of the nurse once the ulcer is healed. While this may be the case in some instances, many patients report intense irritation at this stage and may be seeking to relieve this.

Neurogenic pain

Neurogenic pains are more common in the elderly than other age groups. These include post-herpetic and trigeminal neuralgia, diabetic neuropathy and post-stroke pain which cause continuous inescapable pain. Patients should be referred without delay to a pain clinic where a range of treatments and therapies are available, including nerve blocks, drugs, and transcutaneous electrical nerve stimulation (TENS). However, some of these types of pain can be particularly resistant to treatment, and antidepressant therapy should be considered for all patients with intractable neurogenic pain. Sufferers require a considerable amount of support and encouragement to overcome the difficulties of living with continuous severe pain.

General factors which influence pain control in the elderly

Pain is a potential stressor which can cause anxiety, fear, anger and depression (Walker *et al.*, 1989). Stress is increased by uncertainty, unpredictability and uncontrollability, each of which are likely to accompany pain.

Uncertainty – does the patient understand the pain, what is causing it and how best to handle it?

Unpredictability – can the patient identify trigger factors which will enable him to avoid or control painful episodes?

Uncontrollability – what can the patient do to help control his own pain? Does the patient believe that there is anything s/he can do? Are there treatments or analgesics which will provide relief when the pain gets really bad? Are there actions which the patient can take to reduce or avoid pain? Are there any self-help or alternative measures which the patient might try?

Clearly some people are less able to cope with pain and stress than others because of factors relating to personality and past experiences. Some individuals may cope differently because of their cultural background. Some have fewer resources in terms of motivation or social support. Other problems do not disappear because someone has pain and these will compete for coping resources. Each of these issues needs to be considered in relation to pain management.

The following have been identified as key factors which influence pain control in the elderly (Walker *et al.*, 1990). Each of these is amenable to nursing intervention.

Feeling informed

The importance of information has been demonstrated in relation to acute postoperative pain (Hayward, 1975) and in relation to chronic benign pain (Marcer *et al.*, 1990). It appears to be of equal importance to elderly people with all types of persistent pain. In fact pain is rarely controlled when the patient is anxious about the cause.

Walker (1989) identified that about 20% of the people interviewed felt they lacked information about their pain. Several people clearly suspected that they might have a malignancy. One lady aged 80 described low abdominal pain accompanied by vaginal bleeding. The pain, though moderate, was totally out of control and the patient said 'I think that I have cancer. The doctors have never really told me what the results of the tests were'. Not all patients had such urgent cause for concern but were still dissatisfied. One lady aged 88 said 'The doctor fobs me off. I have told the doctors about my backache . . . but the GP passes it off. The hospital X-rayed it but I heard no more'. An elderly gentleman said 'the GP does not give me the results of anything he does. I worry because I don't know what to do'.

People who are worried about their condition do not necessarily ask the doctor for information (Ley, 1988). Fears of the imagination are frequently worse than those of reality and it really does help to share them. Subjects were asked 'if you had something seriously wrong with you, would you wish to be told all about it, even if the outlook was not good?' Eighty per cent answered yes. Comments included 'you can only deal with what you know about' and 'I could put up with it if I knew what it was'. Only 8% said that they would prefer not to know.

Personal strategies for pain control

It has already been suggested that elderly patients should be encouraged to develop their own strategies to control their pain. One of the reasons that individual strategies work so well in promoting pain control, even though some may appear to have little medical validity, is that the patients are doing something to help themselves. This gives them a sense of personal control over the pain, whereas taking tablets on a regular time basis confers no real sense of control unless the pain-reducing effects are quite marked. TENS is a relatively recent treatment for acute and chronic pain, which is outlined in another chapter in this book. It can prove effective for a variety of conditions, although it does not work for all patients. Not all elderly patients will cope with the electrodes and controls, particularly those with poor vision or function. However, for those who are able, it is something that they can do for themselves and which enhances their sense of personal control.

Patients who are advised to 'try this' and 'try that' often end up with a sense of total failure and hopelessness when treatment after treatment fails. Perhaps patients could be invited to test a particular treatment and report upon the results for the benefit of the nurse and other patients. If the treatment has no positive effects, the patient has still succeeded in providing useful information and should not feel any personal sense of failure.

Keeping occupied

Coping is an active process and having some kind of occupation provides distraction from pain. Pain and accompanying disability in the elderly reduce the potential for keeping occupied which in turn increases the focus on pain.

When elderly patients were asked what was the worst thing about having pain, the overwhelming majority said that it stopped them from 'doing things'. Conversely pain was not considered too bad if 'it doesn't stop me from doing things'. 'Doing things' implies being able to maintain independence and being able to fill time.

Active involvement is more effective in promoting coping than passive occupations, although activity does not necessarily have to involve physical exercise. Thus knitting, sewing, crochet and other crafts, in addition to household activities such as cooking and cleaning, emerge as the most effective means of keeping occupied. Watching television and reading the newspaper are among the least effective, although it may be helpful to engage elderly patients in discussion of favourite programmes, books or news items to enhance active involvement.

Elderly patients who were cared for by a spouse or relative were found to be among those with least to do and who felt most depressed. This in turn reduced their ability to control their pain. Nurses are in a position to encourage relatives to allow patients to do more. One elderly lady had had her leg amputated and was confined to a wheelchair. She experienced phantom limb pain and was quite severely depressed. In conversation she said that she longed more than anything else to make scones. The niece, with whom she lived, said that she would immediately arrange for her to gain access to the kitchen – she had never thought of this before.

Aids to independence and occupation are of vital importance to all elderly people in hospital and at home. One post-stroke patient told of how she had discharged herself from hospital because she could no longer tolerate sitting for hours beside her bed feeling useless. Once home, the district nurse had encouraged her husband to allow her to participate in cleaning and meal preparation. This helped her to overcome pain, disability and depression. The role of the occupational therapist is particularly valuable where occupational and household activities are restricted through disability, including poor vision.

It may be possible to target pain relief in order to promote occupational activities. If an elderly person has a variety of pains it may be necessary to identify the patient's priorities for pain relief rather than attempting a global approach. This may well relate to the type of activity the person wishes to pursue. Many elderly women are happy as long as they can continue to knit. Advice about changes in position of the needles are often all that is required to relieve some of the pain in arms and shoulders. Simple measures are often the most effective and observing an elderly person going about daily activities can provide useful clues. An elderly friend recently developed a painful shoulder. The cause was found to be the height of the arm of the chair in which he spent much time sitting and a change of position rectified the problem.

Having regrets

It is difficult to cope with present problems if those of the past remain unresolved. Regrets about the past are associated with negative mood and loss of well-being, and also appear to be directly associated with inability to cope with pain. Coleman and McCulloch (1985, p. 2532) observed 'It is easy to see how one's inner thoughts and feelings can assume greater importance as one is cut off from the outer world through factors common to old age, such as loss of occupation, physical disability, sensory deprivation/attentional difficulties, bereavement, isolation . . .'.

Regrets may be pain-related. Some people look forward to retirement as a time to fulfill leisure ambitions only to find that a painful and disabling condition has ruined their plans. A variety of other incidents or circumstances may cause regret, such as childhood abuse, unhappy marriages, divorce, early loss of spouse or children, unfilled ambitions or past misdeeds. One lady had just celebrated her golden wedding anniversary. She had a lovely home and an attentive husband. Her pain, though only moderate, was not under control and there was no apparent reason for the depression she reported. However, when her husband went out to make the tea she leant forward and said 'my father asked me on the day we were married "are you sure that you are doing the right thing?" I started to cry and I have been crying ever since'. In the absence of this knowledge it would have been tempting to believe that she was exaggerating her pain.

Nurses cannot alter the events of the past, but having someone to share past memories with can often be therapeutic. At least the patient knows that someone understands their feelings and is sympathetic. Research is currently being designed to investigate the impact of life review on pain control for those with regrets.

Religious involvement can be an important source of practical and spiritual support which helps people to come to terms with pain and disability. However, a minority see pain as a punishment and cannot understand how their God could inflict such suffering on them.

Sharing these feelings may help some individuals to come to terms with their plight.

Non-pain-related problems

Patients who have chronic pain are not exempt from having other problems to contend with. The elderly are particularly vulnerable to certain stressors, notably bereavement through the loss of spouse, close family and friends. If coping is regarded as a finite resource, then the presence of other problems will influence pain coping (and vice versa).

People who have experienced the loss or illness of someone close to them often express loneliness, depression and poor pain control. There is little doubt that supportive visits are particularly important after bereavement. One lady had suffered from continuous severe pain from trigeminal neuralgia for 30 years and had been disabled with arthritis for the last 10 years. She reported that she had been able to cope well until recently when her husband and daughter had both died. Her son-in-law had lived with her after her daughter's death but was now remarrying. She likened herself to 'a dog that has been abandoned'. Her pain was totally uncontrolled and she expressed suicidal thoughts. She was not short of practical support but lacked anyone who would sit with her and help her come to terms with her unfortunate situation. She had many happy memories which may have helped in this process.

It is not unusual for elderly patients to be worried by financial problems. Many have to exist on a low income. Most can manage until there is a need for large expenditure, for example household repairs or maintenance. Some may be able to obtain the necessary help either from statutory or voluntary sources, but referrals for help can only be made if these problems have been detected or assessed in the first place.

Loneliness

Nurses commonly report loneliness as a cause of coping difficulties in the elderly. However, loneliness appears to be a consequence of problems which include loss of close family and friends, lack of occupation, regrets, and not just being alone. Regrets are particularly important for those who are alone. Coleman commented 'Loss of contact can be hard to bear, but far worse is an inability to be content in one's own company' (Coleman, 1986, p. 79). Many elderly people benefit from visits to day centres, luncheon clubs or church groups. Those recently widowed probably benefit most from close social support in the home. However, being alone does not inevitably imply loneliness and many are quite content in their own company provided they can keep occupied and reflect upon pleasant memories.

Other factors which influence pain

There are one or two other factors which may influence an elderly patient's experience of pain. One is excessive consumption of alcohol which may be undetected. Alcohol sometimes helps to alleviate pain but its long term effects are depressant and it probably reduces overall coping capabilities. Likewise antidepressants, anxiolytics and narcotic analgesia may alter the patient's mood and coping abilities. Anxiolytics play no part in the control of chronic pain, while the role of narcotic drugs and antidepressants (other than for neurogenic pain) remains contentious.

Another possible factor is fear of death or of cancer. The nurse should always be alert to this, particularly if the patient's negative mood is not predicted by either the level of pain or any of the other factors discussed above.

All of the factors considered in this section are closely related to the experience of pain. Any attempt to treat or alleviate pain without reference to them may be destined to fail. There is no doubt that the vast majority of, if not all pain in the elderly has a physical origin. However, it is quite likely that the body's natural pain control systems fail to operate under conditions where the patient has lost overall control over his life. Physical pain cannot be cured by physical means alone when there is a hurt which lies much deeper.

The importance of sympathy and understanding

Most elderly patients report that nurses can help with pain by sympathy and understanding. Individual comments about nursing support include:

'Be someone you can rely on – gives you a feeling of security'

'Be understanding – not just write them off as complaining'

'You can talk to a nurse, but a doctor talks to you'

'When there is no medicament they can give you, then a sense of confidence that you can bear it. She (the nurse) can sustain that strength by her attitude'

The provision of support for elderly patients may be difficult for the nurse who has little time available. However, when faced with a patient who feels resentful and depressed and complains vigorously about pain, it may be futile to refer back to the doctor for stronger analgesics when the cause of the patient's inability to cope lies in other unresolved issues. The fact that the nurse understands this will help her to overcome her own sense of frustration and helplessness in the face of continuing demands. The patient may be helped by knowing that the nurse has taken the trouble to find out about his or her other problems, even if there is little that can actually be done about them.

On the whole nurses do not feel that there is much that they can do for elderly patients with pain and some openly expressed feelings of helplessness. One commented:

'It is easier to be empathetic with someone in terminal pain than listening day after day for years to someone's complaint of, for example, severe and disabling arthritis pain, as the nurse gets stressed, unable to offer curing solutions.'

Nurses who feel helpless in the face of persistent pain complaints may tend to attribute them to exaggeration in order to gain attention. It is important to recognise that although pain may be the focus of distress, management requires a much wider nursing perspective.

The elderly in hospital

If as many as 80% of elderly people suffer from some kind of chronic painful condition it is evident that the majority of elderly patients who are admitted to hospital will have some existing chronic pain. Once in hospital they are routinely separated from their preferred analgesia, which they may then be offered at times of the day which do necessarily afford them maximum benefit. They may also be separated from their own ointments, sprays and other personal methods of pain control, so reducing

the level of personal control they normally maintain over their pain. Self-medication is an obvious solution for patients who are capable of, and wish to undertake this.

Elderly patients face practical worries which often seem trivial to nursing staff, but which generate considerable anxiety. One of the most common difficulties involves getting to the toilet. Some recalled the long painful distance from bed to toilet, and the obstacles encountered en route. These were mostly patients who had gone to great lengths to organise things at home and liked to maintain their independence. Unnecessary difficulties often render them irritable and cantankerous.

A few patients who had undergone surgery remembered having hallucinatory effects after anaesthetic. It was interesting to note their vivid recall of such episodes. They remembered their own words and actions as well as the response of the nursing staff. Elderly patients fear losing their dignity under such conditions which are clearly outside their control.

Patients do not automatically shed all of the problems of home on admission to hospital. Many elderly people worry that they may not be allowed to return home. They are anxious about their finances. They fret over their spouse or their pet. Such anxieties will inevitably interfere with their pain control. Being able to discuss these issues with a sympathetic nurse may help, and there may be practical solutions which the medical social worker could investigate. Being told not to worry is hardly reassuring.

There are many geriatric, rheumatology and pain centres which cater excellently for elderly people. Their patients are well-informed. They are encouraged to express their needs and have their treatment tailored to suit those needs. They appreciate the fact that someone has taken the trouble to find out what is wrong and is trying to help. Under these circumstances they can often accept that there is no cure.

Pain in patients with Alzheimer's disease

Patients with Alzheimer's disease present particular problems for pain assessment. However, patients who are quite markedly confused (unable to remember their age or where they are living) have little difficulty in reporting the

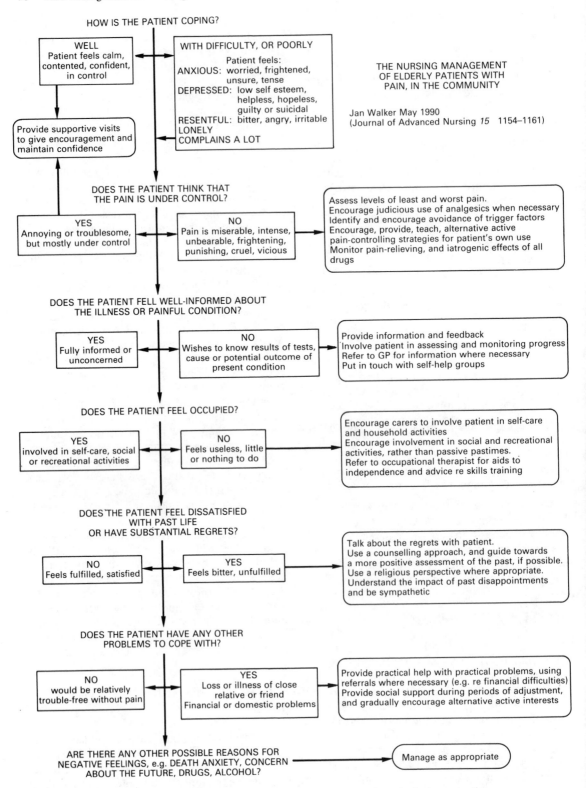

Figure 9.2 The nursing management of elderly patients with pain, in the community

intensity of their pain using Raiman's verbal rating scale, or in describing other aspects of their pain experience. Once verbal reporting becomes vague or communication impossible, it is necessary for the nurse to be alert for other signs of pain such as restlessness or withdrawals, crying out, groaning, rocking, guarding or rubbing particular sites. Treatment and evaluation presents difficulties. Discussion with close relatives or carers may provide useful information about possible causes, past effective treatments for pain and prior personal stagies for pain relief. Special attention should be paid to gentle handling and general comfort measures to minimise pain in this vulnerable group.

Nursing assessment and intervention for chronic pain in the elderly

This chapter has examined a variety of factors which may influence the ability of elderly people to cope with pain. It is clearly necessary to ensure that the patient is receiving the best and most appropriate medical treatment available; however, nurses have much more to offer. Nursing care has a vital role to play in the lives of elderly people who suffer from pain, but opportunities are currently being lost through over-reliance upon medical treatments, failure to recognise the importance of a range of other factors which influence pain control, and failure to adopt an holistic approach to assessment. The flow chart given in Figure 9.2 is offered as a comprehensive guide to assessment and intervention for nurses to use with the elderly who have chronic pain.

References

Coleman, P. G. (1986) *Ageing and Reminisence Processes: Social and Clinical Implications*. John Wiley, Chichester

Coleman, P. G. and McCulloch, A. W. (1985) The study of psychosocial change in late life: some conceptual and methodological issues. In: *Life-span and Change in a Gerontological Perspective* (eds J. M. A. Munnichs, P. Mussen, E. Olbrich and P. G. Coleman), Academic Press, Orlando

Hayward, J. (1975) *Information – a Prescription Against Pain*. RCN, London

Kremer, E., Atkinson, J. H. and Ignelzi, R. J. (1981) Measurement of pain: patient preference does not confound pain measurements. *Pain*, **10**, 241–248

Ley P. (1988) *Communicating With Patients*. Croom Helm, London

Marcer, D., Murphy, E. J. J., Pounder, D. and Rogers, P. (1990) The pain relief clinic: how should we define success? *Journal of Intractable Pain Society of Great Britain and Ireland*, **7(2)**, 9–17

Masi, A. T. and Medsger, T. A. (1979) Epidemiology of the rheumatic diseases. In: *Arthritis and Allied Conditions* (ed. D. J. McCarty). Lea and Febiger, Philadelphia

Melzack, R. (1975) The McGill Pain Questionnaire: major properties and scoring methods. *Pain*, **1**, 277–299

Raiman, J. (1986) Pain relief – a two-way process. *Nursing Times*, **82(15)**, 24–27

Walker, J. M. (1989) *The Management of Elderly Patients with Pain: a Community Nursing Perspective*. Dorset Institute (Bournemouth University), unpublished PhD Thesis

Walker, J. M., Akinsanya, J. A., Davis, B. D. and Marcer, D. (1989) The nursing management of pain in the community: a theoretical framework. *Journal of Advance Nursing*, **14**, 240–247

Walker, J. M., Akinsanya, J. A., Davis, B. D. and Marcer, D. (1990) The nursing management of elderly patients with pain in the community: findings and recommendations. *Journal of Advanced Nursing* **15**, 1154–1161

Walker, J. M. and Campbell, S. M. (1989) Pain assessment, nursing models and the nursing process. In: *Nursing Models* (ed. J. Akinsanya), Churchill Livingstone, Edinburgh

10

Paediatric pain

Patrick J. McGrath, Judith A. Ritchie and Anita M. Unruh

Introduction

Although pain in adults has been recognised as a major health problem for some years, pain in children is only now attracting research and clinical attention. Nurses have played an important role in the understanding of paediatric pain. Observations by nurse-clinicians have been the impetus for research. Nurse-researchers had conducted many of the key studies in paediatric pain. Finally, nurses have instituted new clinical protocols to control paediatric pain.

Eland and Anderson (1977), two nurses, did a very important early study. They found that a group of 18 children received only 24 doses of analgesics, whereas 18 adults received 372 doses of analgesics following surgery. Subsequent studies by another nurse, Judy Beyer (Beyer *et al.*, 1983) and by Neil Schechter (Schechter *et al.*, 1986) have confirmed the earlier findings but found that the gap between adults and children had lessened. These studies increased interest although they did not directly lead to the understanding or solution of any paediatric pain problems.

In this chapter, we will first discuss the role of basic science in understanding pain in children and then examine the assessment and management of pain. Finally, we will focus on the nursing environment that will promote adequate pain management for children.

The basic sciences and pain in children

Clinical sciences need a basic science foundation in order to progress. Unfortunately, the basic sciences relating to paediatric pain, including biology, psychology and epidemiology, have received scant attention.

The biology of paediatric pain

The biology of paediatric pain is concerned with the mechanisms of pain structures, the transmission of pain via these structures, and the impact of maturation on both. Recent research in this area has challenged the once commonly held assumptions about neonatal pain. There is now ample evidence that pain transmission in neonates occurs (Anand and Hickey, 1987). In addition, it appears that the immaturity of the nervous system serves primarily to reduce the neonate's ability to fully activate the descending control mechanisms that reduce pain perception (Fitzgerald *et al.*, 1988). Thus, neonates, and especially premature neonates, do feel pain and may be more sensitive to pain than older babies. Research on spinal cord mechanisms in cutaneous response is progressing but little is known of the development aspects of peripheral mechanisms or non-cutaneous pain. Moreover, critical issues such as the role of early prolonged experience on later pain perception, is unknown. Beyond early infancy, there do not appear to be any essential differences in pain tranmission between children and adults.

The epidemiology of paediatric pain

Epidemiology is concerned with the frequency of occurrence (in this case, pain in childhood) and the cause of that occurrence. There have been numerous epidemiological studies of various pains in children (see review by Goodman and McGrath, in press). Unfortunately, the methodology used in most studies has been poor. It is only in the past year that a proper epidemiological study of pain in hospitalized children has been completed (Johnson, et al., 1992 The epidemiology of the impact of pain on specific behaviours and on the child's social role also has been neglected. Epidemiology is important, not only to ascertain the extent of a pain problem but also to examine the correlates which may provide clues to the cause.

The developmental psychology of paediatric pain

Developmental psychology examines change over time in how children understand and react to pain. Most studies in this area have been questionnaire studies. For example, Gaffney (Gaffney and Dunne, 1986, 1987; Gaffney, 1988) surveyed 680 Irish children aged 5–14 years. They found a developmental trend in the way that children thought about pain. There has been some outstanding work by Grunau and Craig (1987) and Johnson (1989) on the response of young babies to needles. This work is further discussed in the section on measurement.

As yet, there have been no attempts to apply the latest thinking on children's cognitive development, such as theories of mind, to children's conceptualization of pain.

How children cope with pain and other stressful situations has only begun to be examined and most studies focus on the school-aged child. The types of strategies used by children vary according to the type of painful situation and factors such as age, gender, and locus of control (Curry and Russ, 1985; Lamontagne, 1987). Younger children tend to use self-protective behaviours (aggression or efforts to escape to prevent the procedure from occurring), seeking information and control, and/or reaching out to others for support and help (Hyson, 1983; Ritchie et al., 1990). In the postoperative period, older children use controlling behaviours as their dominant coping strategy (Savedra and Tesler, 1981). In other situations older children use a variety of coping strategies including seeking information, attention diversion, seeking support from others, seeking medication, cognitive reappraisal, calming self-talk, imagery, inhibiting motion, relaxation, resting, withdrawing and catastrophising/worrying behaviours (Savedra and Tesler, 1981; Tesler et al., 1981; Curry and

Russ, 1985; Brown et al., 1986; Peterson and Toler, 1986; Ritchie et al., 1988, 1990; Branson et al., 1990; Peterson et al., 1990). Increasing age has been associated with more cognitive and fewer emotion-focused or behavioural coping strategies (Curry and Russ, 1985; Peterson and Toler, 1986).

Assessment and measurement of pain in children

Measurement of pain in children has received a great deal of attention over the past few years. As a result, measures of pain intensity are now better validated in children than in adults.

Measurement and assessment of pain are related but not identical concepts. Measurement refers to the application of a specific metric to an aspect of pain, usually the intensity. Assessment is a much broader endeavour that includes the selection of what aspects of pain to measure as well as the investigation of the variables that impact on the pain experience (McGrath and Unruh, 1987).

A model of pain assessment

We have developed a model for the assessment of pain based on the World Health Organisation's (1980) classification of the effects of disease (see Table 10.1). The first plane of experience is that of the occurrence of an abnormal dysfunction, disorder or disease. The second plane (impairment) refers to the pain. The third plane, disability, occurs when there is any restriction or lack (resulting from the pain) of ability to perform an activity in the normal way. The fourth plane of experience, handicap, occurs when the experience is socialized. Handicaps are concerned with the social disadvantages experienced by the individual as a result of pain and disabilities. It is critical to understand that there is no necessary relationship between the different planes of experi-

Table 10.1 The WHO model of the impact of disease

Disease or disorder	Impairment	Disability	Handicap
Migraine	headache	difficulty in concentration	educational failure
Cancer	body pain	none	none

Revised from WHO, 1980, p. 30

ence. That is, serious pain may result in neglig-
ible or no disability or handicap. Similarly,
minor pain may trigger major handicap.

Discordance within and between planes of experience

Clinicians usually have difficulty in making
assessments when there is discordance within or
between planes of experience. Discordance
between planes of experience occurs when the
assumption that a specific disorder causes a
certain amount of pain, disability and handicap
is violated. For example, a child who is missing
school because of migraine would tend to vio-
late most clinicians' notions of a reasonable
amount of handicap for migraine. Similarly, a
child who is playing and yet reports pain may be
seen as showing discordance within a plane of
experience. Discordance should lead to further
assessment. Unfortunately, discordance often
leads to inappropriate labelling of pain as
psychogenic.

Self-report measures

Self-report measures include descriptions of
pain-relevant feelings, statements and images,
as well as information about the quality, intensity, and temporal/spatial dimensions of pain.
The methods used to measure self-report of
pain include: direct questioning, pain adjective
descriptors, self-rating scales, and pain drawings.

Direct questioning about pain can be useful
with verbal preschoolers and school-age children. Direct questioning may include: asking
the child to make comparisons with previous
pain experiences, providing the child with
temporal anchors for measuring the duration of
pain, or facilitating communication through the
use of objects and gestures. Ross and Ross
(1988) suggest using questions that are open-
ended rather than questions with forced-choice
answers. Direct questioning has some shortcomings. It is open to bias due to demand
characteristics, lacks an associated metric, and
may be biased by inaccurate memory of a
previous experience (McGrath and Unruh,
1987).

Verbal scales or pain descriptors, such as the
McGill–Melzack scale (Melzack, 1975), have
been used successfully with older adolescents to
measure the effective, evaluative, and sensory

dimensions of pain. Children as young as 8
years are able to select simple adjectives from
word lists to describe their pain and assign
intensity values to each (Gaffney, 1988; Tesler
et al., 1988; Abu-Saad, 1990). Pain descriptors,
however, rely on advanced linguistic competence and may not be appropriate for many
children. Pain descriptors better represent the
richness of the pain experience, but these
methods are time consuming and have yet to be
shown superior to simpler methods.

Self-rating scales vary according to the type
and number of anchor points provided. Visual
analogue scales (VAS) consist of either a vertical or horizontal line with verbal, numerical or
facial anchors indicating a continuum from no
pain to severe pain at each end.

Children indicate on the line how much pain
they are feeling. For children over 5 years, the
VAS is a reliable and valid measure of pain
arising from a variety of procedures and conditions. For example, children's ratings of their
pain on a visual analogue scale correlate with
parents', nurses', and physicians' ratings
(O'Hara et al., 1987; Varni et al., 1987). Visual
analogue ratings also correlate with behavioural measures of pain (Maunuksela et al.,
1987). As a VAS has no markers other than
endpoints, they are particularly useful for children with limited language skills. Nevertheless,
the child must have the cognitive ability
required to translate the pain experience into
an analogue format and to understand pro-
portionality. Category scales consist of a series
of words along a continuum of increasing value
(e.g. no pain, mild pain, moderate pain, severe
pain). Category rating scales may be difficult to
interpret as descriptors such as 'moderate' may
have different meanings for different children
(Ross and Ross, 1988). However, Wilkie et al.
(1990) have recently shown that a category
scale may be very useful with children.

The Poker Chip Tool (Hester, 1979) is a
concrete measure requiring the child to evaluate the intensity of pain by choosing one to four
poker chips, representing the 'pieces of hurt'
experienced. This method is appropriate for
younger children between the ages of 4 and 8
years. Children's ratings correlate with overt
behaviour during immunization (Hester, 1979).
A recent study comparing child, nurse and
parental ratings of pain demonstrated adequate
convergent validity and partial support for dis-

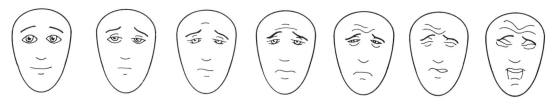

Figure 10.1 'Faces' scale (reprinted from Bieri *et al.* (1990) with permission)

criminant validity of this tool (Hester *et al.*, 1990).

In faces scales, which consist of faces expressing varying amounts of distress, each face is assigned a numerical value reflecting its rank order within a series of facial expressions. Several variants of the happy-sad faces scales have been used to measure children's level of pain. The Oucher (Beyer, 1984) is a faces scale designed to measure pain intensity in children 3–12 years. The scale is in a poster format and consists of a vertical numerical scale (0–100) on the left and six photographs of children in varying degrees of pain positioned vertically to the right. Validity studies indicate that children are able to classify the pictures in the correct sequence (Beyer and Aradine, 1986) and that scores correlate highly with visual analogue scores and results from a poker chip measure (Beyer and Aradine, 1987). Scores on the Oucher are sensitive to analgesia-caused reduction in pain (Aradine *et al.*, 1987).

Perhaps the best developed faces scale is one developed by Bieri and her colleagues (1990) to assess pain intensity in children ranging between 6 and 8 years (Figure 10.1). The drawings used in the scale's development were derived from those generated by children themselves. Strong agreement was demonstrated among children in the rank ordering of the faces according to pain severity, as well as their perception of the faces as representing equal intervals. Finally, the scale demonstrated adequate test–retest reliability.

Numerical rating scales use numbers (i.e. 0–10 or 0–100) to reflect increasing degrees of pain. Children must understand number concepts in order to use this type of scale. The intervals along the scale cannot be assumed to be equal.

Pain thermometers consist of a vertical numerical rating scale ranging between 0 and 10 or 0 and 100. Anchors at each end point indicate no hurt and most hurt possible. The child is asked to point to the place on the thermometer that represents the intensity of his or her pain. Scores on the pain thermometer correlate with scores on other rating scales and predict changes in pain associated with burns.

Diaries (see Figure 10.2) are a type of numerical rating scale with repeated ratings of pain. Pain diaries have been used for the measurement of headache, abdominal pain and limb pain. Typically, ratings range from 0 to 5 and each number corresponds to a verbal description of pain severity. The scale requires a minimum of instruction and has satisfactory inter-rater reliability when comparisons are made between parent and child ratings (Richardson *et al.*, 1983).

Children's pain drawings provide the clinician with a non-verbal description of the child's pain. Typically, children are asked to draw the colour of their pain or to draw pictures of their pain. Drawings can be reliably classified according to content and dominant colour (Unruh *et al.*, 1983). Several studies confirm that children prefer the colours red and black to describe their pain (Eland, 1974; Jeans, 1983; Unruh *et al.*, 1983; Kurylyszyn *et al.*, 1987). However, drawings do not appear to discriminate between different pain intensities (Kurylyszyn *et al.*, 1987). Children over 6 years of age can accurately locate their pain on a pain drawing or body outline (Varni *et al.*, 1987; Savedra and Tesler, 1989). The expressive and detailed nature of children's drawings suggests that they are a useful clinical tool.

Behavioural measures

Behaviours such as vocalization, facial expression, and body movement are typically associated with pain. Behavioural responses are invaluable for inferring pain in children who cannot rate their pain. There is, however, the ever present challenge of distinguishing behaviour due to other forms of distress, such as

**INTRODUCTION WEEK 3
HEADACHE DIARY**

FILL IN THIS FORM AT BREAKFAST, LUNCH, DINNER AND BEDTIME EACH DAY

Name _____   Week beginning _____

Day	Time	Intensity Rating	Other Symptoms	Medication	Possible Cause
	Breakfast				
	Lunch				
	Dinner				
	Bedtime				
	Breakfast				
	Lunch				
	Dinner				
	Bedtime				
	Breakfast				
	Lunch				
	Dinner				
	Bedtime				
	Breakfast				
	Lunch				
	Dinner				
	Bedtime				
	Breakfast				
	Lunch				
	Dinner				
	Bedtime				
	Breakfast				
	Lunch				
	Dinner				
	Bedtime				
	Breakfast				
	Lunch				
	Dinner				
	Bedtime				

Intensity Ratings
0 – No headache
1 – Headache   – I am only aware of it
I pay attention to it
2 – Headache   – but I can ignore it at times
3 – Headache   – I can't ignore it but I can
do my usual activities

4 – Headache   – It is difficult for me to
concentrate; I can only do
easy activities
5 – Headache   – such that I can't do anything

Figure 10.2 Pain diary (reprinted from McGrath *et al.* (1990) with permission)

hunger, thirst, and anxiety from behaviour due to pain. The best evidence for reliability and validity of behavioural measures is for short, sharp pain such as that from needle procedures.

Investigators have attempted to differentiate the pain cry in infants in terms of its psychoacoustic properties (Johnston and Strada, 1986;

Grunau and Craig, 1987). Johnston (1989) reported that a high-pitched, tense, non-voiced, and intense cry is typical in very stressed states. Grunau and Craig (1987) found that both gender and sleep state affected crying behaviour. Although some characteristic cry patterns have been identified during medical procedures (Johnston, 1989), a cry pattern or cry template unique to painful stimuli has not been identified.

Infant facial expression during needle procedures has been examined using facial expression coding systems. Using different systems, Johnston and Strada (1986) and Grunau and Craig (1987) have both found changes in the brow, nose, eyes and mouth. Facial response may be the most consistent response to pain. Facial expressions are relatively free of learning biases and may represent the infant's innate response to pain. Although facial responses may be clinically useful for evaluating pain in healthy babies, they may be of limited use with neonatal infants in distress, given that their faces are often obstructed due to medical interventions.

Others (McGraw, 1945; Craig et al., 1984; Franck, 1986; Johnston and Strada, 1986) have observed more gross body movements in infants and young children. Commonly observed behaviours include: general diffuse movements in newborns, withdrawal of the affected limb in 6-month-old infants and touching the affected area in 12-month-old infants. Kicking and thrashing of limbs, tensing of limbs and a rigid and tense torso have also been observed.

In our survey of neonatal nurses' perceptions of pain, similar behaviours were identified as indicative of pain, but there was essentially no relationship between the various behaviours and nurses' judgements of pain intensities (Pigeon et al., 1989).

Barrier et al. (1989) assessed postoperative pain levels in infants using a clinical, neurological and behavioural scoring system. Fifty-four percent of infants receiving analgesia were judged to have had satisfactory analgesia according to the scale, in comparison to 18% of infants receiving placebo. Unfortunately, the psychometric properties of the scale have not been evaluated.

Behavioural rating scales have been developed to measure pain in children undergoing medical procedures. These scales require that trained raters observe children and record the occurrence of operationally defined, pain-related verbal and non-verbal behaviours.

The Procedural Behavioural Rating Scale (Katz et al., 1980) and the Observational Scale of Behavioural Distress (OSBD) (Jay et al., 1983) measure distress in paediatric oncology patients due to bone marrow aspirations and lumbar punctures. Behaviours include crying, screaming, physical restraint, verbal resistance, requests for emotional support, muscular rigidity, verbal pain expression, flailing, nervous behaviour, and information seeking. The scales have satisfactory inter-rater reliability and distress behaviours on the OSBD correlate with children's self-report of pain and anxiety scores (Jay et al., 1983).

The Children's Hospital of Eastern Ontario Pain Scale (CHEOPS) (McGrath et al., 1985) is a behavioural rating scale developed in the recovery room to measure post-operative pain. It consists of six behaviours (crying, facial expression, verbal expression, torso position, touch position, and leg position). The scale has inter-rater reliability above 0.80 and independent pain ratings by nurses provide evidence for concurrent validity. Also, the scale is sensitive to change in behaviour due to intravenous analgesia. It has excellent measurement characteristics with needle pain (Fradet et al., 1990). However, it is insensitive to pain that is not occurring in the immediate post-operative situation (Beyer et al., 1990).

There is little work on longer lasting pain. Beyer et al. (1990) established that gross behaviours such as grimacing and body movements rarely occurred in children who were suffering from post-operative pain. Barr et al. (1987) found that parents' recording of the frequency and duration of infant crying was correlated with the infants' crying as measured by a voice-recording system. This study, however, did not attempt to determine if the crying was due to pain.

Gauvain-Piquard et al. (1987) developed a 15 item behavioural rating scale for paediatric oncology patients between the ages of 2 and 6 years. The scale consists of three sub-scales: 1) pain behaviours toward the affected area; 2) psychomotor alterations such as slowing down and withdrawal; and 3) anxiety behaviours such as nervousness and irritability. The scale appears to have adequate sensitivity between patients and satisfactory inter-rater reliability (Gauvain-Piquard et al., 1987). Validity studies are ongoing and the scale is being used with other groups such as paediatric burn patients (Gauvain-Piquard and Rodary, 1989). Adults can rate on a visual analogue scale how much pain they think a child is having by observing the child. This approach is efficient and appears to be valid as these ratings correlate well with the child's own self report of postoperative pain (O'Hara *et al.*, 1987). Unfortunately, it is not clear exactly which behaviours these ratings are measuring.

Biological measures

Biological measures are similar to behavioural measures in that the perturbation being measured may be due to causes other than pain. Behavioural measure is therefore better for measuring short sharp pain than longer lasting pain. There are sufficient data on heart rate, transcutaneous oxygen, sweating, EEG, and the stress response to argue for their validity as measures of pain in some circumstances.

Although heart rate is widely used as a pain measure, it is not well understood. Different time samples have been used (Johnston and Strada, 1986) and healthy and ill babies react differently (Field and Goldson, 1984). No studies have evaluated heart rate as a measure for longer term pain.

Transcutaneous oxygen reduces during clearly painful procedures such as circumcision (Rawlings *et al.*, 1980; Williamson and Williamson, 1983), lumbar punctures (Porter *et al.*, 1987), and intubation, but also during other handling of neonates.

Palmar sweating, as measured by an evaporimeter was a sensitive index of pain from heel lance in full-term babies (Harpin and Rutter, 1982). Cruder measures, using palmar sweat index, show less consistent results.

Automated spectral EEG analyses have been used to measure pain during surgery (Meyer *et al.*, 1989) and found to correlate with a clinical pain score (Barrier *et al.*, 1989). This interesting work requires further validation.

The stress response of premature and full term infants to surgery consists of marked increases in plasma catecholamines, glucagon, and gluco-corticosteroids and a suppression of insulin secretion, leading to hyperglycaemia and lactic acidosis (Anand *et al.*, 1987, 1988). Such measures are important in research but, as yet, of limited use in the clinical setting.

The role of parents in pain measurement

Parents have the most intimate knowledge of their children and will be sensitive to changes in a child's behaviour that reflect pain. Children, who may be reluctant to communicate feelings of pain to a nurse because of fear of a needle or of what the pain might mean, may be more likely to tell a parent that they have pain (Alex and Ritchie, 1992).

If the child has impaired speech, expressing pain may be difficult. A nurse may also have difficulty using behavioural pain measures if a child has a motor disability resulting in impaired or atypical physical movement. In both cases, parents will be very helpful in indicating how the child communicates pain.

Nurses' methods of pain assessment

Several studies have demonstrated that nurses use a variety of methods and criteria to assess children's pain. These criteria include vital signs, behavioural cues, knowledge of the child and procedure, verbal cues, and nursing judgment (Bradshaw and Zeanah, 1986; Powers, 1987; Ritchie *et al.*, 1989; Gonzales and Gadish, 1990).

The need for routine measurement

The routine measurement of pain is a prerequisite for good pain management and should become part of the vital signs assessment. Stevens (1990) showed that the taking pain measures leads to better pain control because of better evaluations and more use of analgesics.

Management of children's pain

Preventions

The prevention of pain is the best strategy for treatment. Prevention of pain can take many forms including: education of parents, child care providers, and children about safety issues (car seats, risks of infant walkers, safe toys, helmets for sports); avoidance of unnecessary procedures or surgery; using less painful methods for required procedures; and, use of pharmacological and non-pharmacological methods of pain management in anticipation of pain rather than at its onset.

Much medically-induced pain would be eliminated if unnecessary invasive tests were eliminated. Any test that does not have a reasonable probability of significantly influencing clinical practice should not be done. In addition, non-invasive methods, perhaps by transcutaneous measures or by sampling of bodily fluids such as saliva, should be developed to replace invasive needle procedures such venepunctures, lumbar punctures and bone marrow aspirations.

Unnecessary surgery should be avoided. Once routine, tonsillectomies should now be suggested only to children who have had either seven episodes of tonsillitis in 1 year, five or more episodes in each of the 2 previous years, or three or more episodes in each of the 3 preceding years. Even with these more stringent criteria, a randomised control trial of outcome for children following a tonsillectomy provided suggestive evidence of no long term benefit (Paradise et al., 1984).

For many necessary tests and procedures, there are pharmacological, physical and psychological strategies which can be implemented by practitioners to provide pain relief to children. Incorporating pain management procedures requires assessment and measurement of pain and adjustment of procedures to allow for implementation of pain management.

Our philosophy of pain management

We believe that pain not serving a useful signalling function should be aggressively treated with the aim of abolishing all unnecessary pain. Lack of recognition of pain in childhood has occurred for a variety of reasons. Young children have greater difficulty verbally expressing their pain. Crying and other forms of protest can be taken to mean something other than that the child is in pain. Limited speech and ambiguity about crying and other protest behaviour were thought to make assessment and measurement of pain improbable. Children appear to recover more quickly from tissue damage and they may seem to forget negative life events. Children are generally unable to protest that their pain may not have been taken seriously. Finally, until very recently, infants were not thought to be capable of pain perception due to the immaturity of their central nervous system. These beliefs are no longer tenable.

PRN administration requires the child to be aware that the nurse must be told about the pain and then to convince the nurse that sufficient pain exists to warrant provision of analgesia. PRN schedules provide medication when pain has become severe and more difficult to relieve. Scheduled administration with fixed or titrated intervals is far superior to PRN schedules (O'Hara et al., 1987). If an order is written as PRN nothing prohibits the nurse from giving the drug around the clock in situations where pain is predictable (McCafferey and Beebe, 1989). Addiction, as a result of medication for pain, is a primary concern for many parents and some health professionals. Addiction to medication when medication is appropriately provided for pain has not been documented in the paediatric literature. In adult research, addiction following pharmacological treatment of pain is very rare (Porter and Jick, 1980).

Respiratory depression can be a serious side effect, especially in the neonate. However, titration of dosage, careful monitoring of the patient and the ready availability of reversal agents can make opiate use safe in the paediatric age group.

Approaches to pain management must consider the quality, severity and duration of the pain and the resources of the child and family. All pain management strategies should incorporate ongoing measurement to determine if the strategy is effective in relieving pain and when a change in strategy may be necessary. We will discuss each category of pain management in turn.

Psychological intervention

Psychological interventions include therapeutic milieu and specific behavioural and cognitive strategies.

Therapeutic milieu

Therapeutic milieu refers to the psychological climate or atmosphere that envelops the treatment of a specific child. It may be a milieu of anxiety permeated by mistrust or it may be a positive, therapeutic milieu.

The elements of a therapeutic milieu are many. First of all, only the child with pain can really tell how much pain she experiences. This follows from the definition of pain accepted by the International Association for the Study of Pain (Merskey, 1986). Pain is an emotional and sensory, and therefore, subjective experience. If a child says that she is in pain, then, unless we have very good evidence to the contrary, we should believe her.

The second principle is whenever pain is likely to occur, it should be measured and targeted for intervention. Pain should be routinely measured in children following surgery. Indeed, a recent survey by Johnston and her associates (Johnston *et al.*, 1992) would suggest that pain should be measured in all hospitalised children.

Third, it is better to prevent pain than to treat pain when it occurs. Prevention is better than treatment on humanitarian grounds (Angell, 1982), on medical grounds (see for example Anand *et al.*, 1987, 1988), and on physiological grounds (Woolf, 1989). As a result, pain should always be treated prophylactically (that is before it emerges) by systemic, regional or topical analgesia.

Fourth, when at all possible, children undergoing painful procedures should be accompanied by their parents. Although children may be somewhat more disruptive with their parents present, almost all children indicate that having a parent present is the most important thing that could be done to help them cope with pain (Ross and Ross, 1988). Parents should be given clear instruction about the procedure, its rationale, and honest information about possible pain. Parents should be guided in their role to give support to the child during this procedure.

Fifth, children should be given developmentally appropriate explanations of what is going to happen to them and how it will feel. Explanation should be geared to a child's level of comprehension, using language that the child understands. In addition, children should never be lied to or tricked into a painful experience as this is only likely to increase the child's apprehension and distrust in subsequent procedures.

There is little research to determine how a positive therapeutic milieu would increase coping with pain, or how it may reduce pain. However, from a conceptual perspective, a positive therapeutic milieu would seem more likely to encourage trust and cooperation between child and parents with nursing and other professional personnel. Trust and reduced anxiety are important components for the implementation of most cognitive and behavioural pain management strategies. A positive therapeutic milieu may also increase the nurse's confidence in her ability to more effectively manage the child's pain.

Cognitive and behavioural strategies

Children may vary in their preference for one cognitive or behavioural strategy over another and some strategies may be more helpful for some pain conditions than for others. The nurse should be familiar with the child's preferences, since one strategy may be incompatible with another. For example, a child who prefers to use relaxation may be frustrated if a nurse tries to distract his attention. The nurse should discuss coping strategies with the child and encourage the child to continue to use his own strategies while also learning others if these would be beneficial. The nurse's role in helping a child to learn and use a strategy is that of a coach who will teach specific strategies, prompt their implementation and praise the child for any effort to use the strategy during a procedure or other episode of pain.

Some cognitive and behavioural strategies can be used in combination with each other and with other physical or pharmacological approaches. Increasing the child's control, diversion, guided imagery, positive self-talk, thought-stopping, hypnosis, role-playing, play and art are all forms of cognitive strategies. Positive reinforcement, relaxation, and biofeedback are behavioural methods. We will discuss each strategy in turn.

Children may feel helpless and overwhelmed in the unfamiliar surroundings of the hospital. When they also experience pain, their feelings of helplessness may increase. This may lead to aggressive behaviour or resistance. Giving a child control over aspects of a procedure, where this is possible, is likely to decrease the child's helplessness and increase cooperation (Osgood and Szyfelbein, 1989). Increasing a child's control in the situation may also lead to manipulation and stalling if the limits of the child's control are not specified and increasing control is the only strategy used during a moderate to severe pain situation. The nurse should be specific about factors which the child can control and which factors are the nurse's responsibility.

Diversion involves distracting attention from pain. Diversion may involve: focusing attention on some pleasant aspect of the surroundings during a painful procedure (such as a pleasant picture or playing music which the child enjoys); altering the circumstances of the specific situation in the child's imagination (for example, pretending that one is an astronaut about to take off during the sound of the dentist's drill); or actively engaging in a diverting activity (Ross and Ross, 1988). This last activity is not usually possible during an acute pain such as during a procedure but it may be helpful when the pain is ongoing. Diversion may be more helpful for mild pain.

Guided imagery is a more structured form of imagination that diverts the child's attention away from pain to a more pleasant sensation. It is frequently combined with an initial relaxation procedure. Following the relaxation exercise the child will be instructed to concentrate on a pleasant activity, paying special attention to the pleasant sensory aspect of the activity and its surroundings. Focusing on lying on a beach or eating an ice cream are examples of images commonly used in this exercise. The image used should be something that the child particularly enjoys.

Anxiety due to prior painful experiences may cause the child to anticipate the worst possible outcome for a painful procedure. The child may imagine that the pain will be horrific and unbearable and that the professional will dislike her and be oblivious to her suffering. She may believe that she will be unable to cope and will behave in a way that will later embarrass her. Such thinking is called catastrophising. Catastrophic thinking increases a child's anxiety and fear and is likely to enhance pain. Changing catastrophic thinking involves teaching the child to use positive self-talk to encourage herself through the procedure and to remain as calm as possible. Positive self-talk may include some of the following statements: 'I know this will hurt but I know I can do it'; 'The doctor likes me and will not hurt me any more than is necessary.' 'This will only hurt for a few minutes. I can try thinking about something else until it is over.' The nurse may want to model how she would use positive self-talk to guide herself through a procedure.

Thought-stopping is a form of positive self-talk. It requires the child to have become familiar with his own particular type of catastrophising statements. When such a statement enters his head he imagines a large stop sign flashing into view and imagines telling himself to stop this thought (McGrath et al., 1990).

Hypnosis has been used in the management of pain associated with cancer, burns, migraines, sickle cell anaemia and haemophila. Hypnotic susceptibility in children increases from the age of 4–5 years to a peak at 8–12 years (London and Cooper, 1969). It gradually decreases with age. Hypnosis incorporates relaxation, cognitive imagery and positive suggestions. Children who are receptive to hypnosis may also be able to learn to use self-hypnosis.

Modelling requires that the child is capable of learning through observation of another person's effective coping behaviour (such as a parent, older child, or nurse) and implementing this learning when exposed to a similar procedure or painful episode. Modelling can be conducted by actual demonstration or by videotape or film demonstration of other children or of cartoon characters or puppets. Children are more likely to learn effective coping strategies by modelling if they are demonstrated by a well-liked or admired person or character.

Any cognitive or behavioural strategy will be more effective if role-play of the strategy is used before the actual painful procedure. Role-play allows the child to rehearse what she is going to do to manage the pain prior to the episode. If the child is confident in her ability to be able to use the strategy then it is more likely that she will be able to carry it out when she has pain. The nurse should create the setting and then walk and talk the child through the procedure and prompt the use of a pain management strategy. When the child is sufficiently familiar with the situation, the nurse may want to switch roles and have the child instruct the nurse through the procedure to increase the child's confidence.

Some types of play are not possible when an acute pain is anticipated because the child will need to be still and relaxed. However, quiet play may be used even during a procedure. A child's play can be used in several ways. Play can divert attention if pain is ongoing. The nurse may use play or drawings to encourage the child to share his/her feelings about painful procedures. The nurse may also be able to explain a painful procedure to the child through play. Dolls and doctors kits will be helpful to elicit this discussion. Play can also be used to help a child role-play what will happen during a procedure. Discussion about pain through play will enhance the child's trust in the nurse and will increase his relaxation in her presence.

Trust and relaxation are important components in managing pain.

Positive reinforcement is giving the child positive recognition for having tried to cope effectively in a painful situation. Reinforcement should focus on the child's efforts: 'You worked hard at counting to help make yourself stay still.' The child's efforts are more important than actual success especially when the child is attempting to utilise a new strategy. Positive reinforcement will increase the child's self-esteem, sense of control and the likelihood that the child will try the strategy a second time.

A variety of different types of muscle relaxation have been developed: tension relaxation (Jacobsen, 1938), autogenic suggestion relaxation (Schultz and Luthe, 1959), relaxation with breathing techniques (Benson, 1975), mini-relaxation and differential relaxation.

Tension relaxation typically involves instructions to tense successive groups of muscles for 5–10 seconds concentrating on sensations of tension and relaxation. Instructions often refer to feelings of calm, warmth and heaviness with images of pleasant surroundings. Autogenic suggestion focuses on relaxation of individual muscle groups with feelings of calm and heaviness but omitting prior tensing of each muscle group. Relaxation with breathing utilises muscle relaxation with a focus on slow and deep breathing as part of the relaxation induction. Mini-relaxation is usually taught when the person has become skilled with a longer relaxation method. In mini-relaxation, deep breathing using five slow deep breaths with suggestions of calm and relaxation, is used to trigger relaxation throughout the body. Differential relaxation requires relaxation of one part of the body while maintaining tension in other parts of the body, allowing an individual to relax a painful area while continuing with one's work. .

Relaxation can be used for migraines, muscle contraction headaches, cancer pain, chronic pain, procedure pain and postoperative pain. Cautela and Groden (1978) have published a detailed manual for teaching professionals how to teach children to relax. McGrath *et al.* (1990) have provided a stress reduction programme for adolescents with a patient workbook and a corresponding professional handbook. It includes a relaxation tape as well as instructions for a variety of other cognitive and behavioural strategies. This programme has been shown to be effective in the treatment of migraine headaches in adults and children (Richardson and McGrath, 1989; McGrath *et al.*, 1990).

In biofeedback, physiological responses associated with stress or tension and not normally under voluntary control are measured and displayed to the patient. Biofeedback may use finger temperature, alpha EEG, muscle EMG, or temporal pulse. It is often used with a relaxation procedure; the measurement providing the person with an objective appreciation of the extent to which relaxation has been achieved. Biofeedack has been shown to be effective with treatment of headache, in children and adolescents (Labbe and Williamson, 1984) but it also requires trained instructors and specialised equipment.

Physical interventions

It seems almost instinctive for a person to rub the part of the body which is in pain. Similarly, parents often respond to a child's complaint of pain by a touch, massage or a kiss. It may be that such contact has an effect on pain by giving emotional comfort as well as reducing the immediate sensation of pain by jamming pain signals. Vibration has long been used as a way of interfering with pain transmission. Unfortunately, the impact of message, touch and vibration has not been systematically investigated in children. On the other hand, excessive stimulation may cause distress in premature neonates (Wolke, 1987).

Some pain conditions appear to be relieved more effectively by hot and some by cold. Acute pain is usually treated initially by cold and then by heat. Unfortunately, in some cases, pain may be exacerbated by hot and cold stimulation.

TENS (or transcutaneous electrical stimulation) is a procedure in which electrical stimulation is provided by electrodes which have been placed on the surface of the skin. TENS has a direct inhibiting effect on pain transmission. The procedure has been primarily used in adults demonstrating effective pain relief for a wide variety of pain conditions. Jo Eland, a nurse, (Eland, 1989) has pioneered the use of TENS with children. No controlled trials with children are available.

Acupuncture relies on the insertion of fine needles into specific points on the body. The needles are then manipulated to cause stimulation that reduces or eliminates pain. There is evidence of short-term effectiveness for acupuncture in acute and chronic pain management with adults (Richardson and Vincent, 1986) but research of its use in paediatrics has suffered from numerous methodological flaws (Ross and Ross, 1988). In addition, children may be quite frightened by the use of needles in acupuncture. There is no evidence that low power laser acupuncture is effective (Devor, 1990).

Pharmacological interventions

Pharmacological interventions are an important aspect of pain management in children. The use of pharmacologic interventions in neonates, especially ill neonates, is now beginning to be adequately researched and clinical protocols are just now being developed (Anand and McGrath, in press).

Non-opioid analgesics

Acetylsalicylic acid (ASA) interfers with prostaglandin synthesis and has anti-pyretic and anti-inflammatory action. the recommended dosage for ASA is 10 mg/kg every 4 hours or 60 mg/kg every 24 hours. The side effects from ASA are: blood loss from the gastrointestinal tract and interference with platelet functioning. ASA has been implicated in precipitating Reye syndrome when it is given to vulnerable children with varicella or influenza. Recommended dosages are: 10–15 mg/kg PO q4h.

Acetaminophen or paracetamol has now replaced ASA. It is a prostaglandin antagonist, has little anti-inflammatory action and is less likely to cause bleeding than ASA. Recommended dosages are: 10–15 mg/kg PO q4h.

Non-steroidal anti-inflammatory agents have recently had more widespread use. They may have particular use in pain from bony metastases, headache, dysmenorrhoea and other inflammatory pain. The most commonly used are ibuprofen in a dosage of 4–8 mg/kg q6h and naprosyn 5–7 mg/kg bid or tid.

Opioid analgesics

Opioids are often referred to as narcotics. The commonly used paediatric opioids are all agon-

ists and appear to act mostly in the CNS, primarily at the mu receptor.

Codeine is the most frequently used opioid in children. Codeine is usually administered orally in combination with acetaminophen. The two drugs act at different sites and thus potentiate the analgesic effect of each. Codeine is usually prescribed PO at a dosage of 0.5–1 mg/kg with concurrently administered acetaminophen at 10 mg/kg.

Demerol or meperidine is very commonly used for postoperative pain in children. There are two unfortunate aspects of demerol. First, it is usually delivered by intramuscular injection on a PRN basis. Second, extended use of demerol can lead to central nervous system side effects. Meperidine is similar to morphine in its effects and offers no advantages over morphine. It is used at a dose of 1–2 mg/kg.

Morphine is the standard opioid against which other opioids are measured for effectiveness. It is water soluble and can be given orally, subcutaneously, intramuscularly, intravenously or rectally. It is thought that oral morphine is considerably less potent as parenteral administration (Jaffe and Martin, 1985; Schechter, 1985) although this has also been debated (McQuay et al., 1985). Unlike other analgesics, there is no ceiling effect for morphine. Dosages are determined by analgesic effect and side effects. Starting dosages with children for morphine are 0.1 mg/kg administered intravenously.

Side effects from opioids can be a problem but seldom require discontinuation of opioid therapy. The most limiting is nausea and vomiting. Reducing patient movements and anti-nausea medications may be helpful. Tolerance may, in some circumstances, require increasing dosages to maintain effectiveness. Physical dependence can be controlled by gradual tapering of the drug during withdrawal. Respiratory depression can be problematic and respiration should be monitored during opioid administration. Constipation is frequent but can be managed with stool softeners, laxatives and a high fibre diet. Pruritis may also be a troublesome side effect. Opioid agonists can be reversed by naloxone.

Fentanyl, alfentanyl and sufentanyl are potent synthetic opioids. These drugs are used almost exclusively by anaesthetists. Fentanyl is often used for conscious sedation.

Topical analgesics

EMLA or Eutectic Mixture of Local Anaesthetic is a combination of 5% lidocaine and prilocaine that is in an eutectic mixture. That is, when in suspension, the melting point of the two local anaesthetics is lowered and they more easily penetrate the skin. In repeated double-blind controlled trials, EMLA has been shown to be effective in sharply reducing the pain from needle procedures including venepunctures, lumbar punctures and access to subcutaneous drug reservoirs (e.g. Halperin et al., 1989). EMLA is put on the skin and covered by an occlusive bandage about 1 hour before the needle procedure. The cream is removed and the skin is then cleaned for the needle procedure. EMLA can be left on for at least an hour longer with no diminution of effect. Mottling of the skin may occur but this is not a problem. The most widely cited disadvantage is that EMLA must be in place an hour prior to the needlestick. In rare cases, such as an emergency lumbar puncture for suspected meningitis, this is a problem. With inpatients, placement of EMLA is almost never a problem. For outpatients, parents can be shown how to place EMLA before coming in for a procedure. EMLA is very effective and if widely used can provide an important step forward in reducing children's pain.

Topical anaesthetic sprays or jellies have also been reported. Tree-Trakern and Pirayavaraporn (1985) in a study of 77 boys undergoing circumcision found topical analgesics (lidocaine spray, ointment, or jelly) were as effective as intramuscular morphine or bupivacaine dorsal nerve block in postoperative pain management for circumcision.

Regional blocks

Regional blocks have recently experienced a revival in their use. A full discussion of this topic is beyond the scope of this chapter. The interested reader should consult the regional anaesthesia chapter in a textbook of paediatric anaesthesia (e.g. Sethna and Berde, 1989).

Caudal epidural blocks are probably the most widely used of all blocks and among the technically easiest and safest to perform. Caudals are used alone or in conjunction with a light general anaesthetic. Caudals have been used for lower limb and all types of abdominal surgery. Lumbar and thoracic epidural blocks have received less widespread acceptance but are used in some centres.

Peripheral nerve blocks are numerous and include: brachial plexus blocks, wrist blocks, femoral nerve blocks, lateral femoral cutaneous nerve blocks, inguinal paravascular blocks, sciatic blocks, ankle blocks, ilioinguinal and iliohypogastric blocks, penile blocks, intercostal blocks. Intravenous regional blocks are also possible. Finally, local infiltration of a wound or area may provide valuable analgesia.

DPT cocktail

Intramuscular combinations of Demerol (meperidine) Phenergan and Thorazine (chlorpromazine), although widely used for procedures such as bone marrow aspirations, are ineffective and have significant negative side effects.

Patient Controlled Analgesia (PCA)

Patient controlled analgesia is a new computer-based method of delivering analgesic medication, usually an opioid, based on the individual's specific requirements. A computer driven pump responds to a signal (usually pushing a button) from the patient and a small bolus of analgesic is administered via an intravenous line. The computer controls the size of the dose, the minimum time between doses and the total amount of drug that can be delivered. The biggest advantages of PCA is that the drug is titrated by the patient and a very steady flow of drug is provided. In addition, there is no need for intramuscular injections. PCA may also be supplemented by a low dose continuous infusion. Compared to nurse-delivered injections or IV boluses, PCA may also save nursing time. PCA has been used in sickle cell diseases (Schechter et al., 1988) but probably will find its most widespread use in postoperative pain. Berde et al. (1991) have recently completed a randomised controlled trial comparing PCA, PCA plus low-dose continuous infusions and IM morphine. They found that both PCA strategies were superior in terms of pain relief and satisfaction and equivalent in terms of complications as compared to the IM regimen.

Table 10.2 Pain secondary to disease

Disease	Treatment	Effectiveness	Resources
Sickle cell disease	NSAIDs	May be effective for mild pain	Shapiro, 1989
	Opioids	Effective for severe pain	
Juvenile rheumatoid arthritis	NSAIDs	May be effective	Lovell & Walco, 1989
	Relaxation guided imagery hypnosis	May have short term benefit but long term benefit unknown	
Reflex sympathetic dystrophy	TENS Regional sympathetic blockade		Wilder, *et al.* in press
Cancer	Use analgesic ladder with NSAIDs, mild and strong opioids	A comprehensive programme of pain control is best for assessment and management	Schechter, Altman & Weisman, 1990

Common paediatric pains

Pains common to children and adolescents can be divided into four categories: (1) recurrent pains; (2) pain secondary to disease; (3) pain caused by procedures; and, (4) pain caused by injuries. We have previously discussed the prevention of pain due to injuries.

Recurrent paediatric pain includes colic, headache, recurrent abdominal pain, limb pain and dysmenorrhoea. There is considerable range in the estimate of prevalence for colic in infancy (13% by Carey, 1968 to 49% by Cobb, 1956). Estimates vary according to the definition of colic which has been used by the authors. Limb pain is associated with a number of pathological processes including haemophilia, juvenile rheumatoid arthritis and endocrine or hormonal abnormalities (Bowyer and Hollister, 1984). The prevalence of limb pain as a recurrent, non-pathological pain is not well established. The incidence of growing pains has been reported as 4–12.5% in boys and 4.7–18.4% in girls (Naish and Apley, 1951; Oster, 1972). The prevalence of migraine headache among children aged 7 years is 1.4% increasing to 5.3% at age 15 (Bille, 1962). Girls have a higher rate of migraine once they enter puberty. Recurrent abdominal pain is more frequent than migraine headache, estimates ranging from 12.3% to 16.7% for school aged girls and 9.5% to 12.1% for boys (Apley and

Naish, 1958; Oster, 1972). Dysmenorrhoea is a common problem for adolescent females. Its prevalence has been estimated as 48% in 12-year-old post-menarchal girls and 79% in 18-year-olds (Teperi and Rimpela, 1989). Many children cope well with recurrent pains and do not require active treatment. Others have greater difficulty and often require a combination of psychological and pharmacological treatments with supportive counselling for the child and parents. The treatments for these pains, their effectiveness and resources for further information are presented in Table 10.2.

Pain secondary to disease is a stressful problem for children and for their families. For the child and family, pain may be a more important problem even than the disease itself. This pain may be continual or episodic in nature. Recurrent bouts of acute pain, such as that experienced by children and adolescents with sickle cell disease or juvenile rheumatoid arthritis, are particularly stressful because these painful episodes are often unpredictable and disruptive of normal activities (Shapiro, 1989). The severity of pain also demonstrates considerable variability from child to child. For this reason, management of pain should be considered on a case by case basis. Non-pharmacological methods may be effective alone for mild to moderate pain while providing supportive relief when used in combination with pharma-

Table 10.3 Recurrent paediatric pain

Type of pain	Treatment	Effectiveness	Resources
Colic	Feeding changes	May be effective for severe colic with diarrhoea, otherwise ineffective	Geertsma & Hyams, 1989
	Increased carrying	Not effective	
	Dicyclomine	Effective but not approved	McGrath & Unruh, 1987
Headache	Stress management	Effective	McGrath et al. 1990
	Propranolol	Not effective	Forsythe et al. 1984
	Paracetamol	Probably effective	
Recurrent abdominal pain	Stress management	Unproven	McGrath & Unruh, 1987
	Psychotherapy	Unproven	
	Behaviour therapy	May be effective	
	Fibre supplements	Effective	Feldman et al. 1985
Limb pain	Heat massage	Probably effective	Bowyer & Hollister, 1984
	Paracetamol	Probably effective	
Dysmenorrhoea	NSAIDs, oral contraceptives	Effective	Beard & Pearce 1989

cological treatment for moderate to severe pain. When implementing pain management strategies for a child with a chronic disease, it is helpful to ensure that the child still has time and energy for normal activities (McCaffery and Beebe, 1990). Unfortunately, the problem of pain management in some diseases such as sickle cell disease is exacerbated by prejudice, since patients are usually black and poor whereas health care providers are typically white and middle class (Schechter, 1985). Pain secondary to disease, treatments, their effectiveness and additional resources are outlined in Table 10.3.

In addition to childhood pains or pain due to disease, children also experience pain due to the procedures which are used to treat the underlying condition. These procedures may be conducted by a variety of professionals including technicians, nurses, occupational therapists, physiotherapists, and physicians. Much of procedural pain can be reduced and eliminated by a combination of non-pharmacological and pharmacological approaches. Procedural pain, treatments, treatment effectiveness and resources are presented in Table 10.4.

Clearly, children may experience pain as an inevitable part of childhood. Some pain such as

that from injury or due to procedures can be prevented. Other types of pain, such as colic and reflex sympathetic dystrophy, still have no acceptable, well-validated treatment currently available. For some types of pain disorders, treatment, although effective, is far from perfect. For example, many children with headache and many children with recurrent abdominal pain are not substantially assisted by the best available treatments. A distressing problem remains that for a variety of sources of paediatric pain effective treatment exists but it is not widely utilized. For example, although conscious sedation or general anaesthesia are clearly effective in eliminating the pain from bone marrow aspiration in childhood cancer, these methods are only rarely employed. Similarly, although no one could doubt that circumcision hurts, analgesia or anaesthesia for infant circumcision is almost never practised and is not currently recommended (Schoen et al., 1990). Many children suffer considerable pain from venepunctures. Yet each day thousands of unnecessary tests are performed on children without any attempt to mitigate the pain. Pain due to dressing changes and debridement in burn care is often poorly managed.

Table 10.4 Pain due to procedures

Disease	Treatment	Effectiveness	Resources
Venepuncture	Distraction	Effective	Zeltzer, Jay, & Fisher, 1989
	EMLA	Effective	Halperin, Koren Attias et al. 1989
Sutures	Distraction	Effective	
	Infused lidocaine	Effective	
	EMLA	Effective	
Lumbar puncture	Conscious sedation	Effective	Schechter, Altman
	General anaesthesia	Effective	& Weisman 1990
	EMLA	Effective	Halperin, Koren Attias et al. 1989
	DPT cocktail	Ineffective	
Bone marrow aspiration	Conscious Sedation	Effective	Schechter, Altman & Weisman 1990
	General anaesthesia	Effective	
	DPT cocktail	Ineffective	
Dressing changes and debridement (burns)	Increasing child's control	Supportive	Osgoode & Szyfelbein 1989
	Distraction,	Supportive	
	Hypnosis	Supportive	
	TENS	Unproven	
	Paracetamol	Effective for mild/moderate pain	
	Scheduled opioids	Effective	
Post-operative pain	Regional anaesthesia	Effective	Berde 1989
	Paracetamol	Effective for mild/moderate pain	
	Scheduled opioids	Effective	
	PRN analgesics	Often ineffective	O'Hara et al. 1987

Finally, some pain in childhood, which may be presented as the result of accidental injury, is in fact the unfortunate result of physical or sexual abuse. In addition, sexual abuse in childhood or adolescence is a stressor that has also been linked to subsequent pain problems (Caldirola et al., 1984; Haber and Roos, 1985). The mechanism is not understood but it is thought to follow the pattern of a post-traumatic stress disorder.

Creating the nursing environment for good pain management

Many factors influence a nurse's ability to effectively manage children's pain. Very often, deficits in care are attributed to the individual nurse's inability to assess pain or to the nurse's own attitudes and values in relation to children's pain and its management. However, the factors that influence the extent to which a nurse can manage a child's pain extend beyond the individual nurse. The philosophy and practice of nursing management and of attending physicians are critical components that affect the care given by a nurse.

Nurses in management positions are key in creating work environments that enable nurses in direct care positions to effectively manage children's pain. Nurse managers have responsibility for the establishment and promotion of standards of care. They must provide a working milieu in which a nurse can question procedures and meet the standards of care in paediatric pain.

Education

Most advances in our understanding of children's pain have occurred in the past decade.

Therefore, many practising nurses have been given incorrect information about pain, and may have very considerable misconceptions abut the reality of children's pain. There is some evidence that pain assessment and management improves with greater education (Gonzales and Gadish, 1990). Nurses have a professional responsibility to pursue self-initiated learning opportunities so that their knowledge base is current. Nursing educators and employers share the responsibility to assure that nurses can enhance their knowledge and skills about pain management in both basic and continuing education programmes. Knowledge is an essential ingredient in being empowered to provide high standards of care.

Organisational factors influencing pain management

Many organisational factors remove control and power from the nurse's hands and, thereby, present barriers to providing care. These factors include time pressures, few opportunities for continuity in patient assignments, and the low priority placed on pain management and patient comfort.

Time pressure

Working environments place the nurse under considerable time pressure. Workload measurement systems in hospital settings are sometimes implemented in a way that reduces all of nurse's work to the visible tasks and the expected time to complete them (Colliere, 1986). Nursing units or districts that are managed with efficiency as the top priority by means of workload measurement systems run the risk of fragmenting care. Care may become fragmented to such an extent that the nurse is unable to recognise patterns of pain behaviour in a patient in a way that permits adequate pain assessment and management.

Continuity of care

The way in which nursing care is organised may present barriers to effective care of the child with pain. Nursing care delivery systems such as functional nursing or team nursing require different nurses to be responsible for individual care elements and thus fragment the child's care. Such systems do not provide any conti-nuity for the nurse with the individual patient. Continuity is necessary to enable the recognition of behaviour patterns that are major factors in pain assessment. In addition, the nurse assessing the child's pain is not responsible for the pharmacologic management of it. The nurse will need to rely on another team member to administer analgesics and she will have incomplete information on which to base here assessment of the effect of analgesics. In such management systems, there will be great potential for conflicting assessments about whether the child has pain requiring intervention, and for conflicting priorities for pain relief. More professional models of care delivery, such as primary nursing (Manthey, 1990), where the same nurse plans the patient's care througout the hospital stay, enable nurses to have more continuity with patients, and to accept more accountability for the management of the patient's care.

System priorities and supports for pain management

There are several mechanisms which can be used to give priority to pain assessment and management and to hold nurses accountable. However, management must establish a system that allows the nurse to exercise the authority that is necessary to adequately meet this responsibility.

First, nursing management can help establish a work atmosphere in which the nurse, who is concerned about effective pain management, is supported both for her decisions and in the required staffing. In some settings, a concerned nurse may be ridiculed by other members of the illness care team. If the source of such ridicule is from a physician, who holds a higher power base, there may well be detrimental effects on the patient's care. For example, the nurse may avoid the patient due to her inability to relieve the patient's pain. Sometimes the problems encountered in convincing others of a child's pain are the result of miscommunication caused by the jargon used by different disciplines. Very often, however, the problems relate to a nurse's sense of disempowerment.

Secondly, nursing management can encourage effective problem-solving that is time efficient and uses optimal strategies. Problems nurses encounter in convincing physicians that the child is in pain or requires a stronger analgesia are similar to those that exist in other formats of the 'doctor–nurse game' (Stein 1967; Stein *et al.*, 1990). Deny the problem exists or tackle it? What technique will work in this situation? To successfully obtain an adequate order, the nurse must know which arguments convince and which approaches are effective for each physician (Benner *et al.*, 1990) and she must spend valuable time searching for the physician to obtain the medical order. Another major problem for the nurse may be relying on her anecdotal or vague descriptions of observations rather than on a systematic method of assessment. Given the relative power and authority states in nurse–physician relationships, the debate may be lost because of reliance on what is regarded as personal opinion.

Thirdly, nursing management can support a stance of powerfulness rather than helplessness. In some situations, the nurse may feel powerless to effect any change because of an overwhelming workload, an anticipated extremely unpleasant response from a given surgeon (persistence may be tantamount to professional suicide), or the likelihood that other aspects of care will suffer. Perceptions of powerlessness among nurses is related to the status of women in society at large. When women are treated equally in all sectors of society, including in health care, interprofessional interactions will change and some of the problems nurses encounter in attempting to manage children's pain will be solved.

Empowering nurses to provide good pain management

Nurses are in a position to determine the extent of the child's pain and do something about it but they require power and authority to take action. For example, legislative and policy changes that enable nurses to increase analgesic dosages when the current levels provide inadequate relief would provide the nurse with the authority she requires. Indeed, such a change could have a significant effect on many aspects of nursing care as the time saved in not having to pursue an adequate order could be well spent in providing direct care.

With authority and responsibility comes accountability. However, the continued inadequate management of children's pain suggests that lines of authority, responsibility and accountability for pain management remain unclear. When an agency considers an aspect of care to be important, the management team develops explicit systems for dealing with it. For example, all hospitals have some form of graphic chart on the health record to depict the pattern of the patient's vital signs, and forms for the reporting of unusual incidents such as a child falling and bumping his head. Both forms of records are indicators of the hospital's belief that it must accept accountability for those aspects of care. However, there are usually no records, policies, and procedures routinely documenting pain assessment and management. There are few incentives for nurses who spend extra time with a patient trying to intervene to relieve pain, advocate for a decrease in the number of unnecessary painful procedures, or argue for more adequate approaches to pain management. Departmental Quality Assurance programs should designate patient comfort as one of the expected outcomes of care that are regularly monitored. Requiring documentation for pain levels and management effectiveness through such mechanisms as a flow sheet can have a dramatic effect on improved care of children in pain (Stevens *et al.*, 1989).

If we are to reduce paediatric pain we must develop systems that make the institution and the individual health professional responsible for monitoring and ameliorating pain. Models for Quality Assurance and Infection Control are already in place for other aspects of care. Paediatric pain could be incorporated as an important risk with new systems created to control it.

Finally, a system that supports family-centred care will enable nurses to work as partners with parents to assure better care of children in pain. In a family-centred system, priority is given to parent/professional collaboration (Shelton *et al.*, 1987). Working with parents enables nurses to expand their resources in pain assessments and provisions of pain care (McCaffery and Beebe, 1989).

Discussion and future direction

Research

Advances in research knowledge about children's pain over the past decade have been exciting and rapid. However, much remains to be accomplished. The basic science of paediatric pain requires considerable work. We need new tools to enable more accurate assessment of children's behavioural cues in pain other than short sharp pain. Very often self-report is not a feasible approach because of the child's age or condition. We have only rudimentary knowledge about ways of intervening with children to relieve pain. We must pursue studies that will determine which pharmacologic and non-pharmacologic interventions and in what combinations are most effective. Finally, we need more studies that demonstrate the effect of environmental change on nurses' ability to manage children's pain.

Collective and political action

Better management of children's pain extends beyond the boundaries of the particular nurse's scope of practice or the particular agency. Some issues are very broad. For example, if the health care system exercised better control over the activities for which it pays, children would undergo fewer unnecessary procedures. Most issues, however, are related to the need for education, policy change, and the sense of being supported to make change in one's own workplace. All of these can be addressed by working collectively and politically to achieve the goals.

Nurses are not alone in the campaign to provide better care for children with pain. They have great power to effect such change through solidarity with other nurses in their professional associations locally, nationally and internationally. Nurses can collectively work through such organizations to set new agendas for care, to establish standards for nursing care, and to hold each other accountable for meeting such standards. For example, the management of pain is an ethical issue – the failure to prevent pain or the infliction of unnecessary pain is a failure to respect the individual as a human being (Curtin and Flaherty, 1982). The nurses of the world practice under the ethical standards set by the International Council of Nurses (1973) which demand, among other things, that the nurse alleviate suffering, and respect the dignity of man. In Canada, the Canadian Nurses Association (1985) Code of Ethics, obligates the nurse to provide competent care, to advocate the client's interest, and 'as a member of the health care team, . . . to take steps to ensure that the client receives

competent and ethical care' (p. 11). With the setting of such standards, professional associations undertake the responsibility to support the nurse who endeavours to meet such obligations.

In addition, nurses share their goal with members of other health disciplines and the members of organisations such as the International Association for the Study of Pain (IASP). Such multidisciplinary groups have great potential through research and through their advocacy efforts to influence, not only individual approaches to pain management, but also the standard of care for pain. By participating in collectives such as professional associations or pain associations, nurses can empower themselves through the powers of numbers and diversity, and through unity with others to work to create change for children with pain.

References

Abajian, J. C., Mellish, R. W. P., Browne, A. F. et al. (1984) Spinal anesthesia for surgery in the high-risk infant. *Anesthesia and Analgesia*, **63**, 359–362

Abu-Saad, H. H. (1990) Toward the development of an instrument to assess pain in children: Dutch study. In: *Advances in Pain Research and Therapy: Paediatric Pain* (eds D. C. Tyler and E. J. Krane), Raven Press, New York, pp. 101–106

Alex, M. R. and Ritchie, J. A. (1992) School-aged children's interpretation of their experience with acute surgical pain. *Journal of Paediatric Nursing*, **7**, 171–180

Anand, K. J. S. and Hickey, P. R. (1987) Pain and its effects in the human neonate and fetus. *New England Journal of Medicine*, **317**, 1321

Anand, K. J. S. and McGrath, P. J. (1993) Pain in the neonate. Elsevier, Amsterdam (in press).

Anand, K. J. S., Sippell, W. G. and Aynsley-Green, A. (1987) Randomized trial of fentanyl anaesthesia in preterm babies undergoing surgery: effects on the stress response. *Lancet*, **1**, 243–247

Anand, K. J. S., Sippell, W. G., Schofield, N. M. and Aynsley-Green, A. (1988). Does halothane anaesthesia decrease the stress response of newborn infants undergoing operation? *British Medical Journal*, **296**, 668–672

Angell, M. (1982) The quality of mercy. *New England Journal of Medicine*, **306**, 98–99

Apley, J. and Naish, N. (1958) Children with recurrent abdominal pains: a field survey of 1000 school children. *Archives of Disease in Children*, **33**, 165–170

Aradine, C. R., Beyer, J. E. and Tompkins, J. M.

(1987) Children's pain perception before and after analgesia: a study of instrument construct validity and related issues. *Journal of Pediatric Nursing*, **3**, 11–23

Barr, R. G., Kramer, M. S., Leduc, D. G. *et al.* (1987) Parental diary of infant cry and fuss behaviour. *Archives of Disease in Children*, **63**, 380

Barrier, G., Attia, J., Mayer, M. N., Amiel-Tison, C. and Shnide, S. M. (1989) Measurement of postoperative pain and narcotic administration in infants using a new clinical scoring system. *Intensive Care Medicine*, **15**, S37–S39

Benner, P., Tanner, C. and Chesla, C. (1990) The nature of clinical expertise in intensive care nursing units. *Anthropology of Work Review*, **11(3)**, 16

Benson, H. (1975) *The Relaxation Response.* Morrow, New York

Berde, C. B. (1989) Pediatric postoperative pain management. *Pediatric Clinics of North America*, **36**, 921–940

Berde, C. B., Lehn, B. M., Yee, J. D. *et al.* (1991) Patient-controlled analgesia in children and adolescents: a randomized, prospective comparison with intramuscular morphine for postoperative analgesia. *Journal of Pediatrics*, **118**, 460–466

Beyer, J. E. (1984) *The Oucher: A User's Manual and Technical Report.* The Hospital Play Equipment Co, Evanston IL

Beyer, J. E. and Aradine, C. R. (1986) Content validity of an instrument to measure young children's perceptions of the intensity of their pain. *Journal of Pediatric Nursing*, **1**, 386–395

Beyer, J. E. and Aradine, C. R. (1987) Patterns of paediatric pain intensity: a methodological investigation of a self-report scale. *Clinical Journal of Pain*, **3**, 130–141

Beyer, J., deGood, D. E., Ashley, J. C. and Russell, G. A. (1983) Patterns of postoperative analgesic use with adults and children following cardiac surgery. *Pain*, **17**, 71–81

Beyer, J. E., McGrath, P. J. and Berde, C. (1990) Discordance between self report and behavioural pain measures in 3–7 year old children following surgery. *Journal of Pain and Symptom Management*, **5**: 350–356

Bieri, D., Reeve, R. A., Champion, G. D. *et al.* (1990) The faces pain scale for the self-assessment of the severity of pain experienced by children: development, initial validation, and preliminary investigation for ratio scale properties. *Pain*, **41**, 139–150

Bille, B. (1962) Migraine in schoolchildren. *Acta Pediatrica Scandinavia*, **51 (suppl 136)**, 1

Bowyer, S. L. and Hollister, J. R. (1984) Limb pain in childhood. *Pediatric Clinics of North America*, **31**, 1053–1081

Bradshaw, C. and Zeanah, P. (1986) Pediatric nurses' assessments of pain in children. *Journal of Pediatric Nursing*, **1(5)**, 314–322

Branson, S., McGrath, P. J., Craig, K. D. *et al.* (1990) Spontaneous coping strategies for coping with pain and their origins in adolescents who undergo surgery. In: *Pediatric Pain, Vol 15, Pain Research and Therapy* (eds D. Tyler and E. Krane). Raven, New York, pp. 237–245

Brown, J. M., O'Keefe, J., Sanders, S. H. and Baker, B. (1986) Developmental changes in children's cognitions to stressful and painful situations. *Journal of Pediatric Psychology*, **11**, 343–357

Caldirola, D., Gemperle, M., Guzinski, G. *et al.* (1984) Chronic pelvic pain as related to abdominal pain in childhood and to psychosocial disturbance in the family. In: *Pain: Proceedings of the joint meeting of the European chapter of the International Association for the Study of Pain* (eds R. Rizzi and M. Visentin), Piccin and Butterworth, Padua, pp. 291–297

Canadian Nurses Association (1985) *Code of Ethics for Nursing.* Ottawa

Carey, W. B. (1968) Maternal anxiety and infantile colic: Is there a relationship? *Clinical Pediatrics*, **7**, 590–595

Cautela, J. R. and Groden, J. (1978) *Relaxation: A Comprehensive Manual for Adults, Children, and Children with Special Needs.* Research Press, Champaign, Ill

Cobb, J. C. (1956) Family tension as a cause of colic in infants. *Pediatrics*, **18**, 835

Colliere, M. F. (1986) Invisible care and invisible women as health care providers. *International Journal of Nursing*, **23(2)**: 95–112

Craig, K. D., McMahon, R. J., Morison, J. D. and Zaskow, C. (1984) Developmental changes in infant pain expression during immunization injections. *Social Science in Medicine*, **19**, 1331

Curry, S. L. and Russ, S. W. (1985) Identifying coping strategies in children. *Journal of Clinical Child Psychology*, **14**, 61–69

Curtin, L. and Flaherty, M. J. (1982) *Nursing ethics: Theories and Pragmatics.* Bowie, MD: Robert J. Brady

Devor, M. (1990) What's in a laser beam for pain therapy? *Pain*, **43**, 139

Eland, J. M. (1974) *Children's Communication of Pain.* Master's Thesis, University of Iowa, IA

Eland, J. M. (1989) The effectiveness of transcutaneous electrical nerve stimulation (TENS) with children experiencing cancer pain. In: Key aspects of comfort (eds S. G. Funk, E. M. Tornqvist, M. T. Champagne *et al.*) Springer, New York, pp 87–100

Eland, J. M. and Anderson, J. E. (1977) The experience of pain in children. In: *Pain: A Sourcebook for Nurses and Other Health Professionals.* Little Brown and Company, Boston, pp 453–473

Ellerton, M. L., Caty, S. and Ritchie, J. A. (1985) Helping young children master intrusive procedures through play. *Children's Health Care*, **13**, 167–173

Field, T. and Goldson, E. (1984) Pacifying effects of non-nutritive sucking on term and preterm neonates during heelstick procedures. *Pediatrics*, **74**, 1012–1015

Feldman, W., McGrath, P. J., Hodgson C. *et al..* (1985). The use of dietary fibre in the management of simple childhood idiopathic recurrent abdominal pain: results in a prospective double blind randomized controlled trial. *American Journal of the Disabled Child*, **139**, 1216–1218

Fitzgerald, M., Shaw, A. and Macintosh, N. (1988) Postnatal development of the cutaneous flexor reflex: Comparative study of preterm infants and newborn rat pups. *Developmental Medicine and Child Neurology*, **30**, 520–526

Forsythe, W. I., Gillies, D. and Sills, M. A. (1984) Propranolol (Inderal) in the treatment of childhood migraine? *Developmental Medicine and Child Neurology*, **26**, 737–741

Fowler-Kerry, S. and Ramsay-Lander, J. R. (1987) Management of injection pain in children. *Pain*, **30**, 169–175

Fradet, C., McGrath, P. J., Kay, J. *et al.* (1990). Prospective survey of reactions to blood tests by children and adolescents. *Pain*, **40**, 53–60

Franck, L. S. (1986) A new method to quantitatively describe pain behaviour in infants. *Nursing Research*, **35**, 28–31

Gaffney, A. (1988) How children describe pain: A study of words and analogies used by 5–14 year olds. In: *Proceedings of the Vth World Congress on Pain* (eds R. Dubner, G. F. Gebhart, M. Bond), Elsevier, Amsterdam, pp. 341–347

Gaffney, A. and Dunne, E. A. (1986) Developmental aspects of children's definition of pain. *Pain*, **26**, 105–117

Gaffney, A. and Dunne, E. A. (1987). Children's understanding of the causality of pain. *Pain*, **29**, 91–104

Gauvain-Piquard, A., Rodary, C., Rezvani, A. and Lemerle, J. (1987) Pain in children aged 2–6 years: A new observational rating scale elaborated in a paediatric oncology unit-preliminary report. *Pain*, **31**, 177–188

Gauvain-Piquard, A. and Rodary, C. (1989) Evaluation de la douleur. In: *La Douleur Chez L'Enfant* (eds E. Pichard-Leandri and A. Gauvin-Piquard), Medsi/McGraw-Hill, New York, pp 38–59

Geertsma, M. A. and Hyams, J. S. (1989) Colic – A pain syndrome of infancy? *Pediatric Clinics of North America*, **36**, 905–919

Goodman, J. E. and McGrath, P. J. (1991) Epidemiology of pain in children and adolescents: a review. *Pain*, **46**, 247–264

Gonzales, J. and Gadish, H. (1990) Nurses' decisions in medicating children postoperatively. *Advances in Pain Research Therapy*, **15**, 37

Grunau, R. V. E. and Craig, K. D. (1987) Pain expression in neonates: facial action and cry. *Pain*, **28**, 395–410

Haber, J. D. and Roos, C. (1985) Effects of spouse abuse and/or sexual abuse in the development and maintenance of chronic pain in women. In: *Advances in Pain Research and Therapy*, vol. 9 (eds H. L. Fields, R. Dubner and F. Cervero), Raven, New York, pp. 889–895

Halperin, D. L., Koren, G., Attias, D. *et al.* (1989) Topical skin anesthesia for venous, subcutaneous drug reservoir and lumbar punctures in children. *Pediatrics*, **84**, 281–284

Harpin, V. A. and Rutter, N. (1982) Making heel pricks less painful. *Archives of Disease in Children*, **8**, 226–228

Hester, N. K. (1979) The preoperational child's reaction to immunization. *Nursing Research*, **28**, 250–255

Hester, N. O., Foster, R. and Kristensen, K. (1990) Measurement of pain in children: generalizability and validity of the pain ladder and the poker chip tool. In: *Advances in Pain Research and Therapy: Pediatric Pain* (eds D. C. Tyler and E. J. Krane), Raven Press, New York, pp. 79–84

Hyson, M. (1983) Going to the doctor: a developmental study of stress and coping. *Journal of Child Psychology and Psychiatry*, **24**, 247–259

International Council of Nurses (1973) *Code for Nurses: Ethical Concepts Applied to Nursing*. Geneva

Jacobsen, E. (1938) *Progressive Relaxation*, University Press, Chicago

Jaffe, J. H. and Martin, W. R. (1980) Narcotic analgesics and antagonists. In: *The Pharmacological Basis of Therapeutics*, MacMillan, New York, pp. 245–283

Jay, S. M., Ozolins, M., Elliott, C. and Caldwell, S. (1983) Assessment of children's distress during painful medical procedures. *Journal of Health Psychology*, **2**, 133–147

Jeans, M. E. (1983) Pain in children: a neglected area. In *Advances in Behavioral Medicine for Children and Adolescents* (eds. P. Firestone, P. McGrath, W. Feldman), Erlbaum, Hillsdale, NJ, pp. 23–38

Johnston, C. C. (1989) Pain assessment and management in infants. *Pediatrician*, **16**, 16.–23

Johnston, C. C. and Strada, M. E. (1986) Acute pain response in infants: a multidimensional description. *Pain*, **24**, 373–382

Johnston, C. C., Jeans, M. E., Gray-Donald, K. and Abbott, F. V. (1992) *A Survey of Pain in Hospitalised Patients Aged 4–14 Years. Clinical Journal of Pain*, **8**, 154–163

Katz, E. R., Kellerman, J. and Seigel, S. E. (1980) Distress behaviour in children with cancer undergoing medical procedures: Developmental considerations. *Journal of Consulting and Clinical Psychology*, **48**, 356–365

Kurylyszyn, N., McGrath, P. J., Capelli, M. and Humphreys, P. (1987) Children's drawings: what can they tell us about intensity of pain? *Clinical Journal of Pain*, **2**, 155–158

Labbe, E. L. and Williamson, D. A. (1984) Treatment of childhood migraine using autogenic feedback training. *Journal of Consulting and Clinical Psychology*, **52**, 968–976

Lamontagne L. (1987) Children's pre-operative coping: replication and extension. *Nursing Research*, **36**, 163–167

Lawson, J. (1990) The politics of newborn pain. *Mothering*, **57**, 41

Leikin, L., Firestone, P. and McGrath, P. J. (1988) Physical symptom reporting in type A and B children. *Journal of Consulting and Clinical Psychology*, **56**, 721–726

London, P. and Cooper, L. M. (1969) Norms of hypnotic susceptibility in children. *Developmental Psychology*, **1**, 113

Lovell, D. J. and Walco, G. A. (1989) Pain associated with juvenile rheumatoid arthritis. *Pediatric Clinics of North America*, **36**, 1015–1027

Manthev, M. (1990) Delivery systems and practice models: a dynamic balance. *Nursing Management*, **22(1)**, 28–30

Maunuksela, E. L., Rajantie, J. and Siimes, M. A. (1986) Flunitrazepam-fentanyl induced sedation and analgesia for bone marrow aspiration and needle biopsy in children. *Acta Anaesthesiology Scandinavia*, **30**, 409–411

McCaffery, M. and Beebe, A. (1989) Pain in children: special considerations. In: *Pain: Clinical Manual for Nursing Practice*. Mosby, St. Louis

McGrath, P. A. (1990) *Pain in Children: Nature, Assessment, Treatment*. Guilford, New York

McGrath, P. J. and Unruh, A. M. (1987) *Pain in Children and Adolescents, vol 1, Pain Research and Clinical Management*. Elsevier, Amsterdam

McGrath, P., Johnson, G., Goodman, J. T. *et al.* (1985) CHEOPS: A behavioral scale for rating postoperative pain in children. In: *Advances in Pain Research and Therapy, vol. 9* (eds H. L. Fields, R. Dubner, F. Cervero), Raven Press, New York, pp. 395–402

McGrath, P. J., Cunningham, S. J., Lascelles, M. and Humphreys, P. (1990) *Help Yourself: A Program for Treating Migraine Headaches*. University of Ottawa Press, Ottawa

McGrath, P. J., Mathews, J. and Pigeon H. (1991) Assessment of pain in children. In: *Proceedings of the World Congress of Pain, vol. 5, Pain Research and Clinical Management*. Elsevier, Amsterdam, pp. 509–526

McGraw, M. B (1945) *The Neuromuscular Maturation of the Human Infant*. Hafner, New York

McIlvaine, W. B. (1989) Perioperative pain management in children: a review. *Journal of Pain and Symptom Management*, **4**, 215–229

McQuay, H. J., Moore, R. A., Glynn, C. J. and Lloyd, J. W. (1985) High systemic availability of oral morphine sulfate solution and sustained-release preparation. In: *Advances in Pain Research and Therapy* (eds H. L. Fields, R. Dubner and F. Cervero), Raven Press, New York, pp. 719–726

Melzack, R. (1975) The McGill pain questionnaire: Major properties and scoring methods. *Pain*, **1**, 277–299

Merskey, H. (1986) Classification of chronic pain: description of chronic pain syndromes and definition of pain terms. *Pain*, **Suppl. 3**, S58

Meyer, P., Bensouda, A., Mayer, M. N. and Barrier, G. (1989) Analyse spectrale continue de l'EEG lors de l'anesthesie et du reveil chez l'enfant de moins d 1 an. *Agressologie*, **30**, 581–584

Miser, A. W. and Miser, J. S. (1989) The treatment of cancer pain in children. *Pediatric Clinics of North America*, **36**, 979–999

Naish, J. M. and Apley, J. (1951) 'Growing pains': a clinical study of non-arthritic limb pains in children. *Archives of Diseases in Childhood*, **26**, 134–140

Offsay, J. B. (1989) The pain of childhood leukaemia: a parent's recollection. *Journal of Pain and Symptom Management*, **4**, 174

O'Hara, M., McGrath, P. J., D'Astous, J. *et al.* (1987) Oral morphine versus injected meperidine (Demerol) for pain relief in children after orthopedic surgery. *Journal of Pediatric Orthopedic Surgery*, **7**, 78–82

Osgood, P. F. and Szyfelbein, S. K. (1989) Management of burn pain. *Pediatric Clinics of North America*, **36**, 1001–1013

Oster J. (1972) Recurrent abdominal pain, headache and limb pain in children and adolescents. *Pediatrics*, **50**, 429–436

Paradise, J. C., Bluestone, C. D., Bachman, R. N. *et al.* (1984) Efficacy of tonsillectomy for recurrent throat infection in severely affected children. *Pediatrics*, **62 (suppl.)**, 877

Peterson, H. A. (1977) Leg aches. *Pediatric Clinics of North America*, **24**, 731

Peterson, L. and Toler, S. M. (1986) An information seeking disposition in child surgery patients. *Health Psychology*, **5**, 343–358

Peterson, L., Harbeck, C., Chaney, J. *et al.* (1990) Children's coping with medical procedures: a conceptual overview and integration. *Behavioral Assessment*, **12**, 197–212

Pichard-Leandri, E. and Gauvain-Piquard, A. (eds.) (1989) *La Douleur chez l'enfant*. McGraw Hill, New York, 263

Pigeon, H., McGrath, P. J., Lawrence, J. *et al.* (1989) Nurses' perception of pain in the Neonatal

Intensive Care Unit. *Journal of Pain and Symptom Management*, **4**, 179–183

Porter, J. and Jick, H. (1980) Addiction rare in patients treated with narcotics. *New England Journal of Medicine*, **302**, 123

Powers, D. M. (1987) Rating of pain from postoperative children and their nurses. *Canadian Journal of Nursing Research (Nursing papers)*, **19(4)**, 49–58

Rawlings, D. J., Miller, P. A. and Engel, R. R. (1980) The effect of circumcision on transcutaneous pO_2 in term infants. *American Journal of Diseases of Children*, **13**, 676–678

Richardson, G. M. and McGrath, P. J. (1989) Cognitive-behavioural therapy for migraine headaches: a minimal-therapist-contact approach versus a clinic-based approach. *Headache*, **29**, 352–357

Richardson, G. M. and McGrath, P. J., Cunningham, S. J. and Humphreys, P. (1983) Validity of the headache diary for children. *Headache*, **22**, 184–187

Richardson, P. H. and Vincent, C. A. (1986) Acupuncture for the treatment of pain: a review of evaluative research. *Pain*, **24**, 15

Ritchie, J. A., Caty, S. and Ellerton, M. L. (1988) coping behaviors of preschool children. *Maternal-Child Nursing Journal*, **17**, 153–171

Ritchie, J. A., Caty, S., Ellerton, M. L. and Arklie, M. (1990) Descriptions of preschoolers' coping with finger pricks from a transactional perspective. *Behavioral Assessment*, **12**, 213–222

Ross, D. M. and Ross, S. A. (1988) Childhood pain: current issues, research and management. Urban & Schwarzenberg, Baltimore, 400 pp

Savedra, M. C. and Tesler, M. D. (1981) Coping strategies of hospitalized school-aged children. *Western Journal of Nursing Research*, **3**, 371–384

Savedra, M. C. and Tesler, M. D. (1989) Assessing children's and adolescent's pain. *Pediatrician*, **16**, 24–29

Schechter, N. L. (1985) Pain and pain control in children. *Current Problems in Pediatrics*, **15**, 1

Schechter, N. L., Allen, D. A. and Hanson, K. (1986) The status of paediatric pain control: a comparison of hospital analgesic usage in children and adults. *Pediatrics*, **77**, 11–15

Schechter, N. L., Berrien, F. B. and Katz, S. (1988) the use of patient controlled analgesia in adolescents with sickle cell pain crisis: A preliminary report. *Journal of Pain and Symptom Management*, **3**, 109–113

Schechter, N. L., Altman, A. and Weisman, S. (eds) (1990) Report of the consensus conference on the management of pain in childhood cancer. *Pediatrics*, **86(5)**, Suppl.

Schoen, E. J., Anderson, G., Bohon, C. *et al.* (1989) Report of the Task Force on Circumcision, American Academy of Pediatrics. *Pediatrics*, **84**, 388–391

Schultz, J. H. and Luthe, W. (1959) *Autogenic Training: A Psychophysiologic Approach to Psychotherapy*. Grune & Stratton, New York

Sethna, N. F. and Berde, C. B. (1989) Paediatric regional anaesthesia. In: *Paediatric Anaesthesia*, (ed. G. Gregory). Churchill Livingstone, New York, pp. 647–651

Shapiro, B. S. (1989) The management of pain in sickle cell disease. *Pediatric Clinics of North America*, **36**, 1029–1045

Shelton, T. L., Jeppson, E. S. and Johnson, B. H. (1987) *Family-Centred Care for Children with Special Health Care Needs*. Association for the Care of Children's Health, Washington

Slotkowski, E. L. and King, L. R. (1982) The incidence of neonatal circumcision in Illinois. *Illinois Medical Journal*, **162**, 421–426

Smith, R. P. (1988) Primary dysmenorrhoea and the adolescent patient. *Adolescent Pediatric Gynaecology*, **1**, 23

Stein, L. I. (1967) The doctor–nurse game. *Archive of General Psychiatry*, **16**, 699–703

Stein, L. I., Watts, D. T. and Howell, T. (1990) The doctor–nurse game revisited. *New England Journal of Medicine*, **322**, 546–549

Stevens, B. (1990) Development and testing of a paediatric pain management sheet. *Paeadiatric Nursing*, **16**, 543–548

Teperi, J. and Rimpela, M. (1989) Menstrual pain, health and behaviour in girls. *Social Science and Medicine*, **29**, 163–169

Tesler, M. D., Wegner, C., Savedra, M. *et al.* (1981) Coping strategies of children in pain. *Issues in Comprehensive Pediatric Nursing*, **5**, 351–359

Tesler, M., Savedra, M., Ward, M. *et al.* (1988) Children's language of pain. In: *Proceedings of the Vth World Congress on Pain* (eds R. Dubner, G. F. Gebhart, M. Bond) Elsevier, Amsterdam, pp. 348–352

Tree-Trakarn, T. and Pirayavaraporn, S. (1985) Postoperative pain relief for circumcision in children: comparison among morphine, nerve block and topical analgesia. *Anesthesiology*, **62**, 519–522

Unruh, A., McGrath, P. J., Cunningham, S. J. and Humphreys P. (1983) Children's drawings of their pain. *Pain*, **17**, 385–392

Varni, J. W., Thompson, K. L. and Hanson, V. (1987) The Varni/Thompson paediatric pain questionnaire: 1. Chronic musculo-skeletal pain in juvenile rheumatoid arthritis. *Pain*, **28**, 27–38

Wilder, R. T., Wolohan, M., Masek, B. J. *et al.* (1993) Reflex sympathetic dystrophy in children and adolescents: follow-up of a cohort of 70 patients and development of a treatment algorithm. *Journal of Bone and Joint Surgery* (in press)

Wilkie, D. J., Holzemer, W. L., Tesler, M. D. *et al.* (1990) Measuring pain quality: validity and reliability of children's and adolescents' pain language. *Pain*, **41**, 151–159

Williamson, P. S. and Williamson, M. L. (1983) Physiologic stress reduction by a local anaesthetic during newborn circumcision. *Pediatrics*, **71**, 36–40

Wolke, D. (1987) Environmental and developmental neonatology. *Journal of Reproductive and Infant Psychology*, **5**, 17

Woolf, C. J. (1989) Recent advances in the pathophysiology of acute pain. *British Journal of Anaesthesia*, **63**, 139

World Health Organization (1980) International classification of impairments, disabilities and handicaps. World Health Organization, Geneva, Switzerland

Zeltzer, L. K., Jay, S. M. and Fisher, D. M. (1989) The management of pain associated with pediatric procedures. *Pediatric Clinics of North America*, **36**, 941–964

11

The psychological aspects of pain

Linda Edgar

'Man is disturbed not by things, but by the appearance of things.'

— Epictetus

Introduction

This chapter is about the psychological aspects of pain from the patients' and caregivers' perspective. An integrated approach to dealing with pain is now accepted as the most likely way to succeed. In fact, the National Institute of Health (NIH) in the United States held a consensus development conference on pain which they called very appropriately for this chapter, 'The Integrated approach to the Management of Pain.' As pain involves the physical and psychological aspects of individuals, so must its management.

We have learned much about how important the psychological aspects of pain are from knowledge of the physiology of pain. The gate control theory proposed by Melzack and Wall (1965) integrates the physiological, psychological, cognitive and emotional aspects of pain. There is some evidence that there may even be memory circuits that interact between the periphery of the body and the spinal cord. In support of that theory, research has found that patients who received only general anaesthesia required much more postoperative analgesia than those who received local anaesthesia in addition to the general anaesthesia. Wall concluded that pain is a response to a 'series of controls acting in the context of a whole integrated nervous system.' Pain, then, is much more than the stimulus alone. To further complicate the complexity of pain, we are aware that interactions with others, with the environment and also culture also influence how pain is felt, experienced and managed.

In spite of this complexity, there are useful definitions of pain that can guide our approach to management. Margo McCaffery's (1968, 1979) definition of pain, 'Pain is whatever the experiencing person says it is, existing whenever and wherever he says it does,' continues to be an excellent working definition that integrates the complex nature of pain in a clear and straightforward way.

If we accept that pain is both a physical and psychological phenomenon, then we are more likely to be successful in treating patients with pain. If we continue to deny that belief, then pain relief will continue to elude us. We know that pain causes strong emotions in its sufferers. Fear, anxiety, depression and anger are frequently common companions to both acute and chronic pain. What we are only now beginning to appreciate is the impact of these and other emotions on the perception and control of pain.

Let us start at the beginning when pain is felt, and observe how people cope.

Psychological aspects of pain

Although there are many definitions of coping, all of us intuitively know when we observe a good coper and we can usually differentiate between a good and a poor coper. For the purposes of this chapter we will define coping as active problem solving (Weisman *et al.*, 1980). Good coping or active problem solving consists of:

Optimism or an expectation that positive change is possible.
Practicality about the kinds of solutions that are feasible.

Flexibility in approach to any problem.
Resourcefulness in finding support or additional information that helps implement behaviour

Another way of looking at coping is to see it as the means by which we succeed in gaining a sense of personal control over the effect that pain has on us. The degree to which the patient succeeds in gaining a sense of control over the ways pain is interpreted and responded to may be a measure of how well that individual handles the changes wrought by pain in his life. Many people express the notion that their life is out of control when they are dealing with pain. Irritability, impatience and anxiety are three ways in which a loss of control is expressed.

The concept of personal control embodies the belief that people need to avoid the feelings of powerlessness that accompany illness and pain, and maintain a sense of options and belief in their own capacity to control their fate (Stone, 1979). In other words, personal control suggests that people can affect how outcomes are handled (Mills and Krantz, 1979). Although the impact of personal control has been studied in a variety of situations, only recently has attention been directed to the effect of increasing perceived personal control in people with pain.

How do we learn the ways we cope? According to social learning theory, all behaviour is a result of a learned response. Individuals develop an understanding about the relationship between their actions and the results of their actions. Thus, coping with events such as pain can be viewed in different ways.

The degree to which people attribute events to their own actions, or to circumstances beyond their control is referred to as locus of control (Rotter, 1966). Although attributions of control occur along three dimensions, the most common one is called the internal–external dimension. The internal–external dimension of locus of control is believed to be an important factor in understanding the extent to which people perceive the events that happen to them as internal, that is, dependent on their own behaviour, and thus under personal control, or as external, meaning a result of luck, chance, or fate.

To illustrate the internal–external dimension, consider the person who views the responsibility for total pain relief as resting completely with his/her physician or health care team. This person would have a strongly external locus of control. Another person with a strongly internal locus of control may feel that their pain should be able to be controlled purely by his/her own actions. A more logical approach might be to feel that some of the pain control can be achieved by the subject, while some is dependent on external activities, such as the appropriate analgesic prescription. In any event, people in pain feel they have lost a sense of control over their bodies and events in their lives, and one of our major roles in nursing is to find ways to return this sense of control to them.

The perception of uncontrollability has been directly related to the feeling of helplessness. In the theory of helplessness, Seligman (1975) suggested that individuals exposed to uncontrollable events become passive and unable to exert control over their environment. Individuals exposed to uncontrollable events became motivationally, cognitively and emotionally passive. Motivationally, the incentive to respond is reduced, since previous attempts have not led to relief of the stress; cognitively, the individual has not learned that successful responding can lead to stress reduction; and emotionally, the individual is bothered by fear and inhibition (Maier and Seligman, 1976). Seligman (1975) contends that even death from helplessness is real. Therefore, understanding the psychological basis of pain, and the implications of control may allow us to build instrumental control into the lives of those who are in pain.

Cognitive appraisal, perception of control, and degree of helplessness influences a person's ability to cope with, or manage pain. The specific strategies used to cope with pain depend upon both the individual's appraisal of the situation, and the degree of personal control that can be exercised (Ray *et al.*, 1982). They contend that a person may choose coping strategies consciously, or make responses without self-awareness and deliberation. Since stress implies inadequacy in actual or anticipated control, a repertoire of coping strategies may be needed to restore or maintain control at different stages of a situation.

Anecdotal reports suggest that patients with pain develop beliefs not only about their disease, but also about whether or not they can control it. Such beliefs may include the degree to which the pain can be influenced by the patient, the physician, or the prescribed treatment. Therefore, if the patient believes he can control neither the situation nor his response to it in such a way that positive outcomes are possible, he may see himself as having no control at all, and may suffer anxiety, low self-esteem, and heightened pain.

When pain first occurs, the patient appraises the situation to determine the significance and meaning of the pain to his/her well-being. The significance and meaning determines whether the event is perceived as benign, challenging or threatening. This first appraisal is called primary appraisal (Lazarus and Folkman, 1984). Secondary appraisal follows next as the expectation for the potential for action is evaluated. We each have our own individual expectations concerning how effectively we can cope with the demands as we assess them.

The notion of expectation draws heavily from work by Bandura (1977) on self-efficacy. He noted that one must first believe that an action will have the desired outcome, and then that one is able to perform the actions required. Perceived self-efficacy affects what people choose to do, how hard they will work at the task, and how much stress they will experience with the process.

In summary, the degree to which people attribute events to their own actions, or to circumstances beyond their control may determine the reactions of an individual to stressful situations. However, it may not be the situation itself that produces helplessness, rather the belief that one lacks control over the situation. In attempting to retain, or maintain control across the situation, and feel that one's actions will be successful, an individual may utilize a variety of coping strategies, which nursing can readily facilitate.

There are important differences between the sensation of pain and the reaction to pain. Pain threshold or the lowest level of pain that produces a recognizable feeling of pain is remarkably similar for us all. Pain tolerance or the amount of pain one can accept without seeking relief, and pain reaction or what one feels, thinks or does, however, differ widely from person to person.

Thus, pain tolerance and pain reaction depends not only on the pain intensity, but also on how one appraises the pain and the surrounding circumstances, how one evaluates his/her likelihood of coping well and what coping strategies are actually used.

If you have followed this fairly complicated discussion on coping and control, you may have realized that if we can teach patients with pain ways of coping, and means of restoring a sense of personal control we may help them to manage their pain and their reactions to it so that pain is lessened. The gate control theory also supports this assumption by suggesting that thoughts can act to close the gate as they enhance good coping and perceived control.

Nursing approaches to help deal with the psychological problems caused by pain which will be discussed in this chapter include cognitive appraisal, music, imagery, humour, distraction, goal setting, problem solving and relaxation. The nursing strategies in the following section are techniques that are in current use with patients in acute and chronic pain. As far as possible, we have attempted to present these techniques in a practical way so that implementation and understanding can be facilitated. For these approaches to be effective, the nurse needs to feel comfortable with them, and best of all, to have tried them or even use them routinely as part of good coping.

Nursing strategies for patients with pain

Cognitive reframing

Cognitive reframing is a skill that helps us to deal in a different way with thoughts, feelings, and beliefs. This technique offers an opportunity to alter the cognitions or thoughts that contribute to the stress response in the body by changing the perception that we have of a situation. A sizeable amount of research shows that 'self-talk,' or the messages one tells oneself, can dramatically influence an individual's performance of widely varying tasks (Meichenbaum, 1974, 1977).

Cognitive reframing is defined as the ability to change the way one thinks or more specifically, to enable one to think more positively and even more importantly, less negatively. Other names for this approach are cognitive appraisal and cognitive therapy.

It is well established that thoughts influence moods and feelings. Thoughts may be illogical or distorted, thus leading to increased anxiety or depression. Patients can be taught that the first step to changing negative moods and feelings is to be aware of the type of thought processes that are occurring. In our experience with patients who had a helpless–hopeless disposition, the simple awareness of the control they held over their thoughts was frequently sufficient to provide positive change and improved mood. Actively participating in cognitive reappraisal has been an effective tool to help patients regain some of the control that they had lost with the onset of their pain. We provide a brief explanation and simple examples of the interaction between *facts, thoughts* and *feelings*.

Facts are events; reality; something *known* to exist or to have happened.
Thoughts arise directly from a fact or event.
Feelings come from the thought processes, and thus only indirectly relate to the fact.

Facts cannot be changed, and we have, by and large, little control over most of the facts in our lives. It is, however, possible to *control* the feelings by changing one's thoughts.

We present neutral examples of cognitive restructuring to illustrate the process. Try this exercise yourself before you share it with your patients.

Example

Picture yourself walking down a street and observing someone you know coming towards you. As you approach the person, you smile, expecting a greeting. Instead, the person looks at you but continues to walk past without either a greeting or sign of recognition.

How does this make you feel?
Why do you feel this way?
What thoughts went through your mind when you were ignored?

You are encouraged to practise separating the fact from the thought, and the thought from the feeling.

If you are *feeling* angry, rejected, disappointed, you may have been *thinking* that the person was aware of you yet chose to ignore your presence, or doesn't like you.

On the other hand reflecting a little, you

might *think* that your friend may be preoccupied with family concerns and you will *feel* sympathetic instead of angry. You might realize she wasn't wearing her glasses and even *feel* amused and plan to tease her about her vanity.

It is important to understand that the uncomfortable feelings emerged not from the facts but directly from the thought processes. Recognise that it is not the *fact* that gave direct rise to your *feelings*, but the *thoughts* arising from the *fact* that caused you to feel the way you do.

The next step in this process of cognitive reappraisal involves the issue of personal control. Examine the three states of facts, thoughts and feelings to determine where personal control continues to exist, and how it can be strengthened. Patients are informed that while they may have little control over most of the facts in their lives, they continue to have total control and choice over the thoughts which arose from the facts.

A typical approach to patients that we might make is as follows, 'You can *control* the way you feel by *controlling* the way you think. Choosing to *think* positively by changing or reframing your negative thoughts will allow yourself to *feel* positively.'

When your patient finds him/herself feeling negatively, encourage him/her to step back and ask, 'What am I thinking? Do I need to think this way? Can I choose to think differently and feel better?'

Every feeling has a thought behind it

Examples of cognitive appraisal and self-efficacy beliefs are self-statements such as, 'You are doing fine, you're coping, just keep on top of the pain.'

Guidelines for use

Whether the nurse's role is to suggest cognitive strategies, to work directly with the patient on them, or to simply 'plant seeds' (Scandrett, 1985) about what may help, the following guidelines may be useful:

1. Don't forget that the patient is the most important person in the process.
2. It is essential to develop a collaborative team approach with the patient as director of the team. Patient centredness and team collaboration are important whenever one treats pain.
3. The patient must always be in control of the

process, since his feedback determines the next step. The patient is central to the pain, the process and the control.

4. Encourage the patient to observe his own behaviour and thought processes, and at the same time be aware of your responses too.
5. Help the patient identify cues in his environment that will prompt him to talk to himself differently.

If the patient is reluctant to 'buy' into these approaches, suggest that he is actually enduring two kinds of pain, physical and emotional. Whether or not the physical pain can be readily eliminated, the other pains can be minimized (Ciccone and Grzesiak, 1988).

People with chronic pain often have puzzling and confusing feelings to contend with. The following are examples of thoughts that patients may have, coupled with some more positive thoughts that can help regain that sense of control and hopefulness.

Not helpful	*Helpful*
'I feel powerless that I can't stop the pain.'	'I do have control over my thoughts, and the pain isn't so much of a threat.'
'I'll never get better.'	'There are still things I enjoy and can do.'
'I just didn't have any energy.'	'I will make an effort.'
'What if I lose my job . . .'	'I can work within my limitations.'
'I will always have pain.'	'The pain may go away, and I can reduce it to a level I can cope with.'

Here are some examples of common thoughts that prevent good coping with pain. These thoughts are illogical and distorted and can be readily disputed and changed.

1. In order to feel happy, I must be cured completely of my pain.
2. Everyone must act the same way to me as they did before I became ill.
3. I should be able to do everything I used to do.
4. I will not be able to bear the pain.
5. I must be dependent on others in order to be happy or to solve my problems.
6. My doctor always knows what is best for me and my family.

7. My family should not be tense or scared, or worried.
8. Everything is horrible in my life when I have pain.

Imagery

Although guided imagery as a therapeutic tool for pain control has seen renewed interest in recent years, imagery can be traced back thousands of years to ancient cultures. Imagery is a mental representation of reality or fantasy, and may use all five senses in its creation.

Guided imagery is generally preceded by some form of relaxation which is thought to facilitate image development. Imagery is an effective way to help people actively participate in gaining relief from pain.

There are several reasons why guided imagery helps people deal with pain successfully. One explanation is that the distraction which results from focusing on a pleasant relaxing image adds to its effectiveness. Another is that patients who use guided imagery regain a sense of personal control, especially when they are encouraged and directed to create their own images. The relaxation that either precedes and/or accompanies imagery also contributes to reduced muscle tension, anxiety, and pain.

Perhaps the key function of guided imagery lies in its ability to alter how patients perceive the sensations of pain. Guided imagery varies in whether the patient chooses the image or whether someone else directs it. Other guided imagery occurs when the nurse guides the imagery development explicitly by leading the patient through a prepared description of the scene to be imagined, while with self-guided imagery patients are instructed to use their own imagination to remember or create pleasant images. It is often helpful for the nurse to know that there is no one right way to teach guided imagery, or any other cognitive–behavioural interventions. Each nurse must learn and practice a technique so that she feels comfortable with it before employing it with patients. The nurse and the patient become partners in a collaborative relationship in selecting the imagery that the patient will develop, and when and how he will use it, and practicing and providing feedback.

Specific strategies that focus on the pain and change it into a less painful sensation are:

1. Converting the pain to non-pain, e.g. turning the painful area into ice, rushing water, trickles of sand, or pressure caused by imaginary animals sitting on the area.
2. Imagining the pain to be a colour and then converting it to another colour, by switching from a warm to a cool colour, or vice versa.
3. Determining the pain level on a 0–10 visual analogue scale, and then slowly moving the indicator lever to a slightly lower number, while breathing slowly and deeply with each incremental decrease in the pain rating.

The following are two relaxation images that can be easily practiced by people in pain. As you have noticed, they differ from the preceding examples as they focus away from the pain. Both methods of focusing on and transforming pain, and focusing away from the pain are useful.

Find yourself a comfortable place to sit or lie down, and pay attention to your breath. Just notice how you are breathing, do not attempt to change anything. Simply be aware of the rhythm of your breathing, and how effortless it is to breathe. Let the air breathe you. Then imagine one of the following:

(a) You are like a pad of butter melting in the warm sun. Feel the warmth of the sun on your body. The warm rays feel soothing and nurturing. Your body releases tension and gently relaxes.
(b) You are in an elevator that is slowly descending floor by floor. At each floor you become more and more relaxed. Feel the gentle sensation as the elevator takes you safely and gently into a deep state of relaxation.

Music

Music has long been known for its soothing and relaxing qualities. As a therapy, music is used to restore, maintain, and improve mental and physical health. Music can encourage distraction or dissociation from unpleasant or painful stimuli through the development of imagery, increase the production of endorphins (Goldstein, 1980), and serve as a cue for relaxation. All of these processes are well in keeping with our understanding of the mechanisms of the gate control theory. The potential of music as a practical measure has only begun to be recognized. According to Bailey (1986), the goals of music therapy in pain management are to improve the patient's comfort level, to assist him or her to regain a sense of perceived personal control, and to become actively involved in the management of his/her pain.

Although music is an easy-to-use modality, it is not enough to simply present the music to the patient and insruct that he/she listen to it. A clear set of instructions is required so that the patient will become an active participant in his/her own care. The following guidelines from McCaffery (1979) are particularly helpful:

1. Listen only to the music.
2. Feel the music lifting you upward.
3. Let each measure rhythmically flow through your body and relax the muscles.
4. Let yourself float through the air with the melody.

It is best to introduce the patient to music therapy before pain becomes intense, or prior to commencing a painful procedure, (Angus and Faux, 1989). With portable tape recorders and head sets, music is readily available to patients at home or in the hospital. Remember to encourage instrumental music over music with words. Other than that instruction, let patients choose their favourite type – from classic to rock!

Distraction

Almost everyone has used distraction at one time or another for pain relief. McCaffery and Beebe (1989) has defined distraction as simply focusing attention on stimuli other than the pain sensation. Using that definition, almost any activity can qualify as distraction, from talking on the telephone to studying a favourite painting.

Distraction may increase pain tolerance (Scott and Barber, 1977) or raise the perception threshold (Fellner, 1971). Distraction places pain at the periphery of awareness so that the patient can 'tune out' the pain for the time distraction is being used. Whatever the exact mechanism may be, distraction does not make the pain disappear but makes it more tolerable.

Like all techniques, there are some disadvantages associated with distraction. Others may doubt the existence or severity of pain if distraction is a successful intervention. However, the very fact that distraction works indicates that pain is present and has been only temporarily relieved. Distraction is fatiguing, and therefore is most useful for brief periods of time (less than 2 hours). Distraction requires energy and concentration, which results in a return of pain, irritability, and fatigue after its termination. However, the many benefits of distraction far outweigh the disadvantages, and an explanation of its efficacy and rationale should be provided to every patient in pain and their caregivers and family members.

Humour is a highly successful distraction strategy which has been shown to improve the release of the body's natural endorphins. The therapeutic uses of humour in pain control have only begun to be recognized in the last few years. Norman Cousins (1989) discovered that 10 minutes of genuine laughter gave him 2 hours of pain-free sleep. Cousins has written extensively on the importance of positive emotions, including laughter, in pain management. Laughter has been described as internal jogging and a way to promote simplicity in living, delight, optimism and hope. It may alter the brain's perception of hope through the stimulation of endorphins. Health care professionals can suggest the use of books, records, movies, songs, games and stories to patients and families. Humour is a form of communication that has therapeutic value when used with appropriateness, timing and sensitivity in consideration with the patients' degree of discomfort and individual characteristics. Some patients may claim they need to feel pain relief before they can laugh, but we respond that they need to laugh first, and then they can feel some relief.

Problem solving

Problem solving is one of the critical dimensions of effective coping. When people are in pain, their problem solving ability is reduced. Coping is an act of flexible and re-sourceful problem-solving, but unfortunately most of us do not really ever learn how to become good problem solvers. Because we often do not take time out to consider a systematic method for dealing with problems, we may experience a great deal more distress than is really necessary. This seems to occur when we are confronted with a situation that is painful, frightening, different, anxiety-producing, or even life-threatening. Learning to solve problems in a step-by-step approach can signifi-

cantly help a patient to cope with his or her situation. Obviously, there are many way to make decisions and to solve a problem. The following is one method which we have used with patients.

Step 1 is to define the problem clearly and attempt to separate it from all the subsidiary concerns which spring up around the major problem. We make it a point to encourage patients to stop and to define the predominant problem which they are experiencing.

Step 2 is to identify and recognize how one feels about the problem. Thinking, feeling and behaving are all closely related and it is important not to ignore any one of these three dimensions. In the same way that thinking can affect the decisions which are carried out, many of the feelings about a problem may lead to some creative solutions. This step allows feelings to be very carefully considered. People with pain begin to feel concerned about such things as finances, work or what will happen to them and their families in the coming years.

Step 3 is a time not to think about solutions or coping strategies for a particular task or concern. This phase of problem-solving is used to take time out and to get away from what is on one's mind, and to relax for a while. We use it as a kind of no-think step. By getting away from concerns for a brief period of time, sometimes a new and creative solution may be uncovered.

Step 4 is the step where one thinks of as many different solutions as possible for a given problem, task or concern. Often patients who are experiencing a great deal of distress want to focus only on one solution. Step 4 requires a consideration of many alternatives including some which could be thought of as poor decisions. By coming up with some poor solutions and some good solutions, it is possible to compare and contrast different avenues towards the resolution of the problem.

In Step 5, imagine or consider how other people would respond to a particular issue. In other words, sit back and say, 'How might my friend solve this problem?' or 'How might my spouse deal with this illness-related task?' In this way, one can shift attention from one's approach or style and suddenly become aware of a totally different new perspective.

In Step 6, begin to list the pros and cons, the advantages and disadvantages of each of the solutions which were generated previously. It is a time to evaluate, to perceive the possible consequences of all the different solutions. Be conscious of the fact the actual decision still has not been made. What one has been doing is going through a very systematic step-by-step process to problem-solving.

Step 7: now that the pros and cons of each proposed solution have been analyzed, it is fairly easy to take all the solutions and put them in order, starting from the least practical or least desirable solution all the way up to the best solution or those solutions which seem to have the most likely chance at resolving the critical concern.

In Step 8, a decision is taken. It is time to make a choice. The actual choice is usually quite simple to make if all of the preceding steps have been followed carefully.

Step 9 is a re-examination and re-definition. Go back to the original concern or problem and ask 'Can it be thought about differently?' or 'Is there anything positive which I can understand about this situation?' Many patients can go back to their original concern and see it from a different perspective. For example, one may go back to a particular problem and discover that one of the positive things which comes out of the situation is that there is more closeness to people or one is better able to understand a particular person. It is possible, through effective problem solving, to discover at least one positive dimension to a difficult situation. This is a vital dimension of flexible coping.

Coping through problem solving seems to be a practical help for patients in pain. However, most of us are not always good problem solvers when events in our life become increasingly stressful or taxing. Furthermore, we may not have learned how to approach specific tasks in a manner which leads to effective resolutions. It is useful to begin to observe how one typically approaches tasks or problems and then try to incorporate this new method of problem solving. An important component of effective coping is how much personal responsibility each one willingly takes for observing behaviours, listening to thoughts and planning an active problem-solving strategy.

It may be the most helpful strategy to work through a simple, neutral example of problem solving when the patient's pain is not severe. Like all cognitive strategies, problem solving takes practice and is best learned when pain is absent or mild.

Goal setting

People in pain often lose sight of their goals, and have feelings of hopelessness. Thinking about and setting goals is a useful coping mechanism because goal setting accomplishes all of the following:

1. Helps to re-establish a normal daily schedule,
2. Helps to prioritize at a time when there may be many demands,
3. Constitutes a realistic means of accomplishing tasks that are important to the patient,
4. Enables the patient to think more clearly on a day-to-day basis,
5. Increases self-esteem (sense of accomplishment) and self confidence,
6. Reaffirms a belief in a better future,
7. Gives meaning and purpose to life,
8. Encourages better use of the imagination.

We adapted goal setting from work in counselling services, from the area of time management, and from behavioural medicine in regard to pain management.

Goals should be personally relevant, realistic and achievable. Examples vary from simply getting dressed in the morning, returning to work part time, to taking off on a motorcycle jaunt, and world travelling.

Thus we invite patients to set goals for tomorrow, next week, for 3 months, and for a lifetime. Some patients are unable to look far ahead and are more comfortable setting goals for tomorrow and next week. A few can only manage initially on a day-to-day basis. In these cases, the concept of thinking and planning ahead can be established. We do not find that the time frame is as significant as the actual behavioural setting of the goal. Goals can be broken down to a series of smaller, graded steps that are seen as possible, and readily achievable.

Goal setting can encourage patients in pain to remain hopeful. Although hope is part of our everyday vocabulary, we sometimes discredit its importance in sustaining us through crises and painful experiences. Hope reinforces the belief that there is a way out of difficulty and distress. In the face of uncertainty, there is nothing wrong and everything right with hope. There are many different kinds of hope and what is hoped for may change with each situation, but there is always room for it. Hope has been found to energize, motivate and sustain.

Setting goals, whether large or small, can stimulate hope and vice versa. For example, hoping to have a good night's rest can direct a person with pain to make that a goal. He or she can plan for it by arranging adequate medication at bedtime, practising some relaxation, avoiding energetic exercise before sleep, and having a warm drink and bath in the evening. Looking at this example another way, setting a goal of sleeping well one night can encourage the emergence of hope.

Relaxation training

The research literature on the use of relaxation techniques is now in the hundreds. As a treatment strategy for stress and pain related conditions, relaxation has been clearly shown to be effective. Relaxation training can be introduced to all patients as a coping strategy and as a step in problem solving, i.e. taking time out in order to look at a problem or concern from a different perspective. In addition, there are other uses for relaxation training that the patient may suggest.

It is important not to rush or short change the patient's introduction to relaxation training. We begin by reviewing the patient's previous experience with relaxation. Patients who are currently using or who have used a method of relaxation successfully in the past should be encouraged to continue with that method. The training then centres on discussing the following points and reinforcing the patient's techniques, making modifications if necessary.

Categories of relaxation

We explain that there are two specific categories of relaxation. The first uses techniques such as meditation that focus primarily on the brain. Relaxation using these methods is more difficult to achieve at first, particularly with people who are very stressed.

The second category of techniques works from the 'outside-in', that is, by relaxing the muscles of the body which then facilitates the relaxation response of the brain. Examples of this method are yoga, autogenic training, deep breathing and progressive muscle relaxation.

Benefits of relaxation

Relaxation is a general, calming, anxiety-alleviating response, which becomes an inoculation against future stress. It is thought to be a potential anti-pain agent by increasing the production of endorphins. Most importantly, relaxation is a way to regain self-control, especially since it is an active coping strategy which can be used at any time. Physiologically, relaxation lowers the respiration and heart rate, lowers blood pressure and muscle contraction. It promotes creativity and enhances problem solving due to the predominance of alpha waves in the brain.

A major benefit is that many patients use audio tapes in their own homes and may already have some background in kinds of relaxation training. Relaxation can readily be practised with the use of such tapes in a very inexpensive way. Most hospital settings also have access to portable tape players through purchase or donations, and relaxation tapes are either commercially available or can easily be made by the nurse.

General information

The positive effects of relaxation are usually not experienced immediately. In fact, it is a response which most of us must learn, allowing for adequate practice over time. We recommended that patients practise a minimum of 20 minutes 3 times a week for several weeks. After this time they should be able to elicit the relaxation response by breathing deeply and using a cue word such as 'Relax.'

Relaxation training requires a passive, 'let it go' attitude. We explain that an effort to relax is usually a failure to relax. Relaxation is a part of each of us. The major task involved is to allow the process to occur, by retraining the body and mind to recognise the difference between tension and relaxation. It is important that the patient understands he/she is always in control.

Medical contraindications

Individuals with a history of cardiac irregularities, severe depression, or psychosis should have medical approval before learning relaxation. Though there are no hard data to substantiate the risk, it is possible that the autonomic changes associated with systematic relaxation could permit increased cardiac irregularity. It is also possible that a depressed or psychotic individual who is exerting tremendous energy to remain in control could decompensate with profound relaxation. Interestingly, both depression and cardiac irregularities have been shown to respond favourably to relaxation therapy specifically designed to treat these conditions.

Those who have experienced respiratory problems in the past need not be excluded. However, they generally do not respond well to any focus on respiration, so that it is preferable to eliminate or minimise the breathing aspects of relaxation. Individuals with musculoskeletal disorders require additional attention and modification of the technique to provide adequate support to painful areas. Contact lenses should always be removed, since the reduction in blinking and tearing which accompanies relaxation can cause discomfort.

Preparation for relaxation

It is important to set the scene carefully, to be free of distractions, turn off the phone, be prepared to ignore the doorbell and let people around know that for the next 20 minutes disruptions are unwelcome. The patient's comfort is important and he should be encouraged to sit comfortably in a chair with support for the head. Resting in bed is also possible, but the patient should be reminded not to fall asleep during practice (unless insomnia has been a problem, in which case sleep is a sign of success!). Avoid practising right after mealtimes.

Relaxation can be taught in many different ways, whether in small groups or on an individual basis, and if the nurse is not able to provide the time necessary, the patient can be referred to yoga classes or other groups that provide instruction. Specific instructions for nurses can be found in Bernstein and Borkovec (1973), Bulechek and McCloskey (1985), and Trystad (1980).

We use a fairly formal, dynamic procedure adapted from progressive muscle relaxation to relax the body; formal, in that we do it in a set way to begin with, dynamic in that, as we progress, the technique evolves to become a more flowing, more automatic one.

We begin by closing our eyes and concentrating on feeling what our body is like when it is at rest. Secondly, we impose tension upon it and

feel the difference. Then we relax the body and feel a third quality – that of deep relaxation. Finally, it is possible to discover another state, what we call a 'letting go', when the body feels different again.

As the relaxation progresses breathing is likely to slow down automatically. There is no need to emphasise breathing after an initial focus on it at the start of the exercise.

When contracting the muscles, it is advisable to hold the tension just long enough to feel it strongly, and then to let it go.

Thoughts are the most difficult to control and let go, although nearly everyone can learn to relax their bodies. Our attitude to unwanted thoughts should be that of an uninvolved observer. Allow them to just roll on, to come and to go. They do just that – and soon stop.

To conclude the section on nursing approaches to psychological strategies to lessen and control pain, remember that it is important to provide as much information as patients want and require about their pain and the relationship between psychological, cognitive behavioural strategies, and the nature of pain. A comprehensive education programme can assist patients to understand the mechanisms of pain and pain control in a realistic way, and help them view the role that all strategies, including pharmacological ones, can play in the successful management of pain.

Psychological aspects of the caregiver

From a different perspective, consider some psychological barriers to pain control that can arise with the caregiver. Pain is a multidimensional and complex phenomenon and requires a flexible, collaborative team approach which includes the patient as head of the team. Suppose that caregivers, family members or the patient have some of the following characteristics:

1. A powerful need to take care of others,
2. Rigidity and perfectionism,
3. Poor communication skills,
4. Difficulty adjusting to changes,
5. Need to control situations and people,
6. Denial and distortion of anger,
7. Dependence on others for approval, and
8. Low self worth.

These are the characteristics of a set of behaviours called codependency (Cauthorne-Lindstrom and Hrabe, 1990).

Codependency develops as a result of prolonged exposure to, and practise of, a set of rules that prevents open expression and direct discussion of feelings and problems. The word codependency did not appear in the literature until the late 1970s. According to Subby and Friel (1984), it was originally used to describe a person whose life was affected by being involved with someone who was chemically dependent. As professionals began to understand codependency better, more groups of people other than those in close relationships with compulsive people appeared to be affected, including those in helping occupations. One currently accepted definition that incorporates the wider meaning states, 'A codependent person is one who has let another person's behaviour affect him or her, and who is obsessed with controlling that person's behaviour.'

We may not realize that we have internalized rules like these (Cauthorne-Lindstrom and Hrabe, 1990):

1. It is not safe to talk openly about problems.
2. Feelings should never be expressed openly.
3. Don't talk to the person you're having problems with directly. Talk to a third party about it.
4. Don't make mistakes; always be perfectly good.
5. Don't be selfish.
6. Do as I say, not as I do.
7. Always follow the rules and be respectful to authority.
8. Don't rock the boat.
9. Don't talk about sex.

Codependents react to the behaviours of others in habitual ways. While some of these ways involve compulsive behaviours such as substance abuse, others involve a strong work ethic and an intense desire to respond to the needs of those around them.

In order to control pain, a whole new approach is needed, whether one is a professional caregiver, patient, family member, or close friend. That is, we must trust the patient's description of pain and allow a free expression of feelings between patient and caregiver that permits two-way communication. Feelings of frustration

and helplessness in finding the right approaches to control pain are uncomfortable, but only temporary. There is frequently a place for trial and error as a variety of strategies are tried until the right combination is found. Pain control is a challenge that can be met through teamwork, open communication, flexibility, true collaboration, and mutual respect.

Although we cannot change the complex and subjective nature of pain or simplify the variety of strategies available for its management, we can impact on almost every other aspect. In doing so, we may discover that neither the nature of pain nor its management continue to be as problematic as they have been in the past.

References

Angus, J. E. and Faux, S (1989) The effect of music on adult postoperative patients' pain during a nursing procedure. In: *Key Aspects of Comfort: Management of Pain, Fatigue, and Nausea* (eds S. G. Funk *et al.*), Springer, New York, pp. 166–172

Bailey, L. M. (1983) The effects of live music versus tape-recorded music on hospitalised cancer patients. *Music Therapy*, **2**, 17–28

Bandura, A. (1977) Self-efficacy: toward a unifying theory of behavioral change. *Psychological Review*, **84**, 191–215

Bernstein, D. B. and Borkovec, T. D. (1973) *Progressive Relaxation Training: A Handbook for the Helping Professions*, Research Press, Chicago, IL

Bulechek, G. M. and McCloskey, J. C. (1985) *Nursing Interventions: Treatments for Nursing Diagnosis*, W. B. Saunders, Philadelphia, PA

Cauthorne-Lindstrom, C. and Hrabe, D. (1990) Codependent behaviors in managers: A script for failure. *Nursing Management*, **21(2)**, 34–35; 38–39

Ciccone, D. S. and Grzesiak, R. C. (1988) Cognitive theory: An overview of theory and practice. In: *Persistent pain: Psychosocial Assessment and Intervention* (eds N. Lynch and S. Vasudevan), Kluwer Academic Publishers, Boston, MA, pp. 133–177

Cousins, N. (1989) *Head first: The Biology of Hope*, E. P. Dutton, New York

Fellner, C. H. (1971) Alterations in pain perceptions of multiple sensory modality stimulation. *Psychosomatics*, **12**, 313–315

Goldstein, A. (1980) Thrills in response to music and other stimuli. *Physiological Psychology*, **8**, 126–129

Lazarus, R. S. and Folkman, S. (1984) *Stress, Appraisal, and Coping*. Springer, New York

Maier, S. F. and Seligman, M. E. P. (1976) Learned helplessness: theory and evidence. *Journal of Experimental Psychology (Gen)*, **105**, 3–46

McCaffery, M. (1968) *Cognition, Bodily Pain, and Man–Environment Interactions*. University of California Student Store, Los Angeles, CA

McCaffery, M. (1979) *Nursing Management of the Patient with Pain*, 2nd ed., J. B. Lippincott, Philadelphia, PA

McCaffery, M. and Beebe, A. (1989) *Pain Clinical Manual for Nursing Practice*. C. V. Mosby, St. Louis

Meichenbaum, D. (1974) *Cognitive Behavior Modification*, General Learning Press, Morristown, NJ

Meichenbaum, D. (1977) *Cognitive Behavior Modification*, Plenum, New York

Melzack, R. and Wall, P. D. (1965) Pain mechanisms: a new theory. *Science*, **150**, 971–979

Mills, R. T. and Krantz, D. S. (1979) Information, choice, and reactions to stress: A field experiment in a blood bank with laboratory analogue. *Journal of Personality and Social Psychology*, **37(4)**, 608–620

Ray, C., Lindop, J. and Gibson, S. (1982) The concept of coping. *Psychological Medicine*, **12**, 385–395

Rotter, J. B. (1966) Generalised expectancies for internal versus eternal control of reinforcement. *Psychological Monographs*, **80(1)**, 609

Scandrett, S. (1985) Cognitive reappraisal. In: *Nursing Intervention: Treatment for Nursing Diagnoses* (eds G. M. Bulechek and J. C. McCloskey), W. B. Saunders, Philadelphia, pp. 49–57

Scott, D. S. and Barber, T. X. (1977) Cognitive control of pain: effects of multiple cognitive strategies. *Psychology Record*, **2**, 373–383

Seligman, M. E. P. (1975) *Helplessness*, W. H. Freeman, San Francisco, CA

Stone, G. C. (1979) Patient compliance and the role of the expert. *Journal of Social Issues*, **35(1)**, 34–59

Subby, R. and Friel, J. (1984) Codependency: a paradoxical dependency. In: *Codependency: an Emerging Issue*. Health Communications, Pompano Beach, FL

Trygstad, L. (1980) Simple new way to help anxious patients. *RN*, **43(12)**, 228–31.

Weisman, A. D., Worden, J. W. and Sobel, H. J. (1980) *Psychosocial Screening and Intervention with Cancer Patients*, (Project Omega, Grant No. CA-19797). Harvard Medical School, Department of Psychiatry, Massachusetts General Hospital, Boston, MA

12

Alternative nursing interventions

Carol Horrigan

If I can stop one heart from breaking,
I shall not live in vain;
If I can ease one life the aching,
Or cool one pain,
Or help one fainting Robin,
Unto his nest again,
I shall not live in vain.

Emily Dickinson.

Introduction

The title of this chapter is open to discussion. What are 'alternative' interventions; are they really alternative methods of care or are they complementary? Are they 'holistic' – in the sense that nurses are considering the patient as a whole person with social, spiritual and psychological needs, and not simply as a 'case' presenting with typical or atypical symptoms? (Rogers, 1970).

A resurgence of 'hands-on' nursing care in the 1980s has been noted, with a growing interest in the use of touch as therapy and an increased awareness by nurses of the importance of 'being with' their patients. This is in response to the growing gulf between nurses and patients created by the technology that must be used for their safety but which can easily de-personalise contact with them.

There is an encouraging increase in the interest and enthusiasm shown by doctors for the use of methods of pain relief which are non-invasive and may complement other methods.

As we have become more 'civilised', human beings have forgotten, (or suppress) the natural instinct to withdraw, rest and sleep when we are tired or unwell. We allow ourselves to be drawn into a spiral of exhaustion and ill-health but often find it difficult to change our lifestyle unaided (Nixon, 1989).

Of the many alternative and complementary therapies available in the United Kingdom, only a small selection are used by nurses, especially in the NHS. They all have a relaxation component, and the direct nurse-patient interaction can be used to help the patient to learn how to avoid the spiral. Some therapies, such as relaxation, can eventually be carried out without the nurse.

The knowledge base and training required in order to practise complementary therapies varies widely. The discrepancy and apparent lack of formality and validity concerns not only doctors but also the nurses who practise them. The arguments surrounding this issue will be offered for consideration by the reader.

Orthodox or alternative?

Nursing has always been underpinned by the philosophy of caring for people as individuals. (Turton, Penson 1989; and Holloway, 1989). However, since 1858 when what is now known as biomedicine became the official healing mode, nursing has been under the powerful influence of doctors who have created an artificial dichotomy between mind and body (Husband, 1988; Stacey, 1989.)

Orthodox nursing care has therefore become reductionist too. There are now clinical nurse specialists who concentrate their studies on a small area, and because of the increase in the importance of the use of technology in medicine, there has been a parallel need for nurses to understand and participate in its application.

With the need to acquire post-registration certificates and 'high-tech' skills, the fundamental skills of nursing are lost or become devalued. These skills have gradually been adopted and developed by other branches of the health care team, for example dietetics, physiotherapy and occupational therapy. Threads of these disciplines remain in nurse education but for the patient they are nearly always dealt with by a therapist, not a nurse.

Of course nurses could not possibly provide the very special skills that these therapists bring to patients. However, the common denominator is that they all require a high degree of one-to-one interaction and patient education. If nurses are to support patients through their pain, they can achieve their objective, in part at least, by teaching them how to recognise and utilise their bodies' own recuperative powers, by encouraging their natural help-seeking instincts, and strengthening their willpower and the wish to be well (Berliner, 1984; Penson and Holloway, 1989).

So what is 'alternative' nursing? Is it completely divorced from orthodoxy or is it complementary to it? What does it have to offer the patient that orthodox nursing cannot provide?

Occasionally it could be said to be alternative; as an example, reflex zone therapy (which works in a similar manner to accupuncture but uses pressure instead of needles), can be used as a single means of pain control prior to wisdom teeth extraction. In most situations however, pain control is achieved by the use of different methods being used simultaneously, or intermittently, when they can then be regarded as complementary (Gibson, 1988).

Sometimes they are complementary to pharmaceutical control, for example visualisation and relaxation used by patients with rheumatoid arthritis. At other times they can be used as an alternative to orthodox nursing, aromatherapy or reflex zone therapy being employed to relieve the pain of constipation or urinary retention. Both therapies encourage relaxation and natural evacuation, thereby removing the cause of the pain (Marquardt, 1983; Tisserand, 1985; Worwood, 1990).

Individualised care and alternative nursing

Contrary to popular belief, it is ·very easy to include massage or any other alternative therapy into a patients' daily care. The day can be planned by the patient, his nurse and whoever practises the therapy. This person may be his nurse, a practitioner or nurse from another team or ward, a volunteer or a professional therapist employed by the patient or his family.

Assessment should ideally include defining the patients' specific problems, preferably by using a recognised method of pain assessment, such as a pain chart. This will enable the therapist to devise a programme for that particular patient, allowing for other daily activities and therapies, so that pain relief is optimised from every source. Simple therapies such as basic massage can be included in other care times such as during a bed bath, whereas visualisation and guided imagery sessions need clear spans of time when interruptions can be minimised or prevented.

The patients' interaction with his environment should not be ruled out, and a peaceful, calming atmosphere is the aim of all alternative therapies. When patients are in pain and under stress from orthodox treatment such as chemotherapy, their sympathetic nervous system is in a constant state of arousal.

It may only take a further small increase in this state of arousal to take the patient to the point where his coping mechanisms are seriously affected (Nixon, 1988).

Patients need to feel that they are in control of their situation, thereby gaining a sense of security in which they can become active in their care, even if only to a limited degree (Sims, 1987). A sense of commitment to their own health status and involvement in their destiny can help prevent the pain – depression cycle which can be overwhelming and difficult to break (Seedhouse and Cribb, 1989).

There is an increasing awareness of individual responsibility for health and well-being, but it is often seen as something that can be purchased: witness the recent interest in and consumption of so-called 'health-foods' – organically grown vegetables, muesli and vitamin supplements. Products such as these are only marginally beneficial unless used within a total concept of healthy living (Penson and Holloway, 1989).

Nurses are in an ideal position to inform patients about lifestyle changes which will not only help them through an acute period of stress or pain but will enable them to feel more in command during any future episodes. The patients' ability and enthusiasm for learning pain and stress-reduction techniques can be assessed by a trained nurse soon after admission.

The nurse can then plan and implement the method so that the patient can become proficient whilst in the supportive care of the nurse. Willingness to undergo passive therapy is usually easier to assess and does not require a period of learning and adjustment by the patient.

Patients who are helped by learning visualisation can carry the 'original photograph' used when learning the method. They can then use the technique not only to control pain, but any other stressful situation in which they find themselves.

Planning care which includes periods set aside for non-orthodox treatment calls for diplomacy and tact if the idea is new to a ward. Evenings and weekends are often suitable times to carry out alternative therapies. Those most useful for chronic pain relief all require a calm and if possible a quiet atmosphere, but it very much depends upon the shift system in operation, the therapist carrying out the treatment and most importantly, how the therapy fits in with the patients' overall plan of care. Acute pain would obviously be treated immediately.

Pain control using alternative therapies can be utilised before, during or after painful procedures, and can be nurse or patient controlled. If the doctor, physiotherapist or other health care worker is unfamiliar with the therapy, a few minutes explanation is usually all that is required before the procedure can go ahead.

If a patient is to have physiotherapy or osteopathy, the relaxation therapy should be implemented before any manipulation so that they derive as much benefit as possible from it by being relaxed.

Implementation of alternative therapies is sometimes difficult, the main problems usually being related to timing and the amount of detail that has gone into planning the coordination of them with the patients' daily activities and orthodox therapies.

Nurses are the main workforce on any ward and are therefore responsible for whether or not the atmosphere is therapeutic in as many ways as possible. Support for the patients by voice, sound and touch are vital to recovery (Nixon, 1989). When carrying out therapy, whichever method is used, the warmth, care and non-verbal communication involved will soothe the patient towards a sense of well-being, and a feeling of uplifting of the spirits. They are then more able to cope with pain even if it is of the same intensity (Turton, 1989; Farrow, 1990; Fisher, 1990).

Evaluation of therapy is often immediate, as in the relief experienced by patients suffering from chronic pain who have received massage and are comfortable for the first time in many months. Other therapies such as reflex zone therapy or visualisation technique may take more than one session before the patient can state positively that their pain is diminished or bearable (Turton, 1989).

As a general rule, the therapies which takes longer to learn and implement have a longer-lasting and deeper effect.

Sometimes the patient fails to derive any benefit. According to Nixon, they may be people who are suffering from what he terms 'self-defeating levels of anger or indignation, those who want to drop out and use illness as an excuse' (Nixon, 1989.) Experience has shown that they are usually those who wish to present the 'stiff upper lip' so revered by the British, as the way to behave in the face of any adversity, or those who consider alternative therapies as 'weird', 'something to do with the occult' or having sexual connotations!

The teamwork of alternative nursing

The 'team' consists of anyone who can contribute to the patients' pain control if such control consists of something – anything – other than drugs, surgery, or radiotherapy alone.

Some hospitals have pain control or palliative care teams. These lean towards orthodoxy but nowadays also refer patients to osteopaths, chiropractors, hypnotists or acupuncturists on a regular basis, and doctors have been allowed to recommend nurse 'healers' who use therapeutic touch since 1977 (Husband, 1988).

Recommendations to nurses who practice massage, reflex zone therapy, or guided imagery tend to be from doctors who have witnessed or experienced the benefits of these therapies themselves.

Britain has a very high proportion of anaesthetists to other doctors, many of them working in pain clinics (Payer, 1990). Many of the patients attending pain clinics suffer from chronic, idiopathic pain, and complementary or alternative interventions are becoming recognised by doctors as useful for such patients. The trend in pain control clinics is moving away from invasive treatments that often need to be repeated, and towards those which have an element of self-help and patient control.

Obviously the patient is the most important member of the 'team', his cooperation and enthusiasm being fundamental to the success of self-help techniques, and highly desirable although not imperative to those that use touch.

Finally, relatives can derive a great sense of satisfaction from giving, or supporting the patients through their orthodox treatments by using complementary therapies.

When a patient is experiencing pain that is all-consuming, sometimes they cannot see an end to it, and yet if it is a shared, supportive experience, it can be enriching for both (Fisher, 1990).

This is especially true of parents with sick children and of couples enduring the nightmare of an admission to ITU. When learning how to use guided imagery, visualisation and simple massage, they are usually enthusiastic students, keen to learn skills that can help in any way. The effects of their involvement are many. The patient is calmed and supported, the relative feels useful and involved and the nurses have more time for patients who do not have visitors.

Training to use alternative therapies

It must be stressed at the outset that training courses in alternative therapies are extremely varied in academic and practical content. They range from a 1 or 2 day course in simple massage to a degree in osteopathy. Aspiring practitioners should ask the following questions before embarking upon what may be a very time and money-consuming course.

1. What are the entry requirements for the course?
2. Are there any exemptions for nurses? Sometimes the anatomy and physiology lectures can be omitted although it may be a requirement that exams are taken in the subjects. This may reduce the fees.
3. How long is the course?
4. What proportion is the theory to practice?
5. How much study time is required?
6. Is there a distance-learning component?
7. When are the classes held? Weekdays or weekends?
8. How much does it cost?
9. Will the ward or department be able to support me? Some hospitals are now funding nurses to take courses.
10. Which therapy will be most valuable to the patients/for my own development and personal use?
11. Will it be possible to teach other nurses to use the method?

Following a course of training does not automatically make one proficient in using a therapy. There will be something to learn with every patient that is helped, even for those nurses who have been using these methods for decades!

Some courses are especially designed for and only accept nurses or other professionally trained people, such as physiotherapists and doctors. It may be preferable to enter this type of course, as less time will be wasted in theory lessons and there is the added advantage of a shared background and working environment where case histories can be explored under professional codes of conduct.

Nurses can use alternative therapies within their work provided that they abide by the UKCC code of conduct. If they also wish to use the therapy in a private practice then they are advised to seek individual or group, private indemnity insurance. This can be obtained for many forms of therapy against professional qualifications, and enquiries should be made before commencing a course to see whether such insurance is possible, available and that the premiums are reasonably priced.

Having undertaken a course of training and gaining experience by treating friends and relatives, the nurse can negotiate the use of the therapy for the good of her patients.

In the first instance this must always be via the doctor. This is because occasionally there are contraindications to the use of some therapies with which a nurse may be unfamiliar, for example, some types of mental illness, unstable pregnancy, epilepsy, and cardiac diseases. Having demonstrated to the doctors that alternative nursing has something positive to offer to patients, recommendations will come faster than you can cope with them!

Some health authorities have already drawn up policies regarding the practice of alternative therapies; any nurse wishing to use a non-orthodox therapy in patient care should abide by any such existing document.

It is important to note that alternative nursing interventions must always be given with the individual patients' preferences borne in mind. Some therapies, such as massage, can be seen as a very intimate and personal treatment, and patients may have completely the wrong idea about its use and implications. Clear explanations of how the therapy can help, and exactly what it entails are vital. If the nurse/therapist is already known to the patient, the patient may be more at ease with the therapy in a shorter time, but not every ward has trained therapists and they may need to come from another ward or department. The most important factor in the therapeutic relationship is that the patient trusts the therapist.

At the present time nurses are mostly using the following therapies: massage, aromatherapy, reflex zone therapy, shiatsu, guided imagery, visualisation and relaxation.

What do alternative therapies have to offer the patient in pain?

Each of the therapies has guidelines and treatment schedules that have been arrived at over many, (sometimes thousands), of years, and there are detailed textbooks and courses available for the aspiring therapist.

The following overview of the seven therapies mentioned will give the reader some indication of the background, modalities and potential value of each, although it must be appreciated that the information given here is an outline and should not replace adequate training and study of the subject.

Massage

Massage can be slow, gentle and relaxing or vigorous and stimulating. The patient may wish to have the deeper tissues manipulated or only be able to tolerate the lightest touch. Pain can be helped by either method; it depends upon their physical stamina, the type of pain and their perception of their own body fragility. (An interesting observation made recently by a staff nurse caring for AIDS patients was that they could tolerate and benefit from deep, stimulating massage until late in their terminal care.)

Acute pain which has been caused by trauma such as a sports injury will respond to moderately deep massage, but patients with chronic pain or with terminal cancer pain will appreciate a gentler method. For one young patient suffering from severe graft versus host disease, it was his only relief from the constant wearying pain in his skin and muscles. Following massage he was able to sleep. Receptors for pain and touch in the skin transmit both sensations at once, but it has been found that caring touch of less than 1 second has the power to make a person feel better (Doerhing, 1989).

Oil, talc or even the soapy water during a bed bath can be used as a lubricant for massage, the only criteria for choice being the condition of the patients' skin, and their preference for the texture of the preparation used.

Aromatherapy

Aromatherapy is fast becoming the most popular and widely practised therapy in hospitals and hospices. Nurse are implementing many of the ways in which this delightful therapy can be used. The use of aromatic essences has been known to be beneficial for thousands of years and some doctors were investigating their antibacterial effects in the last century. However, during the last 40 years there has been a rapid increase in the use of essential oils, at first by French aromatherapists, and now all over the world.

Aromatherapy centres around the use of essential oils which are distilled or obtained by other natural methods from plants. They are not only (mostly) pleasant to use because of their fragrance, but many have specific therapeutic actions, including relief of several types of pain because they each have an affinity to specific body sites.

Most aromatherapy oils are safe to use and are available from reputable suppliers by post or retail shops. However, some are better quality than others, and some are *very* costly. Occasionally patients are sensitive to them, even when correctly diluted. Nurses wishing to use aromatherapy are advised to consult a qualified aromatherapist before purchasing or using oils for the first time.

Aromatherapy can be used for pain relief by using the appropriate method. Some oils are effective because they are relaxing and evocative of happy memories, (rose, lavender, jasmine,) some have a local warming effect (black pepper, rosemary [with caution], juniper), and are useful for muscle pain.

They can be mixed into a carrier oil, such as sunflower oil, and used for massage. In vapourised form, they can relieve sinusitis, bronchitis, (eucalyptus, benzoin, ti-tree) and insomnia (neroli, sandalwood). Patients who are deprived of sleep are less able to tolerate pain, but aromatherapy affects the limbic system, and encourages relaxation.

Essential oil will evaporate when dropped onto hankies or pillows, in hot water or diluted in water and used in a room spray (rose geranium, bergamot and lavender to create a 'garden' fragrance). *The use of electric or candle heaters which also vapourise the essential oil may not be permitted by Fire Officers and they should be consulted before use.* Judicious addition to the bath water can ease aching joints and muscles (rosemary, bergamot, camomile), gentle massage and warm compresses applied to the abdomen can ease dysmenorrhoea, or constipation (camomile, marjoram [with caution], and lavender), or in a more serious case, camomile oil compresses for pancreatitis. Cold compresses can be used for headache (lavender, peppermint), or for sprains and bruises (lavender, camomile).

As a general rule, essential oils should be used as follows:

Massage oil. Mix 25–50 drops essential oil to 50 ml carrier oil. Aromatherapists often use costly base oils, but sunflower oil is quite suitable, inexpensive and is the least likely to cause an allergic reaction. Olive oil has a strong unpleasant smell of its own, and baby oil is unsuitable as essential oils will not mix with it.

Bath oil. Two to six drops of essential oil added after the bath has been filled to the correct temperature. If added when hot they will quickly evaporate and their benefits lost. The essential oil is less likely to irritate the perineum if mixed with a dessertspoonful of milk first.

Inhalation. No more than six drops of essential oil in a bowl of very hot water. Take all precautions against the patient being scalded.

Slow evaporation. Put two to three drops of essential oil onto a tissue or bedlinen. (Tissues are not suitable for children or confused patients.)

Compresses. Six to eight drops of essential oil added to cold or warm water as required, a thick cloth wrung out in it and applied to the appropriate area.

A word of caution

Aromatherapy is both a science and an art: treat it with respect and many patients will benefit from its myriad uses. *However, some essential oils are not suitable for use with pregnant, hypertensive or epileptic patients; check before treating them.*

Reflex zone therapy

Otherwise known as reflexology, when the practitioners are not trained in orthodox medicine.

Based on an ancient skill that has been developed by several cultures simultaneously, it has been formalised and used as a therapy in the west since the 1950s.

The reflexes referred to in the name are responses elicited by the therapy. Every part of the body has a reflex point on the foot, and by sedating or stimulating the reflex points a balancing and normalising of the body's functions will occur. The patient experiences a sense of well-being and relaxation which can be pain relieving in itself or can be a prelude to a session of manipulation by physiotherapy or osteopathy, useful for patients with sports injuries and long term back problems. The effect has been likened to acupuncture without needles, and many of the pressure points used are the same, but it is not invasive and, following suitable training, it is a safe method for nurses to use.

Treatments take the form of a detailed progression of thumb and fingers across the feet or hands of the patient. The practitioner is trained to feel for changes in texture and tone in the tissues of the feet. These changes coincide with sensations experienced by the patient, ranging from normal awareness of being touched to exquisite tenderness, with the feet being withdrawn from the therapist.

When areas of tenderness are found the therapy is concentrated on that area by pressure in a specific manner so that stimulation or sedation of the reflex is obtained. The therapy can be used to encourage normal functioning of organs and glands which can bring pain relief (dysmenorrhoea, constipation, irritable bowel, retention of urine), and as direct relaxation and pain control (muscle spasm, graft versus host disease, migraine). This can take the form of a series of treatments, during which the number and intensity of the painful points will diminish, or it can be used as a first aid measure to calm damaged muscles and nerves (sports injuries) and stop hiccoughs.

Relaxation

There are several methods of relaxation. They include awareness and control of breathing and contraction and relaxation of muscle groups in sequence. The method also concentrates the mind on a specific physical function and by so doing distracts the patient from his pain. The exercises can be performed in any comfortable position but the patient will be able to relax more muscle groups if lying on a soft but supporting surface. Always support painful or weak joints and muscles with pillows before beginning the exercises (Cook, 1986; Levin *et al.*, 1987; Sims, 1987; McCaffery, 1990).

The patient may wish to use additional methods such as visualisation, music (Cook, 1986; Fisher, 1990), or a particular configuration and colour of light. Quiet, non-vocal classical music and low, pink or peach coloured light is very comforting.

Guided imagery

Guided imagery, and to a lesser extent, visualisation, make use of methods of distraction that most small children are familiar with, but adults fail to develop. The methods are now used extensively for cancer patients to help them with the various painful experiences they may have, from investigations to terminal pain (Simonton *et al.*, 1978; Sims, 1987; Moorey and Greer, 1989).

Initially this will have to be nurse-led, but soon many patients can take themselves on imaginary journeys to their favourite real or fictional places.

The method involves concentration on breathing and relaxation of muscles but also distracts the mind through memory or imagination. A suitable mixture of photographs, music, sounds such as birdsong, and aromas aid the patients' imagination with this method.

Sometimes they have happy, peaceful memories that they wish to think about. These

evoke the most powerful and useful visualisations, and they can be repeated at will, simply by memory or by using the 'props' mentioned.

The main advantage of the method is that the components can be manipulated to be totally positive, wheras some distractions such as television, books, or radio can inadvertently interject poignant, or unhappy memories which would destroy the pain-relieving effect (Hendricks and Willis 1975; Keable, 1989; Moorey and Greer, 1989).

Visualisation

This is the most difficult of all the therapies described because, although it is initially nurse-led, the power of the patients' imagination is the most important factor and it is his belief in the method which will decide on its efficacy. It is a controversial method and should not be used for patients who also have serious psychiatric problems such as schizophrenia or manic-depressive psychosis. The patient should not be led to believe that he will be 'cured' of his disease (Moorey and Greer, 1989).

The method can be used in two ways. the first is by asking the patient to describe his disease in his own imagination; he then describes how he sees his orthodox therapy and his natural body defences fighting the disease. Some proponents believe that the more bizarre the images, the more powerful the effect (Simonton *et al.*, 1978). Children, and some adults, find it useful to draw or paint their images.

The second style, more useful for patients with pain, is to ask them to imagine the pain as a colour. When they have described the 'colour' of their pain, they then imagine the colour fading or changing to another colour that they imagine to be less painful. Finally, they imagine it to be moving to another part of their body, usually from a central organ or a joint out to the periphery, and that it is changing colour to the 'less painful' colour as it moves. Pain is usually perceived to be less important and threatening when it is less central. If the patient is very skilled at using his imagination he will even be able to visualise the pain 'flowing out' of his fingers or toes.

Experience with this method has shown that it is enhanced by the added distraction of massage of the feet or hands and by the use of quiet music.

Shiatsu

A traditional Japanese therapy based on promoting the body's own powers of healing. Pressure points are used but in this case, the fingers, elbows, knees and feet can be used to apply it. There are many levels of skill, ranging from everyday first aid to high levels of Oriental diagnosis and healing. It is a powerful relaxation and pain-reducing therapy that can be utilised in any situation. The patient remains clothed, no oils are used and treatment can be carried out with the patient lying in bed or on a carpeted floor.

Nurses as therapists

Nurses carrying out these therapies need to feel confident in their use. In order that their concentration is at optimal level they should undertake some form of relaxation themselves. Therapies should never be carried out under stressful conditions; the practitioner must feel at ease with the therapy and herself. Kreiger describes it as, 'a mental state of being centred – a place of quietude within oneself where one can feel truly integrated, unified and focused' (Kreiger, cited Jurgens *et al.*, 1987).

Which patients can benefit from these methods?

There are few restrictions to the use of the therapies described in this chapter. Nurses undertaking courses of training will be informed of the restrictions placed upon the therapy that they are studying. They also have their orthodox training which will alert them to potential risks for the patient. For example, patients with a history of deep vein thrombosis should not be massaged, and patients undergoing chemotherapy should not have aromatherapy if they are vomiting, as they will always retain a negative memory of the fragrance, and may even vomit the next time they smell it!

All nurses like to make people feel comfortable, and because it enhances job satisfaction there are now nurses in every type of ward using these gentle interventions.

Where do we go from here?

There can be no doubt that anxiety and feeling vulnerable make the experience of pain worse (Fisher, 1990). It has been proposed that children should learn relaxation techniques in school as part of their general education. It could reduce the amount of stress-related disease in the population and would also enable the individual experiencing pain to have a coping mechanism upon which he could draw in times of crisis (Nixon, 1989).

Offers of alternative nursing are very seldom refused, patients enjoying the 'low tech' nature of the treatments which gives them time to be with their nurse under relaxed circumstances (Turton, 1989).

Practitioners of alternative and complementary therapies in the United Kingdom are allowed to do so under Common Law, by which anyone can provide any service that is not deemed illegal under the Act. Much of the freedom that we enjoy as independent practitioners in the UK is denied our European counterparts unless they are also doctors.

At present, there are no ratified UK examinations for the majority of complementary therapies, the exceptions being chiropractic and osteopathy. Other degrees and diplomas awarded are not yet recognised by orthodox practitioners and the State as a licence to practice, and there is little substantiated research to support claims of efficacy. Since 1992, some universities and the Royal College of Nursing offer the BSc in Nursing which has options of hypnotherapy, massage and aromatherapy in the 3rd year. These academic and practical skills-based options allow nurses to use these therapy skills within their care as nurses, but as they may not call themselves masseurs, hypnotherapists or aromatherapists, this maintains the academic credibility of the course content, based on the amount of time spent on these three sections.

There are no regulating bodies except those self-appointed by interested groups. There is no umbrella organisation that controls or sets standards, and for the concerned member of the public who wishes to consult a therapist, their only means of knowing whether the practitioner is safe, and has a standard of ethics, is to go to one who is already deemed 'safe' by the state, i.e. a nurse, physiotherapist or doctor, and preferably by personal recommendation.

In 1986 an investigation into alternative therapies was carried out by the British Medical Association. They condemned almost everything except the few therapies that could 'prove' effectiveness, e.g. osteopathy. The resultant report was concerned with the exploitation of a vulnerable public as there are so few safeguards against charlatans. Their main concern, and rightly so, was the lack of proven efficacy of treatments, and standards of training in their use (Penson, 1989; Hargreaves, 1990). The point is accepted by those who practise alternative and complementary therapies, and yet orthodox medicine has its tragedies and failures caused by inadequate research (Martin, 1989; McCeoin, 1990). A complete reversal of view has occurred. In 1993, the BMA made recommendations regarding the general public choosing a complementary practitioner (BMA, Report on Complementary Therapies, 1993). These included:

- Being a member of a recognized state registered group, i.e. doctors, nurses etc.
- The group should have rights of discipline and sanctions against their members as a professional body.
- That the practitioner carries indemnity insurance.

No single system has all the answers. Unfortunately the Government has stated that it does not wish to enter into a dialogue upon the subject. Their advisors support the orthodox because they have no experience of anything else, and so that is the stand that the Government takes (Thomas, 1990).

Alternative and complementary practitioners must therefore stand together and set their own standards and research (Sharps, 1989; Stacey, 1989). Hostility between Government and the alternative practitioners and indeed, between the practitioners themselves will only produce one loser – the patient.

The enthusiasm and continued support by a public who are often willing to pay for treatments, in addition to their National Health subscriptions, cannot be ignored – and neither, it seems, will the nurses!

'There are those who make things happen, those who watch, and those who wonder what happened'

John Newber

References

Berliner, H. S. (1984) Scientific medicine since Flexner. In: *Alternative Medicines* (ed. J. W. Salmon), Tavistock Publications, New York

Cook, J. D. (1986) Music as an intervention in the oncology setting. *Cancer Nursing*, **9** (1)

Dickinson, E. (1957) Poems by Emily Dickinson. Little Brown and Co., Boston

Doehring, K. M. (1989) Relieving pain through touch. *Advancing Clinical Care*, **Sept/Oct**, 32–33

Eardly, A. (1989) Changing the agenda – the role of the cancer self-help group. In: *Changing Ideas in Health Care* (eds D. Seedhouse and A. Cribb), John Wiley, Chichester

Farrow, J. (1990) Massage therapy and nursing care. *Nursing Standard*, **14**, No. 17

Fisher, E. (1990) *Behavioural Sciences for Nurses – Towards Project 2000*, G. Duckworth Co., London

Hargreaves, A. (1990) Education – a way through the maze. *Journal of Alternative and Complementary Medicine*, **Nov**, 23–25

Hendricks, G. and Willis, R. (1975) *The Centering Book – Awareness Activities for Children and Adults to Relax the Body and Mind*, Prentice Hall, New York

Husband, L. (1981) The therapeutic touch: a basis for excellence. In *Recent Advances in Nursing* 21, Longman Group UK Ltd, pp 25–42

Jurgens, A. *et al*. (1987) Therapeutic touch as a nursing intervention. *Holistic Nursing Practice*, **2(1)**, 1–13

Levin, R. F. *et al*. (1987) Nursing management of post-operative pain: use of relaxation techniques with female cholecystectomy patients. *Journal of Advanced Nursing*, **12**, 463–472

Keable, D. (1989) *The Management of Anxiety*, Churchill Livingstone, Edinburgh

MacCeoin, D. (1990) The myth of clinical trials. *Journal of Alternative and Complementary Medicine*, **Aug**, 15–18

Marquardt, H. (1983) *Reflex Zone Therapy of the Feet*, Thorsons Ltd, Wellingborough

Martin, S. (1989) Who's protecting who from what? *Journal of Alternative and Complementary Medicine*, **Aug**, 21–22

McCaffrey, M. (1990) Nursing approaches to non-pharmacological pain. *International Journal of Nursing Stuties*, **27** (1), 1–5

Moorey, S. and Greer, S. (1989) *Psychological Therapy for Patients with Cancer: a New Approach*, Heinemann Medical, Oxford

Nixon, P. G. F. (1989) Human functions and the heart. In: *Changing Ideas in Health Care* (eds D. Seedhouse and A. Cribb) John Wiley, Chichester

Payer, L. (1990) *Medicine and Culture*. Victor Golancz Ltd, London

Penson, J. and Holloway, I. (1989) Fringe benefits:

alternative medicine in patient care. *Senior Nurse*, **9(8)**, 9–10

Sharps, W. (1989) Taking a positive line. *Journal of Alternative and Complementary Medicine*, **May**, 18–19

Sims, S. E. R. (1987) Relaxation training as a technique for helping patients cope with the experience of cancer: a selective review of the literature. *Journal of Advanced Nursing*, **12**, 583–591

Simonton, S. *et al.* (1978) *Getting Well Again*, Bantam Books, New York

Stacey, M. (1989) Alternatives should negotiate their own research terms. *Journal of Alternative and Complementary Medicine*, **May**, 35

Thomas, R. (1990) Sorry, but we'd rather not know. *Journal of Alternative and Complementary Medicine*, **Dec**, 14–18

Thompson, I. E. *et al.* (1988) *Nursing Ethics*, 2nd edn, Churchill Livingstone, Edinburgh

Tisserard, R. (1985) *Aromatherapy for Everyone*. C. W. Dawie and Co.

Turton, P. (1989) Touch me, feel me, heal me. *Nursing Times*, **85(19)**, 42–44

Wormood, V. A. (1990) *The Fragrant Pharmacy*. Macmillan, London

13

Physiotherapy for the relief of pain

Robert A. Charman

Introduction

This chapter is concerned with the various ways in which physiotherapy may help to relieve acute and chronic pain. The methods discussed are those employed by physiotherapists whose courses and qualifications entitle them to be state registered and become members of the Chartered Society of Physiotherapy. These are the physiotherapists that nurses meet in hospitals, pain clinics, health centres, industry, and domicilary practice. This distinction is made because anyone may call themselves a physiotherapist, whether or not they have any qualifications, but no one may call themselves a state registered physiotherapist (SRP), or chartered physiotherapist (MCSP), unless they have successfully completed a 3 or 4 year graduate diploma or degree course in physiotherapy at an approved higher educational establishment.

Physical therapy procedures fall into four main categories:

1. Electrical therapy
2. Massage and manipulative procedures
3. Exercise therapy, including hydrotherapy
4. Relaxation procedures

Each category contains certain techniques that can be used to combat pain. The first two categories are comprised of techniques that are *applied to* a patient who passively receives them and subjectively assesses their effectiveness in relieving specific aching or pain. The third and fourth categories require active cooperation from the patient and are therefore *applied with* the patient who, again, subjectively assesses the resulting degree of pain relief.

Physical therapy may be applied either to help cure, or alleviate, the tissue source of pain, or to reduce the intensity of pain which the patient is experiencing. In many cases the two aims are combined in that treating the pain source simultaneously activates central nervous system pain gates.

Physical therapy, however, cannot be separated from the physiotherapist, any more than nursing procedures can be separated from nurse practitioners. Physiotherapists, like nurses, interact with each patient to form a personal bond. This therapeutic bonding is extremely important where pain relieving procedures do not directly anaesthetise pain endings.

An accurately given local anaesthetic will be just as effective in blocking the nerve whether given by a person or a robot. It does not matter whether the dentist is liked, or disliked by the patient, the injected gum will be just as numb because the pharmacological effect of procaine, or its equivalent, on pain endings is the major physiological variable. This is not true of those pain relieving measures which obtain a variable degree of pain relief depending upon how well they activate central nervous system pain suppression mechanisms. These are inextricably linked to personal experience of pain and mind/brain interactions, so a major variable is the mind to mind interaction between the physiotherapist, or nurse, and the patient. If it is one of mutual dislike, however well disguised, the CNS bias will be set against adequate pain relief as the procedure is seen by the patient as an extension of the disliked physiotherapist or nurse. If the mind to mind interaction is one of constructive rapport then the CNS bias will favour, or enhance, the pain relief derived from the therapy precisely because it is experienced as an integral extension of the liked therapist. This must never be forgotten because it is often the key to success. Physiotherapy, like nursing, is more than the sum of its textbook procedures.

Pain gate theory

The working hypothesis adopted in this chapter is that the central nervous system contains an ascending series of pain gating mechanisms, from the spinal cord, through midbrain and thalamus, to conscious limbic system and cerebral cortex levels. These mechanisms can be activated by ascending and/or descending control systems to both suppress incoming and ascending pain impulses and reduce the intensity of consciously experienced pain. The neurophysiological mechanisms involved are discussed elsewhere in this book and will receive only brief reference in this account. Throughout this chapter the term 'pain pathway' or 'pain impulses' will be used as it is consistent with the term 'pain gate' which is used to discuss pain relief at all levels of the CNS. It is, however, very important to distinguish between *nociceptor impulses and pathways*, and *pain impulses and pathways*. The *nociceptor system* extends from the nociceptor endings in the tissues to the thalamus. It is *non-conscious neural activity*. Once these pathways are active between the thalamus and the receiving limbic system and cerebral cortex they enter *conscious experience* as *pain*. As long as this distinction is held in mind then the shorthand of *pain system* can be used.

Physiotherapy as a whole

It cannot be overstressed that whatever physiotherapy treatment, or combination of treatments, are employed, they are only decided upon after a full and careful case history has been taken, a full physiotherapy examination performed, and treatment objectives decided upon in full cooperation with the patient within the overall context of medical care. From this point onwards the treatment programme is planned and initiated, and therefore modified, according to patient response and consequent change of treatment objectives. This must be borne in mind throughout the rest of this chapter as no one type of treatment, in itself, is automatically prescriptive for a given diagnosis.

Physiotherapy will be discussed under the following three headings:

1. *Physiotherapy modalities.* That is, the range of pain relieving techniques employed by the physiotherapist.
2. *The physiotherapist as therapy.* Outlining the interaction of physiotherapist and patient.
3. *The physiotherapy synthesis.* Integrating the physiological effects of the modalities and the psychological effects of the physiotherapist into a model of a pain relieving whole. In saying this it must be emphasised that physiotherapy is therapeutically open ended in that it takes place within the greater therapeutic whole of the medical, nursing and allied professional context.

Physiotherapy modalities

Electrical therapy

Electrotherapy involves the application of electrical currents, electrical or magnetic fields, ultrasound, infra-red radiation, ultraviolet radiation and low level laser beams. By tradition it also includes cold therapy, using ice or icecold packs, and hot therapy, using wax or hot packs. Only brief comment on electrical theory will be given as what is required here is an understanding of what each modality does, when it is used, and how the physiotherapist uses it. TENS will be discussed first as it is probably the most widely used application of electricity to relieve pain

Transcutaneous electrical nerve stimulation (TENS)

As the name implies, a TENS unit applies an electrical current to the skin to stimulate the sensory cutaneous nerve endings. The TENS unit supplies such stimuli as a series of tiny electrical impulses to the skin that feels like a buzzing, pricking sensation.

Figure 13.1 shows a typical TENS unit in use for back pain. It is about the same size as a personal radio/cassette and can be carried in a large pocket, or a handbag, or attached to a belt as shown. It is battery powered and fitted with controls for intensity of stimulus, pulse width, pulse rate, and choice of continuous pulse stimulation or short bursts of pulse stimuli with a rest period between each burst.

The intensity of each tiny pulse is in thousandths of an ampere (0–50 mA), the frequency

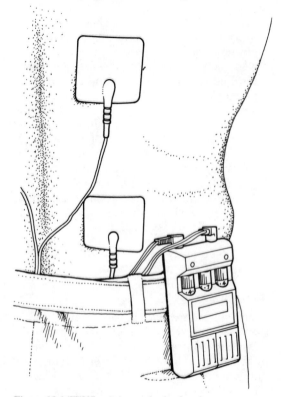

Figure 13.1 TENS unit in use for back pain

of pulses range from 2 to 100 per second (2–100 Hz), the width, or duration, of each pulse is a few millionths of a second (10–120 μs). Intermittent bursts of several dozen pulses last for brief intervals with a corresponding rest period in between each burst, rather like a sensory 'bzzz bzzz bzzz' effect.

Some patients find that they obtain most pain relief by feeling a continuous sensation, others find that intermittent bursts of sensation is more effective, and others, again, regularly change between the two types of sensation as they find the sensory change enhances pain relief.

Application of TENS

TENS units may be fitted with either one socket (single channel) for the plug of a pair of leads, or two sockets (twin channel) for two pairs of leads as shown in Figure 13.1. These insulated leads end in small jack terminals for the attachment of carbon rubber electrodes, either 5 × 5 cm (small), or 10 × 10 cm in size, which conduct the electricity to the skin across their whole

surface. These are attached to the skin, using an electrically conducting gel, by tape strips or adhesive patches. Some electrodes are self adhesive. The procedure is similar to applying ECG electrodes.

When the TENS unit is switched on the output is slowly turned up. At a certain intensity the patient feels a faint prickling, vibratory sensation under the electrodes. This becomes stronger as the output is increased until the sensation is so strong that it can be uncomfortable. At this intensity motor nerves can be stimulated and underlying muscles may show a flickering contraction. This is the most intense that it can feel. There is no risk of electrical burns because between each tiny pulse the current runs in the opposite direction. This prevents any electrochemical reactions building up in the skin.

Probable mechanisms of pain relief

TENS probably relieves pain by several mechanisms. Because ordinary sensory nerves, carrying touch, for example, are more sensitive to electrical stimulation than pain endings they are selectively stimulated. They also conduct much faster and their concentrated impulses arrive at the posterior horn faster, and in larger numbers, than the pain impulses, unless, of course, the pain source is particularly active. This very localised skin sensation then acts in two ways. In the poserior spinal horn, or sensory nuclei of some cranial nerves, this enhanced ordinary sensation strongly inhibits the activity of spinal cord pain neurones whose axons ascend towards the brain. The sensory stimulus, in effect, acts to close the pain gate by nociceptor inhibition. Because the patient can feel TENS sensation under the electrodes, they act as localised sources of skin sensation that demand conscious awareness of themselves in competition with the sources of pain. As the brain selectively concentrates upon skin sensation, rather than deeper sensation, TENS helps to close the conscious gate experience of pain. TENS stimuli may also effect some pain gate closing in the thalamus, where pain endings and normal sensation converge before final distribution to the cortex of the brain. Here they may act in a similar way to gate closure in the spinal horn. Some researchers think that TENS may stimulate the release of extra pain relieving endorphins when applied at a frequency of about 2 per second, especially if what is known as a 'Lo-Tens' unit is used which delivers more intense, sharper pulses.

What sort of pain is best relieved by TENS?

TENS seems particularly helpful in relieving rheumatic type aching in joints and muscles, back and neck pain, postoperative pain, amputation stump pain, metastatic pain, neuralgia and the acutely unpleasant pain sometimes experienced following damage to peripheral nerve or plexus. It has been used with such pain relieving success during childbirth that a special 'obstetric TENS' unit is available with a short extension lead ending in a press button for the mother to hold. As each contraction builds up the mother increases intensity and presses the button to change the pulses from continuous, to pulsed, and back again as desired. This varying sensory response increases the measure of pain relief. The electrodes are applied to the lower back. This pain relieving effect during labour implies that it could be very helpful in painful gynaecological conditions such as menstrual onset pain. A recent, and intriguing, case study on the use of TENS for the treatment of intractable leg pain in a patient suffering from multiple sclerosis (Pert, 1991) not only found considerable relief from pain, but a marked improvement in gait. The combined effect considerably improved the patient's quality of life and personal independence.

Electrode positioning

As figure 13.1 shows, TENS usually work best when electrodes are placed around the painful area with one electrode proximal to the pain and the other distal. If there are four electrodes then they can all be placed around the painful area, or two sources of pain can be treated simultaneously. When the source of pain is deep, as in arthritis of the hip joint, electrodes can be placed in front and behind so that the painful area is in the crossfire of the field.

TENS treatment control

For the first one or two treatments the physiotherapist carefully places the electrodes to discover which positions obtain maximum pain relief and the most effective pulse intensity is

noted. The patient is carefully instructed in the whole procedure of electrode application, use of the TENS unit, and care and maintenance of the apparatus. Once both sides are agreed that everything is understood, the patient uses the unit unsupervised with regular checks. TENS can be used on the wards, in the outpatient departments, at home and at work. The patient is told to use the *minimum* sensation that obtains the most pain relief. This allows some latitude for increasing intensity if there is any habituation to the TENS stimulus.

A TENS treatment programme is decided according to each patient's experience of pain relief. Some find that 20–30 minute sessions, 2 or 3 times a day, is sufficient. Some find that continuous sensation for several hours, or even all day, is best. This sounds vague until it is remembered that the central pain gate mechanisms of each patient respond to differing variables. When the electrodes are removed they can leave red skin patches behind. These are caused by local capillary vasodilatation to the sensory stimulus and are quite harmless. They slowly fade away to normal colour.

TENS and pain relief

The use of TENS for pain relief has generated a considerable literature, with reports ranging from individual case studies to controlled trials. The placebo effect is a strong confounding element, and the drug versus placebo double blind clinical trial is not easily applied to a therapy that relies for its effect on localised sensory stimulus. Overall, the literature indicates that between 30 and 70% of patients experience effective pain relief. A recent in-depth study (Johnson *et al.*, 1991a) of 179 chronic pain sufferers who had been using TENS for more than 3 months produced some interesting findings. Analysis of pain scale records showed that 79 patients (47%) experienced 50%, or more, reduction in pain during the hours of TENS application, including 26 patients (15.5%) who obtained complete relief. Twenty-three patients (13.7%) obtained no apparent relief but still found TENS valuable on the basis that 'TENS does not reduce my pain, but it distracts, or takes my mind off it'. Most patients experienced a steady reduction of pain to base level during the first 30 minutes of application, and a slow return of pain within an hour after switching the TENS unit off. Most patients used TENS for several hours each day, and some used it for up to 60 hours per week. No correlation was found between personality type and degree of reported pain relief, so no assumption of TENS response should ever be made by the professional before application.

In a related study Johnson *et al.* (1991b) found no particular relationship between the pulse frequencies, or pulse patterns, used and the diagnosed cause of pain, or the anatomical site of pain. In other words, osteoarthritic pain, for example, is not specifically relieved by any particular frequency compared to any other. Generally speaking, pulse frequencies between 20 and 80 Hz seemed to be the most effective, but a consistent finding was that each patient determinedly searched for the frequency which gave them the greatest personal relief of pain. In effect, every TENS user 'tunes in' to the frequency which is most effective in operating their own pain gating mechanisms.

An editorial review in the *Lancet* (1991) of the literature on the use of TENS for chronic low back pain concluded that 'TENS can produce some relief in 30% of patients with intractable back pain' and that 'this is an impressive therapeutic result, achieved at little risk'. It therefore advocated that it makes good sense to offer supervised TENS therapy for such patients.

It cannot be overemphasised that much depends upon the patient's understanding and intelligent use of the TENS unit. Some people are simply frightened of electricity and worry constantly in case it goes wrong. Electrode application is deceptively simple, which means that it is often done badly, and lack of adequate pain relief is then blamed upon TENS rather than poor technique. But, when properly explained, understood, and applied, it does give very effective relief in many cases. TENS is always worth trying because there is no way of predicting who might be obtain considerable pain relief or, at least, pain distraction benefit.

Dangers and contraindications

There are a few. It is considered unwise to use TENS on patients with pacemakers or who have heart disease or cardiac arrhythmias, just in case of interaction with the TENS frequencies. It must not be used on skin areas where the patient has no sensation, nor directly upon open wounds or sores. Some patients become allergic to some contact gels. The apparatus must be kept scrupulously clean, the leads and contacts must be regularly checked, and the batteries fully charged. Commonsense maintenance and precautions are the key to hazard free use and maximum effectiveness.

Thermal therapy

Everyone is familiar with the warmth of an electric fire and cooking by microwave. Heating tissues to a comfortable warmth can achieve several useful objectives as follows:

a. Stimulating the thermoreceptors in the skin, and possibly those in the deep tissues, helps close spinal cord pain gates, thus reducing the intensity of pain transmission. The conscious feeling of warmth tends to suppress awareness of pain, and both psychologically and reflexly relaxes uncomfortable muscle tone and spasm.

b. Raising tissue temperature accelerates metabolic processes. This helps to improve local circulation by vasodilatation, assists in the removal of oedema and metabolic waste products, and accelerate healing and repair processes. It also increases phagocyte and other white cell efficiency in combating local infection and removing dead cell debris.

c. Warming connective tissue and scar tissue to around 42–45 °C temporarily reduces its viscosity and tensile strength, thus allowing therapeutic stretching of painful contracted tissues to be more effective. Warming joints also reduces the viscosity of synovial fluid and this helps to reduce painful stiffness during movement and increase joint range.

What type of pain is most relieved by heat?

The deep aching pain and muscle discomfort of many rheumatic conditions, backache and neck pain, and post-traumatic pain arising from scarring and adhesions are typical examples where increased warmth will at least attain temporary pain relief. This use of warmth is almost instinctive. Anyone suffering from the generalised aching heralding the onset of a heavy cold, or influenza, or the localised joint and limb aching of arthritis, automatically applies warmth in the form of hot baths or showers, sitting near the fire, or using a hot water bottle or heating pad.

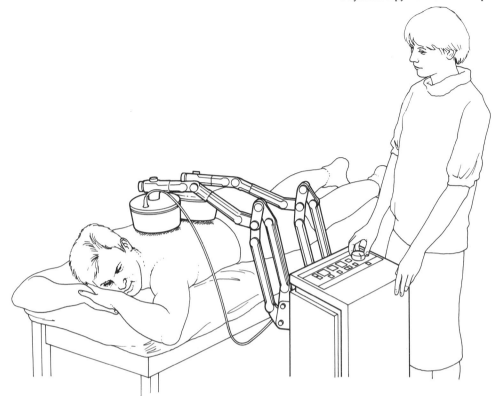

Figure 13.2 Short wave diathermy

Heating by electrical energy

Various methods of heating by electrical and magnetic field energy will now be discussed. It is a standard legal requirement that every patient who is to receive heat treatment is first blind tested by the application of hot and cold test tubes to the skin of the area to be treated. This is done to ensure that their temperature perception is normal. All patients must be legally informed that excess heat can cause burns and must signal their understanding of this fact. This may seem embarrassingly obvious, but some patients have tolerated burning discomfort in the conviction that they are, for example, 'burning the arthritis out'. You do not know what beliefs a particular patient brings with them.

Short wave diathermy (SWD)

Shortwave diathermy is always written in the treatment records as 'SWD'. This apparatus uses high frequency electric or magnetic fields which are applied to the patient. Figure 13.2 shows a typical unit in use for back pain. The frequency is close to FM radio and is fixed by international law at 27 million, 120 thousand cycles per second (27.12 MHz). This means that the atoms and molecules of any object placed within the field, including tissues, will be electrically oscillated one way or the other as they are alternatively attracted or repulsed by the changing negative and positive charges on the electric plates. They oscillate in a similar way when a 27.12 MHz alternating magnetic field is passed through them. This electrically oscillating energy is superimposed upon the normal random movements of molecules and atoms and the absorbed energy is converted to heat. When you consider that the molecules actually oscillate backwards and forwards some 52 million times a second, changing direction at each half cycle, it is not surprising that the resulting molecular 'friction' creates heat. The free field power applied to the tissues can be up to 400 watts. Normally the patient starts to feel the warmth at about 80–100 watts as indicated on the output meters.

Reasons for choosing SWD

Use is made of the fact that both the electrical field and/or the magnetic field radiating from the electrodes passes *through* the tissue bulk between the electrodes, and the field energy heats all of the tissues it passes through. Therefore heating can be obtained at depth, for example, through the hip joint, thigh muscles, knee, shoulder or wherever. This means that the source of pain can be directly treated. It also means that tense muscles around a painful area can be directly warmed and relaxed.

Treatment frequency

Treatment can vary between twice daily to twice weekly, depending upon the condition and the availability of the patient. Acute conditions receive short, 5-minute doses of very mild heating. More chronic conditions receive much warmer heating for between 20 and 30 minutes, by which time the tissues within the field have reached the desired temperature.

Dangers of SWD

Like any heat treatment, if the tissues get too hot they may receive a burn. This is more difficult to detect with SWD as the burn may be in the insulating fat tissue which has become too hot. Therefore the applications of SWD requires great care. The patient *must* have normal heat sensation, *must* hold a safety switch which can turn the SWD off, and *must* clearly understand that 'if it gets too hot it could cause a burn'. During treatment the physiotherapist makes regular enquiry as to the degree of warmth, and at the end of treatment the local pinkness of the skin resulting from heating is checked. Because SWD fields concentrate around metal they should not be applied through tissues with metal implants, such as joint arthroplasties or the screws, wires, plates and nails of orthopaedic surgery.

Pulsed SWD

Like TENS, high frequency energy can be 'chopped up' into a series of pulse bursts with an interval in between each burst. Applying an electric or magnetic field in short, repeated, bursts is a method whereby peak field intensities of up to 1000 watts (1 kW) can be applied without much actual heating, as the heat gener-ated by each pulse disappears during the next interval. The pulse frequency can be varied between 15 and 200 times per second. Many physiotherapists find that pulsed SWD is very effective in reducing the pain and swelling of acute injuries and it is very widely used in outpatient departments and wards treating early trauma patients. Treatment times are around 10–30 minutes per session, and can be repeated ×2 or ×3 times daily.

Infra-red radiation

Many shops sell small heat lamps which rely on their effect by generating infrared radiation (IRR) waves which are invisible because they lie below the deep red that the eye can see. The energy of IRR is completely absorbed in the skin and underlying dermis to a depth of about 5 mm, so it is a superficial heat. IRR can be applied to local areas, such as the shoulder or knee, or to large areas, such as the back. Its pain relieving effect is achieved by concentrated stimulation of thermoreceptors in the skin. It causes superficial vasodilatation and erythema which may reduce deeper congestion by shunting the blood to the surface. With time, and a large treated area such as the back, the whole body temperature can slowly rise as the warmed blood is distributed throughout the body. While the IRR is, itself, invisible, most lamps use one or more red bulbs as the source of IRR, as this both indicates that the lamp is working and red, in itself, is a comforting colour associated with warmth.

When is IRR used?

Usually for chronic aches and pains, especially of small or superficial joints, or so-called fibrositis in the superficial back muscles. Treatment usually lasts about 15–20 minutes and can be repeated daily to ×2 weekly. Localised mild heating of pressure sores and slowly healing wounds can accelerate healing if the underlying circulation system can adequately meet the increased metabolic demand.

Dangers and contraindications

IRR poses no dangers if all the precautions mentioned under SWD are observed. Deep metal implants are not affected as the rays do not go deep, but surface metal is a contraindication, and any eczematous areas are contraindicated. Sustained local heating by home heat lamps, or sitting too close to the fire, will cause unsightly brown mottling of the skin which rarely fades away.

Microwave diathermy

Microwave (MW) has a lower frequency than IRR and a wavelength measured in cms. In this case the wavelength (12.25 cm) and frequency are fixed by law. Microwaves are part of the radar frequency band and, like IRR, are absorbed by water and tissue fluids. MW diathermy is applied by an aerial mounted inside a reflector which directs the beam in the desired direction. It penetrates more deeply than IRR, up to about 2.5–5 cm, so can directly reach deeper structures. Although a very effective heating agent it is much less used now because of unresolved concern that it is just possible that cell chromosome damage may occur on absorption. Patients wear goggles to ensure that it does not penetrate the eyes. Indications for use are as for IRR and, on purely practical terms, it is the halfway compromise in penetration between IRR and effective SWD. Dangers and contraindications are similar to SWD and IRR.

Ultrasound therapy

Figure 13.3 shows ultrasound (US) therapy in the treatment of a knee. Inside the round metal applicator held by the therapist a flat 0.5 inch slice of crystal is stuck to the inside surface of the metal treatment face that is in contact with the patient. Two electrodes are attached to the crystal so that when an alternating current is transmitted along the cable and across the crystal its flat surfaces become alternatively negative and positive. These electrical changes rhythmically distort the crystal structure so that it vibrates at the same frequency as the electrical frequency. In other words, the alternating electrical energy becomes converted, or transduced, to mechanical energy vibrating at the same rate. The metal face is therefore vibrated by the attached crystal. If this face is then pressed in airtight contact against a surface, such as the skin, then a vibrating beam of invisible ultrasound energy will pass into the tissues. This US beam will mechanically vibrate

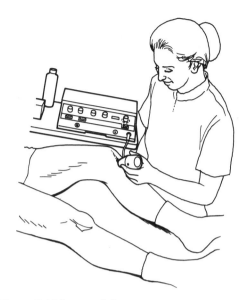

Figure 13.3 Ultrasound therapy

the tissue molecules as it passes through them, and is absorbed by them. This vibrational energy will not only be converted to tissue heat but will also have non-heating physiological effects such as increasing membrane transport.

What frequencies are used?

The answer to this question may be more meaningful if the relationship of ultrasound to ordinary sound is first discussed. Sound is mechanical acoustic energy consisting of a backwards and forwards vibration of whatever structure, or medium, it is passing through, be it air, water, rock, metal or body tissues.

The lowest note that can be heard is between 20 and 30 cycles a second (30 Hz). Low organ notes at this frequency can be both heard and felt as body vibrations. Human speech is around 1000 cycles (1 kHz), and the highest sound that can be heard, such as a mouse squeak, is abut 20 000 cycles (20 kHz). Ultrasound frequencies, meaning 'beyond sound', continue from there. Cats and dogs can hear up to 40kHz, and bats navigate without injury, and catch insects, by emitting 60–100 kHz squeaks and listening for the echo. If the frequency keeps rising above 100 kHz, air is less and less able to transmit it, and it can only be carried by fluids and solids. At these higher frequencies it can easily be focussed into a narrow beam.

Therapeutic US frequencies range between 750 thousand cycles (750 kHz) and 3 million cycles (3 MHz) a second. These frequencies can be imagined as leaving the US metal treatment face like a vibrating torch beam. The energy applied to the tissues is measured in watts per sq cm, and ranges from 0.1 to 3 watts.

Physiological effects of US

US provides a vibratory 'micro-massage' of the tissues as it passes through them and this tends to sedate nerve endings. The vibratory energy is somehow used by healing tissue cells to stimulate repair processes, and it assists reabsorption of exudate and oedema by the local lymphatic and venous circulation. This may be because the vibrating tissue membranes become more porous. If applied as a continuous beam the resulting temperature rise also increases cellular processes and reduces viscosity.

Depth of US beam penetration

This depends upon how rapidly it is absorbed. In general terms, its useful energy penetrates about 10–15 cm. It is more absorbed by fibrous and collagenous tissue than wet tissue such as muscle, and very quickly absorbed by periosteum and bone. When US passes through media of different density, say from fascia to muscle, then some of its energy is reflected from the interface in the same way that light is reflected from glass. This is the basis of ultrasound body scans used, for example, to image the baby during pregnancy.

Application of US

The US head is usually applied in direct contact with the skin, using a coupling gel to eliminate any air bubbles and ensure good transmission. When water is used as the coupling medium, mainly for hands and feet, the US head is immersed with the hand or foot in the warm water container and held about 2 cm from the skin. During treatment the head is moved in small circling movements across the area so that all of the injured tissues receive the US and no area gets too hot. Like TENS and SWD, US can be applied as a continuous beam or 'chopped up' into pulses. When applied continuously care has to be taken that the tissues do

not get too hot. When applied as pulsed US this danger is averted. Generally speaking, US is applied for between 3 and 10 minutes per treatment, depending upon severity of injury and area to be treated, and repeated daily in acute conditions and about ×3 times a week in more chronic conditions.

Therapeutic use of US

US can be used for localised acute or chronic trauma, for example, following an acute ankle sprain. US can be applied in small pulsed doses to assist reabsorption of haematoma and oedema and accelerate healing. In late injury, where tissues are stiff with thickened adhesions and scarring, then continuous US can be used to warm and soften tissue and aid late resolution. Either way, pain is reduced. US may help pressure sore and gravitational ulcer healing, again reducing pain, and some patients have found that pulsed US reduces amputation stump pain when applied over the painful neuromas. Absorption of muscle haematomas is aided by applying the US peripherally around the edge and working towards the centre at each treatment.

Dangers and contraindications

Very few. It is considered unwise to apply US to the lumbar or abdominal area once pregnancy has been confirmed in case of embryo, or fetal damage. This is more a protection against possible litigation than any real known risk. The US scans in obstetric use very much weaker beams than therapeutic US and seem completely safe.

Wax bath

This is a treatment with a long history. In essence, several kilos of paraffin wax is heated in a wax bath unit until it melts like dripping candle wax. Once fully melted at between 110 and 120°F, the patient's hand or foot can be repeatedly dipped into the wax until a thick coating of wax is applied. Alternatively, the part can be held over the wax bath and the wax repeatedly ladled over it. The waxed limb is then wrapped first in plastic and then wrapped in towelling. After about 20 minutes the towelling and plastic sheet is removed and the thick wax coating is then peeled off from the hand or foot and dropped into a separate unit where it can be reheated and sterilised before re-use.

When is wax used?

Patients with stiff, swollen, post-traumatic wrists, hands, ankles or feet, find the warmth very comforting and pain relieving. The skin is much more supple and surface scarring and adhesions feel softer and more pliable. This allows local massage and stretchings, plus active exercise, to be more effective in regaining recovery. Patients in the remission phase of rheumatoid arthritis find that they obtain considerable benefit from wax therapy, and some prefer it to any other form of heat. Treatment can be daily, or less, depending upon the injury itself and the availability of the patients.

Dangers and contraindications

These are mainly obvious ones, such as any skin disorder that might be aggravated by wax heating, and local rheumatoid arthritis, or other arthritis, during periods of exacerbation where the heating may increase the inflammatory activity in the joints and surrounding tissues. As with any heat therapy, acute trauma within the first 36 hours is a contraindication as the tissue will only become more inflamed. Applying the wax is a potentially messy process, so care has to be taken to avoid getting the wax onto the patient's shoes or clothes.

Non-thermal radiation

Low power laser therapy

Everyone is now familiar with the pencil thin rays of light used in laser shows and the military use of laser beams to track targets and guide missiles. High and medium power lasers are used surgically to cut and seal tissues, re-bore clogged arteries and perform delicate eye surgery. Low power laser beams are now used therapeutically to relieve pain and stimulate healing.

Laser light does not look any different from ordinary light but, in a very special way, it is. Ordinary light is a jumble of different frequencies which the eye and brain separates out into different frequency bands and assigns a range of colours and hues to each frequency. The rainbow spectrum of red, orange, yellow, green, blue, indigo and violet is really the brain's way of colour coding increasing light frequencies from red to violet. Below red lie the infra-red frequencies which heat on absorption, and beyond violet lie the ultra-violet frequencies that produce photobiochemical reactions on absorption, such as the skin tan of summer. People and animals that do not have colour vision distinguish frequency bands as shades of grey. White light is an even mix of all frequencies and total black is the absence of light, either because there is no light, or an object has completely absorbed all of the frequencies without any reflection.

Monochromatic light

This is light of one frequency which we would see as a particular colour hue, or shade of grey. All of the wavelengths are the same length. A source of ordinary monochromatic light pours out the wavelength in a random way so that the even length wavelengths are still jumbled in relationship to each other. Imagine, for example, 50 nurses of identical height and stride length all walking at the same speed as they cross a metal catwalk to the wards. Because each would be walking slightly out of step with everyone else the catwalk would rumble with the noise of their shoes. That rumble is like ordinary monochromatic light.

A laser source produces the same single frequency of light with each wave exactly in step with the wave in front and the wave behind. Imagine, again, the same 50 nurses marching with parade ground precision over the same catwalk. Their footsteps would echo in resounding unison as 50 heels hit the bridge in split second precision. That analogy shows the difference between laser light and ordinary monochromatic light. Laser rays can be so intense that their unison wave can melt and vapourise steel.

Low power laser therapy

Figure 13.4 shows the application of a thin laser beam to an injury at the back of the heel from a single point probe, and Figure 13.5 shows treatment to a shoulder using a large cluster probe. In the latter case the central laser beam source is surrounded by a circle of ordinary monochromatic beams of the same frequency. There are controls for treatment time and power, and many units include the choice of

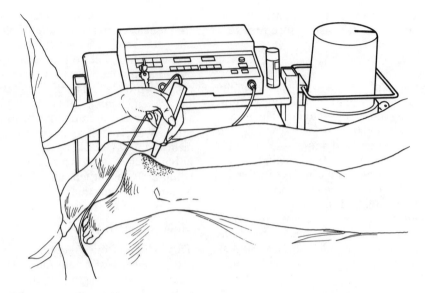

Figure 13.4 Low power laser therapy with single point probe

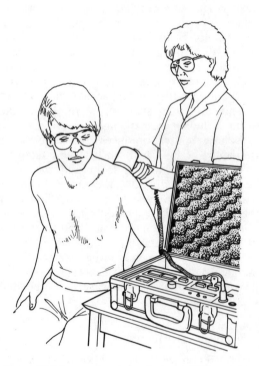

Figure 13.5 Low power laser therapy with large cluster probe

continuous output or pulsed. To prevent un-authorised use a key has to be inserted and turned before laser light can be transmitted.

Patient and physiotherapist wear special glasses, or goggles, to protect the eyes from any chance absorption of laser light, and the area for treatment is carefully localised. The laser head is placed in skin contact, or within 1 cm distance, and the beam applied for several seconds. The beam energy is measured in joules per cm^2 (1 joule = 1 watt) and power is measured in thousandths of a watt (mW). The average power range is about 10–100 mW. This is so small that no heating occurs. Like SWD and US lasers can be applied either as a continuous beam, or in pulses. The beam of energy only penetrates for a few millimetres before its useful energy is absorbed.

Physiological effects of low power laser

This is the subject of much intense research. That cells can selectively absorb and use different frequencies of infra-red, light, and ultra-violet has been known for years. Absorption mainly depends upon the absorption characteristics of the cell components, such as the nucleus, membrane, mitochondria and so on. How they convert this energy into useful purpose is not yet known. It is assumed that laser energy is absorbed in resonance with the regular frequency of its wavelength. Therapeutic lasers are tuned to emit specific frequencies which lie in the infra-red band and nearby visible red band. Research indicates that some frequencies are more effective than others. When the beam is applied at different pulse frequencies, which can range from about 50 to 1200 per second, some researchers have found that, for example, 700 pulses per second, have a better healing effect than 1200 but in each case, the rate of healing is accelerated compared to an untreated area. Because it is a recent development it will take a few years to establish exactly what occurs at cellular level.

What is laser therapy used for?

Its effectiveness in pain relief in, for example, acute trauma, postoperative pain, and superficial joint pain, seems well established, both on an individual experience basis and by clinical trial. Neuralgias, such as post-herpetic neuralgia (shingles), seem relieved, and there is much research into the claims by patients that the application of laser to acupuncture points particularly increases the degree of pain relief. The pain relief is one of reduction of source pain, rather than activating any central nervous system gates, although the latter may be involved in an unexplained way when laser is applied to acupuncture points. Because there is no detectable warmth, or sensory stimulus of any kind, the patient does not feel anything beyond a few seconds of slight contact pressure of the laser head.

Dangers and contraindications

None has been shown. Caution dictates that abdominal treatment is not applied during pregnancy, and that goggles are worn to protect the eyes.

Acupuncture

Many physiotherapists now use acupuncture techniques for the relief of pain. The subject is discussed elsewhere so it suffices to say here that electro-acupuncture is commonly employed, using low frequency currents through the needles to reinforce the mechanical stimulation of needling. That many patients experience pain relief during and after acupuncture is undoubted. The mechanisms still remain speculative. Western medicine emphasises neurophysiological responses, such as opioid release, or pain gating reflexes, rather than the scientifically elusive meridian energy concepts of Eastern thought.

Interferential therapy

Imagine that two pebbles, 1 m apart, have been dropped into a pond at the same time, and that the ripples they have caused are of the same height and the same frequency. When the two circles of ripples meet the combined energy of the crests will double the height of the waves and the combined energy of the troughs will double the depth of each wave. An observer will see the interaction of wave energies as a series of prominent standing waves. In more technical terms their combined amplitude has doubled and they are *in phase* with each other. If they interacted so that the *trough* from one ripple met the *crest* of the other, then their two energies would mutually cancel out and an observer would see a zone of flat water. The waves would be *out of phase*. If the two sets of ripples were at different frequencies then some crests would be amplified, some troughs would be amplified, some troughs and crests would cancel each other out and there would be partial summation and cancellation of other waves and troughs. The resulting interaction would be seen by an observer as a standing series of a few, large, stationary waves. When two, or more, wave systems meet their interaction is known as *interference* and the resulting wave patterns are termed *amplitude modulated (AM)*. Amplitude modulated waves are always larger in size, but fewer in frequency, than the original waves.

For example, if one wave system had a frequency of 100 cycles per second (100 Hz), and another wave system had a frequency of 90 cycles per second (90 Hz), then their interaction would result in 10 amplitude modulated (AM) waves. In other words, the number of AM waves is always the number remaining when the lower frequency is subtracted from the higher frequency. Once formed, these amplitude modulated wave systems now exist in their own right and are called *beat frequencies*.

Interferential therapy (IF or IFT), is based upon the interaction of two different sets of frequencies to produce the required AM beat frequencies to which the tissues respond. In IFT one frequency is *fixed* at 4000 Hz (4 kHz) and the other can be *varied* between 3800 Hz and 4000 Hz. So, if the variable frequency is set

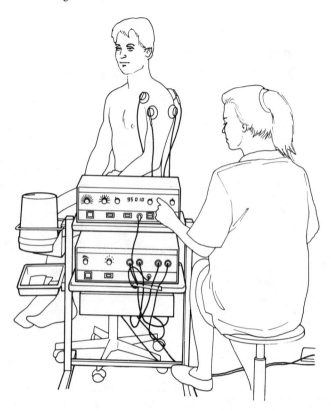

Figure 13.6 Interferential therapy

by the operator at 3900 Hz, the two sets of frequencies will interact deep in the tissues to produce an AM beat frequency of 100 Hz.

Sensory endings, motor nerves, muscle fibres and the autonomic nervous system respond best to frequencies between 2 and 200 Hz, and this is the frequency range used by electrical stimulating currents. TENS, for example, operates in this frequency range to produce a strong sensory skin effect in pain relief. When it is desired to stimulate deeper tissues this sensory effect acts as an uncomfortable barrier at higher intensities. IFT gets around this barrier by using kHz frequencies, that cannot be felt, to interact within the tissues to create the low frequency beat frequencies in the tissues. These beat frequencies can be focussed at different tissue depths and over the last 25 years IFT has come into wide use to stimulate muscles, aid healing, and relieve pain.

Application of IFT

Figure 13.6 shows IFT being applied to the shoulder of a patient. A suction unit is often used, as here, to hold the electrodes in place by placing cups over the electrodes and generating a mild vacuum. This is much more useful than bandaging them on. The circuit for one pair of electrodes is fixed at 4 kHz, and the other can be varied between 3.8 kHz to 4 kHz. This means that the beat frequency can be steadily swept up and down between 0 and 200 Hz over a full sweep, or set to sweep over, say, 10–20 Hz, or set at a continuous beat, say at 70 Hz. A wide variety of stimuli can be given and the intensity increased, or decreased, as required. IFT memory circuits allow the physiotherapist to programme in various sweep patterns during a treatment session.

Therapeutic uses of IFT

On the basis of widespread professional practice IFT is applied for the relief of arthritic and muscular pain; to relieve pain and assist recovery in recent trauma; to strengthen and retrain pelvic floor musculature weakened by the stretching of childbirth, and/or to strengthen sphincter muscle control in incontinence. At the time of writing clinical trials are in progress to evaluate the many claims made for IFT, and it will be some time before the results are known. One undoubted benefit has been the use of IFT to strengthen pelvic floor musculature in cases of stress incontinence and prevention of mild prolapse. IFT is combined with an exercise programme to increase voluntary control of these muscles.

Mechanisms of IFT pain relief

IFT probably operates the same pain gate mechanisms as TENS. There may be an added advantage that mild rhythmic stimulation of underlying muscle, and possibly lymph duct and venous involuntary muscle, may reinforce deep sensory input and mechanically aid removal of trauma debris and inflammatory waste products by stimulating local circulation. Like TENS the pad electrodes are placed so that the area to be treated lies within the field and various combinations of beat frequencies employed to discover whether one set of variables is more effective than another. Treatment times range from 15 to 30 minutes, and can be repeated daily or less often per week.

Dangers and contraindications

None as far as the tissues are concerned, but it is precautionary wisdom not to treat patients with pacemakers.

Cold therapy

It is almost instinctive to cool hot and inflamed tissues, whether caused by burns, trauma, arthritis, infective, or allergic conditions. The more quickly a tissue burn can be cooled the less the secondary damage. Cold therapy has been developed in a systematic manner and there is now a wide range of localised cooling methods that can be used.

Methods of applying cold therapy

Local cold can be applied by using flaked ice folded into terry towelling packs. Commercially available cold packs are gel filled and stored in the refrigerator. Cold wet terry towels can be wrung out and then applied, as can frozen bags of peas on towelling. Intermittent

pressure sleeves can be applied over a limb and filled with cold water. Ice sticks can be used as massage sticks and evaporating cold sprays can be applied for rapid skin chilling. Direct immersion of a limb into a container of chilled water is another alternative.

The skin should be greased to protect it from localised cold spots and to prevent it getting too soggy and liable to injury. Application temperatures are between 18 and 22°C and each application session lasts between 15 and 25 minutes. Apart from ice stick massage, freezing, or near freezing temperatures are not directly applied as there is a real danger of tissue damage through excess chilling and vasoconstriction. Excess cold also creates a very unpleasant aching pain which defeats the purpose of its use.

Physiological effects of cold therapy

Prolonged local cold causes vasoconstriction, reduced metabolism, and reduced nerve conduction. The sensory effect is one of intense cold sensation response from skin thermal receptors registering temperature drop, followed by reduced sensation as the area cools and nerve conduction is slowed. In acute conditions cold reduces inflammatory responses. Following brain and spinal cord injury, application of local cold to the skin over affected muscle groups reflexly reduces hypertonicity and spasticity, sometimes for several hours after treatment.

Following removal of the cold source there is gradual rewarming by incoming blood and periods of changing vasodilation and partial vasoconstriction may follow over several hours. Cold inhibits pain transmission from an underlying pain source, and activates spinal cord gating. Its localised sensory effect directs conscious attention from the pain to the cold itself. The later numbing effect is well known.

Therapeutic use of cold therapy

Recent acute trauma injury and burns benefit from prompt application of cold to reduce further damage and limit the inflammatory response. This also markedly reduces pain. In chronic pain, arising, for example, from arthritis, pain relief is more variable. Some patients find it very effective, others do not, so it is very much one of individual preference. Painful spasticity is often markedly relieved. Ice stick massage is used as a sharp sensory stimulus to reduce hypotonia and stimulate voluntary muscle contraction after, for example, strokes.

Manipulative procedures

Joints and muscles are the main sources of pain for many patients referred for physiotherapy. A careful case history often indicates the tissue source of such pain together with the likely cause. For example, the probability that an attack of acute low back pain is causally linked to a day long session of unaccustomed heavy digging is high. To establish *which* structures are damaged requires considerable skill in physical examination. Physiotherapists specifically learn to compare normal and abnormal joint and soft tissue structures by observation, careful handling and manual testing. In effect, the hands becomes a highly skilled diagnostic aid as the experienced physiotherapist feels the difference between normal tension, shape and movement compared to the abnormal.

The body can display a bewildering ability to present 'obvious' sources of pain and disability, such as a painful knee, pins and needles in the hand, or a painful shoulder, whose actual cause lies elsewhere. For example, a painful shoulder may be the presenting symptom of cervical arthritis. Careful examination may show that the position and angle of the neck has a marked effect on the shoulder pain. Treatment, therefore, must be directed to the cervical joints and structures whose pathology provides the source of such shoulder pain. A detailed knowledge of the musculoskeletal system, its nerve supply, patterns of pain and likely causes, underlies successful physiotherapy diagnosis and treatment.

Physical therapy skills discussed in this section can be grouped under *massage*, *mobilisations* and *manipulations*.

Massage or soft tissue techniques

Contemporary interest in alternative medicine includes massage therapy for the relief of stress, body awareness and interpersonal communication. There is now a wide range of 'How to Massage' books on the health shelves written by non-medical masseurs as part of the holistic approach to self health. That massage plays an important role in this context is undeniable, but the emphasis in this section is upon massage as a therapeutic technique for physical disorders.

Physical disorder, whether from sudden trauma or degenerative joint disease, results in local tissue pathology which is often painful and inhibits normal function. Physiotherapists employ specific soft tissue techniques either to help prevent such pathology, or to aid healing and recovery following damage. Trauma, for example, can cause local swelling, oedema, fibrinous deposits in muscle and joint structures, adhesions in tendon sheaths, and superficial or deep scarring. Massage techniques applied directly to the area can help remove oedema, soften contractures, stretch scar tissue, free tendon adhesions and restore tissue suppleness and extensibility. Techniques that can be employed include the following:

Frictions. These are performed with the tips of one or two fingers across, for example, accurately located scar tissue or tendon adhesions. The movement is a to and fro deep finger pressure applied transversely across the adherent structure. It is uncomfortable for the patient as it mechanically stretches the target tissue, causing a later reactive hyperaemia and accelerating the process of freeing adherent structures. A typical condition is supraspinatus tendinitis, where attempting to lift the arm sideways is very painful through the mid-range of the arc as the inflamed tendon is compressed beneath the overhanging acromion process. The patient is asked to put the affected arm behind them, so that the back of the wrist is in the small of the back. This brings the tendon out from under the acromion and the painful spot is frictioned for 2–5 minutes. Often the initial discomfort becomes numbed as the friction continues. Several treatments, usually accompanied by other treatments such as exercises and/or ultrasound, often bring marked relief.

Kneading. In this technique one or both hands are used to rhythmically grasp, lift, compress and relax muscles. Where both hands are working on the same muscle a 'wringing' action is performed which lifts and stretches the muscle between the hands. this aids venous and lymphatic drainage, helps to stretch contracted soft tissue structures and relieve soreness and tension. One form of two handed kneading is to place the hands either side of the limb, over biceps and triceps for example, and perform the kneading sequence in alternative compressive, lifting and stretching rhythm. Kneading is a very useful technique to help regain function after the immobility of prolonged splintage, or to help maintain soft tissue extensibility in competitive sport. Increased sensory input from the tissues being kneaded helps to 'shut' the spinal pain gate and reinforce conscious awareness of localised ordinary sensation.

Effleurage. This technique consists of a long, firm, flowing, one hand or two hand stroking from distal to proximal, for example, from the hand to the axilla and shoulder region. It follows the venous and lymphatic pathways and helps drain them to relieve oedema and congestion. On the back, a diverging two hand effleurage stroke takes both hands from the lumbar region across the posterior thorax into the axillary area. Effleurage has the double effect of increasing venous and lymph return together with a strong, pleasant, sensory component.

Stroking. Stroking is a light rhythmical movement like effleurage, but it can be applied in any direction. Its effect is entirely sensory and the repetition produces a calming and soothing effect.

Hacking. Less commonly used now than in previous decades, hacking is a fast, repetitious, percussion of the tissues by the little finger edge of the hand. The arms are positioned so that the elbows are out and in front, with the forearms parallel to the front of the body and the wrists in full extension so that the palms and straight fingers face each other some 5 cm apart. The forearms are then rotated so that, for example the left hand is first rotating anti-clockwise as the right hand rotates clockwise, then the rotation is reversed. When applied to the back the alternate left and right palm and little finger edges strike the back in a fast tattoo. This percussive rotating action effect can be moved over the back, or limb, in any direction and creates a very strong and stimulating sensory effect.

Mobilisations

This term applies to techniques used to increase the range of movement of a joint, or joints, whose function is painfully limited by degenerative articular changes and/or contracted surroundings ligamentous or capsular structures.

The patient is passive and relaxed and the physiotherapist first accurately locates the disfunctioning joint and then rhythmically attempts to mobilise the joint to regain the lost range of movement. The technique involves using the hands to both stabilise the joint and repeatedly move the joint surfaces relative to each other to increase the desired range. Gentle manual distraction, or separation, of joint surfaces is applied whilst the manouvre is in progress. The patient is positioned so that he or she is supported and relaxed whilst the mobilisation is in progress. It remains under patient control at all times and can be stopped if unexpectedly painful or uncomfortable.

One well known mobilisation technique for the spine is spinal traction. This can be done manually but it is more common practice to use a motorised traction couch that can apply whatever sustained, or rhythmic, traction is necessary. The patient is placed in lumbar or cervical harness to localise the traction effect. Rhythmic or sustained stretching of tight spinal joint structures often brings considerable pain relief. Manual mobilization of individual spinal joints is a highly skilled procedure that requires considerable practice.

Manipulation

This term is technically applied to the use of an accurate, forceful, mobilising thrust to a joint structure that is applied quickly and cannot be prevented by the relaxed patient in the same way as the more gentle mobilising techniques. It is particularly used in spinal manipulation and is only applied where careful assessment indicates that a particular joint restriction will be released by the application of a controlled, high velocity thrust. Sometimes there is an audible click as the suspected adhesion is stretched, or a malaligned joint angle returned to normal. A patient may find, for example, that they can turn their head, or bend and extend their neck fully without pain after the manipulation.

None of the procedures discussed in this section concerning the various ways in which joints and soft tissues can be stretched and mobilised is an automatic cure of pain caused by physical disorders. However, when skillfully applied after careful case history and examination, they often do offer considerable pain relief associated with improvement of joint function and range of activities.

Exercise Therapy

It may seem odd to use exercise as a potent source of pain relief in so many musculoskeletal disorders where movement is a source of pain. The realistic fact is that we must move in order to do the ordinary, self sufficient, activities of daily life. Many post-traumatic and arthritic conditions become more painful if guarded against all movement as the tissues become tighter, and strength and range of movement decrease. The sheer lack of normal movement sensation throws the sensation of pain into higher relief as pain gating mechanisms are not being operated. Therefore, controlled therapeutic movement is a valuable agent in pain relief and improvement of function.

Exercise therapy can be categorised as follows.

Suspension Therapy

Where limbs are weak, stiff, and painful voluntary movement can be encouraged by placing the limb in a broad canvas sling and attaching the sling by adjustable ropes to an overhead suspension point, or points. The suspended limb will then swing in an arc of movement. The physiotherapist can gently commence a movement that the patient then continues under encouraging guidance. A further advance in effort can be achieved by using calibrated tension springs attached either to the overhead suspension point, or to wall or apparatus points at the sides, so that the patient can move the limb, say bending and stretching the knee, by having to stretch the spring to work the quadriceps muscle when straightening downwards and then controlling recoil of the stretched spring as the knee is flexed upwards.

Hydrotherapy

The use of warm water to regain movement and relieve pain is centuries old as spa towns can testify. The buoyant relief from gravity, and flexible floating and moving of the trunk and limbs in water can bring real relief from pain and improvement of function. Floats can be used both as an aid to buoyancy and as a means of exercise when attempting to move them forcibly through the water. The sensation of water, and relief from the dragging effect of gravity on painful joints, are strong factors in operating pain gates. Swimming is an excellent exercise in itself and mobilises and strengthens movement in a way not possible with any other approach. The use of hot and cold water jacuzzi sprays creates considerable sensory stimulation and has a marked pain relieving effect.

Mobilising and strengthening exercises

Most inpatients and outpatients are carefully instructed in exercises specifically designed to either increase range of movement, increase strength, or both. These can range from the simplest individual joint exercises, such as flexing and extending the wrist 10 times by three sessions daily for post-Colles' fracture, or sitting on the side of the bed, or treatment couch, swinging the lower legs to increase knee range, to full range limb and trunk exercise routines in classwork, and completion of specific tasks in circuit training. Games can be an important element in social cooperation or competition to achieve functional goals.

Task simulation

Where physical risk of further injury is an occupational, sport, or hobby hazard, analysis of the physical demands is the basis of a planned exercise programme, often in circuit format, whereby the patient reduces the chance of injury by improving movement range, strength, and skill to meet task requirements. An injury and pain prevention programme and an important example is learning the techniques of correct lifting and back care. This is part of every nurse training programme and is essential.

In summary, active exercise therapy treats the source of pain by controlled increase in range and strength of damaged tissues, combined with improved control of function in every day life. Often there is increased pain at the commencement of exercise as the affected tissues are used, but the resulting increase in blood supply, temperature rise, stretching of contracted tissues, removal of oedema, and recovery of function brings long term relief. An important pain gating component is the enormous increase in normal sensory stimulation which operates both at non-conscious gating levels and conscious awareness of normal sensation as a balance to awareness of pain.

Relaxation

Relaxation techniques involve the conscious contrasting of uncomfortable bodily tension with active relaxation into bodily non tension. Anxiety and apprehension increase muscle tone and postural tension so that muscles are continuously active and in a state of partial contraction. The shoulder girdle muscles and back muscles are particularly responsive to emotional tension. When worried and anxious the shoulders are raised so that the shoulder elevator muscles, trapezius and levator scapulae, are in a chronic state of tension. Posture tends to be very upright, even when sitting, and movement restless and often clumsy. The opposite extreme occurs in depression when the shoulders are slumped and posture stooped.

Relaxation techniques are particularly used to relieve anxiety states where the non-consciously induced body tension creates conscious awareness of aching tension muscle fatigue which reinforces the anxiety state. They can also be used to help relieve the tension of chronic pain in, for example, arthritis, and are often very helpful for those suffering tension headaches and migraine. A particular system of relaxation exercises is taught during antenatal classes as a preparation for labour.

Relaxation techniques

Following careful discussion and explanation the patient is placed in a comfortable and fully supported position, usually semi-reclined with use of cushions to support the limbs. Breathing slowly and deeply is first taught and the patient asked to imagine themselves to be in their favourite room, or beauty spot, in relaxed security. Then the therapist asks the patient to concentrate on particular limbs, or muscle groups, getting them to first tighten up, for example, making a fist, and then relaxing so that the tightened area 'sinks into the cushion' or stretches into full extension. The therapist speaks slowly and clearly, emphasising the contrast between the tightness and uncomfortable tension and the peaceful bliss of relaxation. Some physiotherapists use background

music and/or soft lighting effects to reinforce the relaxation technique.

Once the patient has learned the idea, and feels in control in the ideal relaxation circumstances, then the same principles are adapted for more ordinary circumstances such as sitting, standing, and walking. In the latter case the emphasis will be upon unhurried walking and breathing.

Relaxation techniques focus the sufferer's mind on body tension control which, in turn, reduces the physical sensation of anxiety and associated aching of prolonged muscle tension. When used for pain relief its purpose is to improve the patient's tolerance of pain, reduce the unhappy emotional tension of pain, and reduce the secondary aching and pain input from associated muscle tension.

In effect, relaxation techniques bridge the gap between the application of physiotherapy modalities to help cure the source of pain, or activate pain gates, and the patient/physiotherapist, person to person interaction, which is the context within which all therapy takes place. This forms the subject of the next section.

The physiotherapist as therapy

The preceding discussion has considered the range of modalities that can be employed by the physiotherapist to either help heal the source of pain, operate non conscious pain gates, and increase conscious awareness of heightened normal sensation as an antidote to pain. In other words, the use of *applied physiotherapy modalities* for their physiological and psychological effects.

This section considers the important mind to mind interaction between the physiotherapist and the patient suffering from pain, in effect, the *applied physiotherapist* part of the therapeutic formula. As mentioned in the introduction to this chapter, treatment cannot be divorced from the person giving the treatment. The patient experiences treatment and treater as a unity. He, or she, tries to understand and accept the explanation for treatment given by the treater, and this explanatory context links therapy and therapist into a therapeutic whole in the patient's mind. Although to the physiotherapist, nurse, doctor or other professional, a patient is one of many, to the patient it is a *one to one* relationship and they will discuss 'their' physiotherapist, for example, in a proprietorial way with relatives, friends and acquaintances on the ward, at home, in shops, pubs, on the streets, or wherever. These discussions will repetitively reinforce the patient's perception of the relationship for good or bad.

For purposes of discussion 'mind' and 'brain' are taken as interchangeable terms, as mind expresses itself through neurological activity and much brain activity expresses itself as mental experience. Therefore, conscious will-power, attitude, understanding and emotion have a neurological substrate. The mechanisms are poorly understood but they exist and express themselves in neural activation or sup-pression of other targeted neural systems. The mechanism may be by excitatory/inhibitory synaptic interactions between neurones, and/or release of neurohormones, such as the large family of neural endorphins or opioids, involved in intrinsic pain relief.

The mind to mind signalling system is com-prised of many components. For example, the empathic rapport of the physiotherapist is expressed in eye contact and facial expression, tone of voice, body posture and gesture, acts of helping and firm gentleness in handling during physical assessment. Ensuring patient comfort, and allowing the patient to talk and explain in a controlled framework of enquiry and response are also important. The friendly ambience should be an oasis of calm, even in a busy department or ward. First meeting is the most crucial moment, as the patient's emotional antennae are highly tuned to detect nuances of acceptance or rejection.

When a positive rapport is established the patient no longer feels that he or she is the passive victim of pain and disability, but can, instead, enter into a constructive liaison with the physiotherapist by seeing pain as an enemy that can be outsmarted and defeated by treat-ment strategy. This adversarial approach profoundly alters the emotional bias of the patient from pain victim to pain manager. This, in turn, has a profound effect on the efficacy of the descending pain gate control systems as cortico-limbic pain suppression gates can be operated by emotional drive and attitude.

Pain tolerance is a subjective assessment of how much the experienced pain interferes with everyday activities. It is very much subject to personality, mood, culture, previous pain experience, social circumstances and the mean-ing of the pain and its cause to the sufferer. In general terms pain tolerance is high in emerg-ency, sport, battle, or where social circum-stances demand stoic acceptance and the fear of 'loss of face' by showing pain is more feared than pain itself. Tolerance is low when alone, friendless, dejected and feeling a victim of circumstance. The relationship of endogenous opioid levels and pain tolerance is not known but it is likely that such levels are lower when depressed than when happy and optimistic.

Whatever the underlying neural mechan-isms, if the physiotherapist and patient can agree on flexible pain coping strategies which demonstrate to the patient that they can ration-ally control the pain, then pain tolerance and improved quality of life are immediate out-comes.

The physiotherapy synthesis

In summary, physiotherapists can apply a range of electrical, manipulative, and exercise modalities, together with relaxation strategies and occupational/sport/hobby pain preventive measures, that can help relieve a wide range of painful disabilities. Just as important is the establishment of a physiotherapist/patient rap-port which can place the chosen spectrum of treatments within an emotionally constructive framework which raises pain tolerance and places the patient as manager of the pain. An essential prerequisite is a careful case history and accurate physical assessment before decid-ing which treatment regime offers the greatest chance of success.

An interesting example of an unusual, and very successful approach to pain relief with patients suffering from the notoriously difficult to relieve problem of back pain is very enlight-ening (Williams, 1989). During the last 10 years hundreds of patients in pain have been referred to the Physiotherapist Department, Doncaster Royal Infirmary. What they all have in common is chronic pain, especially back pain, unrelieved by previous medical, psychological, or physical therapy, and an illness dependency behaviour in whereby whole way of life is centred around their pain. The Doncaster approach, known as the 'School for bravery' acknowledges the pain but ignores it in a firmly sympathetic regime of exercise therapy and games based upon the 'you can do it' approach. Success is measured in pride of achievement and associated restoration of personal dignity and self respect. This, in turn, is reinforced by a real improvement in family, work, and social relationships. The transformation in quality of living has been dramatic and sustained in over 80% of those referred. The 20% whose improvement has been poor appear to share, in common, a strong dependency upon medical authority and hope for a miracle drug. They seem to have accepted the implicit sick role dependency.

Physiotherapy for pain relief ranges from specific treatments to the 'school for bravery' approach and is tailored to the specific circumstances and needs of the patient. This does not mean that it always works, any more than medical or nursing procedures for pain relief, but it is an important and valuable therapeutic resource in pain management.

References

Johnson, M. I. Ashton, C. H. and Thompson, J. W. (1991a) An in-depth study of long term users of transcutaneous electrical nerve stimulation (TENS). Implications for clinical use of TENS. *Pain*, **44**, 221–229

Johnson, M. I. Ashton, C. H. and Thompson, J. W. (1991b) The consistency of pulse frequencies and pulse patterns of transcutaneous electrical nerve stimulation (TENS) used by chronic pain patients. *Pain*, **44**, 231–234

Editorial (1991) TENS for chronic low-back pain. *Lancet*, **337**, 462–463

Pert, V. F. (1991) TENS for pain in multiple sclerosis. *Physiotherapy*, **77** No. 3, 227–228

Swann, P. (1989) Stress management for pain control. *Physiotherapy*, **75** No 5, 295–298

Wells, P. E. Frampton, V. and Bowsher, D. (1988) *Pain: Management and Control in Physiotherapy*. Heineman Medical Books, London

Williams, J. I. (1989) Illness behaviour to wellness behaviour. *Physiotherapy*, **75** No 1, 2–7

Further reading

Bending, J. (1989) TENS in a pain clinic. *Physiotherapy*, **75** No 5, 292–294

Charman, R. A. (1989) Pain theory and physiotherapy. *Physiotherapy*, **75** No 5, 247–254

Forster, A. and Palastanga, N. (1985) *Clayton's Electrotherapy, Theory and Practice*, 9th edn. Bailiere Tindall, London

French, S. (1989) 'Pain: Some psychological and sociological aspects. *Physiotherapy*, **75** No 5, 255–260

Hollis, M. (1987) *Massage for Therapists*, Blackwell Scientific, Oxford

Low, J. and Reed, A. (1990) *Electrotherapy Explained*, Heinemann Butterworth, London

Maitland, G. D. (1986) *Vertebral Manipulation*, 5th edn, Heinemann Butterworth, London

Polden, M. and Mantle, J. (1990) *Physiotherapy in Obstetrics and Gynaecology*, Butterworth, London

Swann, P. (1989) Stress management for pain control. *Physiotherapy*, **75** No 5, 295–298

Wells, P. E., Frampton, V. and Bowsher, D. (1988) *Pain: Management and Control in Physiotherapy*, Heinemann Medical Books, London

14

The pharmacology of analgesics

Susan Tempest

Introduction

Pharmacology is concerned with the characteristics, actions and uses of drugs. An understanding of the basic principles of pharmacology is essential for anyone who is involved with the prescription, administration and monitoring of the effects of drugs.

A drug exerts its therapeutic effect following the interaction of the drug with an appropriate site in the body, usually a 'receptor'. A receptor is an area of cell membrane with special structural features which enable it to bind molecules such as drugs to form a drug–receptor complex. This reaction is analogous to the insertion of a key into a lock. If a drug 'fits' the receptor well it is said to have a high 'affinity' for the particular receptor. The magnitude of the effects produced depends, among other things, on the concentration of the drug at the site of action. Whether or not an appropriate concentration is achieved depends on several factors:

- *dose* given
- *route* of administration
- rate and extent of *absorption* of the drug
- the *distribution* of the drug into the various body tissues
- the site, extent, and products of drug *metabolism*
- the speed and routes of *elimination* of the drug from the body

Dose

The amount, or dose of a drug required to produce a certain therapeutic effect depends on certain characteristics of the drug:

i) The affinity of the drug for the receptor.
ii) The 'intrinsic activity' or ability of the drug to produce a response at that receptor.
iii) the 'efficacy' of the drug. The maximal effect produced by a drug is known as its efficacy and is reflected by the plateau on the dose–response curve. Sometimes it is not possible to give a dose that will produce the maximum effect desired as significant side effects occur before this dose is reached; thus limiting the efficacy of the drug.
iv) The potency of the drug. Potency is a comparison of the ability of different drugs to elicit the same quantitative response.

These concepts are discussed further in the section on opioid analgesics.

Route

Drugs are administered to man by a variety of routes which are partially determined by the physico-chemical properties of the drug, its sites of metabolism as well as patient acceptability.

The *oral* route is convenient and the one most often used. Absorption can take place at various points along the gastrointestinal tract. The extent and rate of absorption depend on the surface area available for absorption, the physical state in which the drug is administered, (solid or liquid) and the pH.

Absorption is maximal when the drug can exist in a unionised (uncharged) form. Thus aspirin (acetylsalicyclic acid, ASA) is well absorbed from the acid environment of the stomach where the low pH ensures that very little of the drug is in the ionised form. Some drugs which irritate the stomach lining or are destroyed in an acid medium are formulated with an enteric coating which prevents them being dissolved by the gastric acid. Oral formulations of prednisolone and diclofenac are available with an enteric coating. Some drugs are formulated in a sustained-release solid dose form which slowly releases the drug over several hours, thus allowing once or twice daily dosing. It may also help to minimise side effects and can improve patient compliance with medication. Morphine as MST Continus/MS Contin and many non-steroidal anti-inflammatory drugs such as indomethacin as Indocid-R/Indocid SR and flurbiprofen as Froben SR are available in a slow release formulation.

The *sublingual* route is very effective for extensively lipid-soluble drugs. Once it has entered the venous blood stream the drug is transported directly to the superior vena cava, thereby avoiding any initial first pass metabolism in the liver. Buprenorphine and dextromoramide are effective when given sublingually.

Administration of drugs via the *rectal* route is not as popular in the United Kingdom as it is on the Continent. As with sublingual administration, this route circumvents initial first pass metabolism in the liver. Although absorption can be erratic and incomplete, the rectal route can be a useful alternative when intractable vomiting or loss of consciousness preclude use of the oral route. Some drugs such as indomethacin can cause irritation of the rectal mucosa.

Intravenous injection of a drug achieves an immediate effect not possible by any other route. It allows the dose of drugs such as thiopentone to be titrated against the effect produced. Certain drugs cannot be formulated to allow intravenous use.

The onset of effect of a drug given by the *intramuscular* route is slower than when given intravenously, as there is no direct access to the circulation. The degree of water solubility of a drug is the main factor which determines the rate and degree of absorption. A drug which is to be given by the intramuscular route must be sufficiently water soluble to remain in solution in the interstitial fluid until absorption can occur. Drugs such as diazepam (Valium, Vivol) and phenytoin (Epanutin, Dilantin) which are not water soluble at physiological pH are formulated in a non-aqueous solvent in order to get them into solution. After intramuscular injection this solvent disperses from the injection site and the drug is precipitated. This results in slow, erratic and often incomplete

absorption of the drug. Maximal blood concentrations of diazepam occur later after intramuscular injection than after oral administration (Martindale, 1989). These drugs are therefore unsuitable for administration by the intramuscular route.

The irritant nature of some carrier solutions used in certain intramuscular injection formulations means that the preparation may only be given over a limited period, as there is the possibility of muscle necrosis.

Local blood flow also influences absorption by this route. Any conditions which decrease cardiac output will diminish local blood flow and lead to a decreased rate of absorption. This may occur following acute myocardial infarction. Blood flow also differs between specific areas of muscle. It has been shown that lignocaine is more rapidly absorbed following injection into the deltoid muscle than into the vastus lateralis and gluteus maximus (Meyer and Zelechowski, 1971).

Non-irritant drugs can often be given by the *subcutaneous* route. The rate of absorption is determined by blood flow to and from the area and the dissolution of the drug from the carrier solution. Diamorphine (diacetylmorphine, heroin) is very effective when given subcutaneously.

The epidural (extradural) and intrathecal (subarachnoid) routes are sometimes used to deliver drugs such as opioids close to their site of action in the spinal cord. The dose required to produce a therapeutic effect is considerably less (especially with the intrathecal route) than by other parenteral means and therefore the potential for side effects is minimised.

Drugs may be applied *topically* to mucous membranes such as conjunctiva or nasal mucosa to achieve a local effect. Sometimes absorption by this route is so efficient that systemic effects can occur as in the case of beta-blocker eye drops. Drugs do not readily penetrate intact skin as the epidermis is an effective lipid barrier. Absorption can be enhanced by use of oily formulations or application under occlusion.

Some drugs, such as salbutamol (albuterol) are given by *inhalation* and thus delivered directly to their site of action in the lungs. The large surface area available for absorption results in a rapid onset of therapeutic effect. Toxic chemicals, e.g. organophosphorous insecticides and cyanide, may also be absorbed by this route. A comparative summary of the routes of drug administration is given in Table 14.1 below.

Pharmacokinetics describes many of these biological processes in mathematical terms by use of various formulae and equations. Such devices may be useful for individualising drug regimens in patients with abnormal hepatic or renal function.

Absorption, distribution, metabolism and *excretion* all involve the movement of drugs across cell membranes. The extent and speed of drug transfer depends on such factors as the shape and size of the drug molecule, its lipid solubility, degree of ionisation (amount of posi-tive and negative charge) and the relative lipid solubility of the ionised and unionised forms.

The extent to which a drug is *absorbed* is largely a reflection of its solubility, with drugs in aqueous solution generally being better absorbed than those in suspension or solid dose form.

Once a drug is present in the bloodstream its further *distribution* into body tissues depends on how extensively it is bound to plasma pro-teins, especially albumin; blood flow to the various organs, and the solubility of its different forms in those structures. The concentration of a drug in liver, kidney or fat will be different and also differ from the concentration of the drug in plasma.

Table 14.1 Comparison of different routes of administration

Route	Absorption characteristics	Special features	Precautions
Intravenous	first pass metabolism circumvented, rapid onset of effect	route of choice in many emergency situations; suitable for administration of large volumes and irritant substances if diluted	give slowly; adverse effects may occur rapidly
Intramuscular	rapid absorption from aqueous solutions; oily solutions may be only slowly and erratically absorbed	can be painful, not more than 4 ml should be given into a single site	some irritant vehicles necessitate deep i.m. injection cannot be used in presence of coagulation abnormalities
Subcutaneous	rapid absorption from aqueous solutions, slow and continual from depot preparations	useful alternative to i.m./i.v. route, suitable for some poorly soluble substances	irritation can occur with some agents
Intrathecal	permits direct entry of drugs into central nervous system, with rapid effect	useful for spinal anaesthesia and administration of antibiotics in treatment of meningitis; only small doses needed minimising potential for side effects	preservative-free solution must be used; onset of side effects can be delayed; technique requires skill
Epidural	effects result from both absorption into spinal cord, paravertebral areas and systemic circulation	extent and duration of action depend on drug, volume & concentration used; doses < for i.m./i.v. route but > for intrathecal route; indwelling catheter can be used for longer duration of action	skill needed to locate epidural space; errors have occurred when topping-up catheters
Sublingual	avoids first pass metabolism, rapid onset of effect for potent lipid soluble drugs	rapid onset of effect.	bitter taste of some drugs unacceptable to some patients
Topical	epidermis acts as lipid barrier, absorption enhanced by oily vehicles, denuded or occluded skin; rapid absorption across mucous membranes	controlled-release patches for sustained delivery of hyoscine and glyceryl trinitrate available	systemic toxicity can result from topical application, e.g. beta blocker eyedrops
Rectal	partially avoids first pass metabolism, absorption can be incomplete and erratic	useful in unconscious and fitting patients	irritant substances can cause pruritus
Inhalation	rapid absorption of gaseous, volatile and atomised substances, avoids first pass metabolism	delivers drug to site of action in pulmonary disease	bulky equipment can be needed, difficult to deliver exact dose, may cause irritation

Every drug has an apparent volume of distribution. This is a theoretical rather than an actual value and describes the total amount of drug in the body if it were present in all body tissues in the same concentration as in the plasma. Drugs such as warfarin which are highly bound to plasma albumin have a small volume of distribution, whereas the tricyclic antidepressants, which are widely distributed in body tissues, have a high volume of distribution.

It is only the free fraction of a drug which is able to cross cell membranes and exert a pharmacological effect. Therefore if a drug is highly protein bound only a small percentage of the total amount of drug in the body is responsible for the effect produced by the drug. Highly protein bound drugs may be displaced from their binding sites by other such drugs. If this occurs an enhanced pharmacological effect is produced. An example of such an effect is the interaction between warfarin and aspirin which results in a markedly increased anticoagulant effect as aspirin displaces warfarin from its binding sites on plasma albumin.

Many drugs accumulate in muscle and fat which then act as a reservoir from which the drug is gradually released, the speed of release being dependent on the blood flow to that organ.

Lipid soluble drugs such as thiopentone are not readily eliminated from the body and in order to be excreted more rapidly must be changed into more ionised i.e. polar compounds. This process is termed *metabolism* or biotransformation. Microsomal enzyme systems in the liver are responsible for the metabolism of the great majority of drugs. Enzymatic activity may be enhanced or inhibited by certain drugs. Drug metabolism is altered in the neonate and in the elderly. Hepatic disease and certain other disease states may retard metabolism and lead to an enhanced drug effect. Dietary factors, pregnancy and alcohol ingestion may also play a role.

Drug metabolites may be either pharmacologically active or inactive. Some drugs such as cyclophosphamide are termed 'prodrugs'. Such drugs are inactive when taken into the body and are then metabolised to a pharmacologically active form, usually by the liver.

The clearance of a drug from the plasma is determined by its volume of distribution, amount of drug present and the half-life. The half-life of a drug is the time taken for the concentration of the drug in the plasma to decrease by half. For the majority of drugs the duration of effect and therefore the interval between drug doses is partially dependent on the half-life of the drug. Drugs with a long half-life such as digoxin only need to be given once daily. If the drug produces pharmacologically active metabolites the half-life of these compounds will need to be taken into account when deciding on the dosage interval.

Some drugs are excreted by the lungs, via bile and faeces or in breast milk, but the most important route of *excretion* is via the kidneys. Elimination by this route depends on the amount of drug entering the kidney tubule by glomerular filtration, the active secretion of positive and negative ions into the proximal tubule and the passive reabsorption into the body of non-ionised molecules. The latter process is very much dependent on the pH, as the cells in the tubules are much more permeable to non-ionised forms.

In an alkaline pH a weak acid will be extensively ionised and thus less susceptible to passive reabsorption. Its elimination will therefore be increased. This phenomenon is exploited in cases of salicylate poisoning where excretion may be enhanced by rendering the urine alkaline.

Renal impairment can substantially decrease the elimination of drugs, especially those that are excreted without being metabolised. Adjustment of dose and dosage interval may be necessary in order to avoid accumulation in these circumstances.

Allergy – fact and fiction

The term 'allergy' is liberally used by patients and physicians alike, many of whom consider it to indicate any type of adverse reaction.

True allergic reactions

The term allergic reaction should only be used to refer to reactions that are immunologically mediated. The true rate of allergies is around 5% but up to 15% of patients believe they are allergic to one or more drugs. Only about 6–10% of all adverse drug reactions (ADRs) are due to immunological mechanisms. Increasing age and atropy are factors which can increase the risk of an allergic reaction. Other criteria may help to alert staff to the possibility of a true drug allergy, these clues are outlined below:

- A reaction unlike any known pharmacological reaction of the drug.
- A gap of 7–10 days following initial drug administration.
- Reappearance of the same reaction following challenge with the same or a closely related drug.

Patients who have an allergic reaction to a drug present with similar symptoms to other classic allergic reactions. These include:

- Urticaria.
- Angioneurotic oedema.
- Cardiovascular disturbances.
- Respiratory distress.
- Rhinitis.
- Diarrhoea.
- Vomiting.

The drug should be immediately discontinued in patients experiencing these symptoms and a doctor summoned straightaway. These reactions can involve one or more body systems. Anaphylaxis is the most serious type of allergic reaction. Cytotoxic agents, muscle relaxants, intravenous anaesthetics and penicillin are the most frequent drugs to cause anaphylaxis.

Non-allergic adverse drug reactions

A non-allergic drug reaction should be considered whenever

- The predictable effects of the drug are exaggerated, e.g. excessive drowsiness following a small dose of benzodiazepine.
- An unexpected event occurs.
- A patient who is receiving appropriate therapy fails to respond to treatment or markedly deteriorates.

The chances of an ADR are increased in certain patient groups such as

- The elderly.
- Patients on multiple drug therapy.
- Patients receiving two or more drugs that are known to interact.
- Patients who have a history of previous ADRs.

- Patients with conditions that result in abnormal drug metabolism or clearance (e.g. renal impairment).

The actual incidence of adverse drug reactions is unknown but may be between 6% and 15% depending on the population sample. Some studies have suggested that about one-third of medical inpatients experience an ADR during their in-patient stay. Approximately 3% of hospital admissions are due to ADRs.

It is vitally important to warn patients about expected initial side effects of drug therapy and to explain that this does not mean that they are allergic to the medication. Classic examples are those of mild to moderate gastrointestinal upset following oral administration of NSAIDS or drowsiness following initiation of opioid therapy. In these cases the patient should be reassured and persuaded to continue with treatment whilst being carefully monitored for any sudden exacerbation of symptoms.

Printed information sheets explaining possible side effects and potentially more serious adverse effects should be given to patients and their relatives and carers whenever possible. They should contain instructions as to the appropriate action that should be taken by the patient in individual instances, especially with regard to when to discontinue treatment and when to call the doctor. Such leaflets act as reassurance, increase patient confidence and encourage compliance with therapy.

Practical aspects of drug administration

The therapeutic effect of a drug depends among other things on the dose given, the route used and the amount absorbed. Drugs are often presented in certain dosage forms such as capsules, slow release tablets or granules for specific reasons. Any attempt to destroy the dosage form or to change the route of administration may affect both the amount of drug absorbed by the body and the rate at which it is absorbed.

Bitter-tasting drugs may be formulated in granules with a specific pleasant-tasting coating in order to aid patient compliance. Drugs which are irritant to the stomach may be presented in a capsule which is not destroyed by gastric acid. Drugs which may be destroyed in the acid medium of the stomach are given an enteric coating so that the full dose of drug reaches the area of the gastrointestinal tract where it is absorbed.

Slow-release preparations must not be crushed before administration as this will partially or completely destroy the slow release mechanism.

Some drugs are inactivated by moisture, heat or light and must be kept in the original packaging in order to maintain their therapeutic efficacy. Glyceryl trinitrate (nitroglycerin), aspirin and papaveretum tablets, and Parentrovite (a high dose vitamin B and C preparation) are some common examples.

Other drugs such as warfarin and tamoxifen are only active in certain stereochemical forms. Inadvertent exposure to heat, light or other chemical catalysts could potentially result in a change or decrease in therapeutic effects. Manufacturers instructions as to storage conditions and reconstitution procedures should be followed explicitly.

The absorption of some drugs such as certain antibiotics and diphosphonates is decreased if they are taken with food. Milk and antacids decrease the absorption of many tetracyclines. The absorption of other drugs such as ketoconazole, propranolol, carbamazepine and phenytoin is enhanced by concurrent administration with food. Drugs which alter the rate of gastric emptying such as metoclopramide and all drugs with anticholinergic effects will influence the rate of absorption of some drugs given concurrently such as paracetamol, ampicillin and digoxin. Gastric emptying is also decreased if patients lie on their left side. Gastrointestinal disease and surgery which removes a significant amount of gastrointestinal tract may have a significant impact on drug absorption.

In certain situations such as the relief of sudden severe acute pain or when rapid termination of a convulsion is required the onset of action of a drug must be fast and safe. Sublingual administration may sometimes be appropriate, but the intravenous or occasionally subcutaneous route is often preferred. Intramuscular administration is unsuitable when a fast onset of action is required. Towards the end of a patient's life significant peripheral shutdown may compromise the efficacy of the subcutaneous route and it may be necessary to consider giving essential drugs intravenously.

Where to go for information and advice

The answers to many of the practical problems outlined above are not always easily available. The pharmacist is the only member of the health care team whose entire training is devoted towards an understanding of drugs, how they act in the body and how disease states influence drug absorption, metabolism and excretion. They are also experts in the formulation, stability and interactions of drugs.

They can help other members of the health care team by formulating a drug in a different presentation, most commonly in a suspension rather than a solid dose form or by suggesting alternative routes of administration.

The likelihood of drug interactions increases with age and the number of preparations being taken. In certain patients these problems are compounded by altered renal, hepatic and haematological parameters, all of which may affect the way the drug is handled by the body. The pharmacist is a valuable source of advice in these situations.

Drug stability can be an important consideration when essential medications have to be mixed in solution and administered to patients by the same route. The administration of analgesics and anti-emetics via a subcutaneous infusion to patients with advanced cancer is a typical example. Although the clinical needs of the patient must remain paramount, doctors often pay scant attention to issues concerning drug compatibility. It cannot be assumed that the absence of a snow storm in a syringe or infusion means that the drugs are chemically compatible. Failure to establish compatability may mean that the patient is not receiving exactly what the doctor prescribed. Significant amounts of either or both drugs in solution may be chemically degraded to inactive compounds, resulting in subtherapeutic doses being administered. When using certain types of syringe drivers a failure to take account of the extra solution needed to prime extension sets can result in significant under-dosing over a designated period.

Many patients with pain have quite complex drug administration schedules which they can find difficult to comply with once they are at home. Physicians, pharmacists and nurses must work together to simplify drug regimens as far as possible by selecting drugs which only require once or twice daily administration. The use of appropriate compliance aids, self-administration schemes prior to discharge and medication record cards which give the name, appearance, purpose and exact times of drug administration, can greatly enhance compliance with medication. The most sophisticated diagnostic and theraeutic interventions are rendered useless if the patient cannot comply with the treatment.

Every nurse and physician should be able to call upon a pharmacist to help them solve these and other drug-related issues. The increasing involvement of clinical pharmacists in acute pain teams, hospice care and many other aspects of acute and chronic pain management is leading to a better understanding of the many issues surrounding drug therapy.

Definition of selected terms

Before moving on to discuss the pharmacology of analgesics in detail, it is important to be familiar with some definitions used in relation to both drug therapy and disease states.

Agonist a drug which combines with a receptor, activates it and produces a characteristic pharmacological effect such as analgesia. (This term is usually restricted to a description of opioid analgesics. Morphine is an example of a pure opioid agonist).

Antagonist a drug which interferes with the action of an agonist. It has no pharmacological effect of its own and can only produce an effect in the presence of an agonist. Naloxone is an example of an opioid antagonist.

Mixed agonist–antagonist a drug which acts simultaneously at two or more classes of receptor and at each one possesses either agonist (complete or partial) or antagonist activity. Nalbuphine is an example of an opioid mixed agonist–antagonist.

Analgesic a drug which modifies the perception of pain without loss of consciousness.

Allodynia pain due to a stimulus that does not normally produce pain.

Ceiling effect term used to describe a situation where at a certain dosage an increase in dosage does not result in an increase in pharmacological effect.

Dysaesthesia unpleasant or abnormal sensation

which may occur spontaneously or after a provoked response.

Hyperaesthesia increased sensitivity to stimulation which results in discomfort or pain.

Hyperalgesia an increased response to a normally painful stimulus.

Hyperpathia severe pain experienced after an initial delay, due to an increased reaction to a repetitive cutaneous stimulus.

Narcotic obsolete term previously used to describe morphine-like analgesics.

Opioid general term which encompasses both synthetic and naturally occurring compounds with morphine-like activity.

Opiate a compound specifically derived from the juice of the opium poppy (Papaver Somniferum), e.g. morphine.

Partial agonist a drug with an intrinsic activity of less than 1, which combines with a receptor. (The largest response obtainable from a partial agonist will always be less than the response elicited by a pure agonist at the same receptor). Buprenorphine is an opioid partial agonist.

Reflex sympathetic dystrophy continuous pain in a portion of an extremity following trauma, which may include a fracture but does not involve a major nerve, associated with sympathetic hyperactivity.

The differences between pure and partial agonists can be seen on the dose response curve in Figure 14.1. Drugs A, B and C are all active at the same receptor. Drugs A and B are both pure agonists but the latter is less potent than the former as a greater concentration of Drug B is required to produce a maximal response. Drug C is a partial agonist and its maximal effect is only about half of that produced by the complete agonists on the graph.

Two effects of partial agonists are important in relation to opioid analgesia:

i) An opioid partial agonist will have a lower ceiling of pain relief than a corresponding complete agonist.

ii) If a partial agonist is added to a pure agonist the effect of the latter may be reduced. (In clinical practice this effect may not result in decreased analgesia if sufficient vacant receptors are available such that the partial agonist does not displace the pure agonist from its opioid binding site).

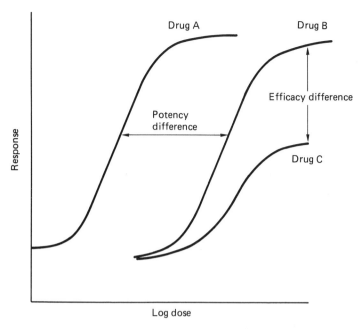

Figure 14.1 Drug potency and efficacy

Opioid analgesics

Historical aspects of opioid use

The therapeutic effects of opium were well known to ancient civilisations and the merits of poppy juice were recorded for posterity as early as the third century B.C. The word opium comes from the Greek word 'opos' meaning juice. The drug is obtained from the juice of the opium poppy, *Papaver Somniferum*. The use of opium spread from Asia Minor to Persia, where opium eating became popular, and from there it extended to India and China. Opium smoking did not become widespread in China until the second half of the eighteenth century. In 1803 Serturner isolated an alkaloid from opium which he named morphine, after Morpheus, the Greek god of dreams. Isolation of other alkaloids quickly followed, with codeine in 1832, and papaverine in 1848. Opium contains some 25 different alkaloids. Alkaloids are naturally occurring plant extracts which react with acids to form salts. The major alkaloids in opium are morphine and codeine.

Mechanism of action of opioid analgesics

Opioid analgesics exert their effect by binding to distinct types of opioid receptors in the body.

These receptors are widely distributed throughout the brain and spinal cord. Attempts have been made to correlate the various pharmacological effects produced by opioids to interactions with the different types of receptor. Drugs which bind to any one of three types of opioid receptor, mu (μ), delta (δ), and kappa (κ), will produce analgesia. The body produces substances called enkephalins and endorphins which can also activate these receptors. A fourth receptor type known as sigma (σ) should also be mentioned as activation of these receptors may be responsible for some of the side effects produced by opioid analgesics. An opioid may bind to a greater of lesser extent with all types of receptor and act as an agonist, partial agonist or an antagonist at each one. Opioids are classified according to their affinity and activity at various opioid receptors. Examples of each classification are shown in Table 14.2.

Absorption, distribution, metabolism and excretion of opioids

Most opioids can be given orally as they are readily absorbed from the gastrointestinal tract. However, first pass metabolism in the liver decreases the amount of active drug reaching the circulation. Therefore a higher oral than

Table 14.2 Classification of opioid receptors

Agent	mu	delta	kappa	sigma
morphine	agonist	agonist	agonist	
naloxone	antagonist	antagonist	antagonist	
buprenorphine	partial agonist	?	antagonist	
pentazocine	antagonist		partial agonist	agonist

parenteral dose is required to produce the same degree of analgesia.

The oral route is not suitable for use in the immediate postoperative period. Surgery and anaesthesia commonly cause vomiting and delayed gastric emptying which slow the passage of opioids into the small intestine where they are absorbed. When these effects subside several doses of opioid may be 'dumped' into the intestine with potentially disastrous results.

Some opioids, such as phenazocine, are given sublingually in order to try to avoid first pass metabolism. Following oral administration, the peak concentration of drug in the bloodstream occurs slightly later than after parenteral administration. The onset of action is shortest when opioids are given by the parenteral route, with the more lipid soluble agents such as diamorphine and fentanyl having a faster onset of action as they penetrate the central nervous system more quickly.

Many opioids have pharmacologically active metabolites which result in prolongation of analgesia. Under normal conditions opioids do not generally accumulate in the body, but if renal function is significantly impaired a pharmacologically-active opioid metabolite may accumulate and the effects of morphine may be prolonged (Aitkenhead *et al.*, 1984; McQuay *et al.*, 1984; Saw *et al.*, 1985).

What kind of effects do opioids produce?

Opioids have effects on many body systems and the magnitude of these effects is not always dose-related. Conditions such as coronary heart disease or respiratory disease may increase the likelihood of related adverse effects in some patients. This means that the nurse should always be alert to the possibility of adverse effects in patients receiving opioids. Vigilant monitoring of *all* patients receiving opioids is essential, especially at the beginning of therapy.

A detailed explanation of opioid effects is given in the following paragraph. Some readers may wish to proceed to the summary of important effects given in Table 14.3 under the section on monitoring of opioids.

Central nervous system

Respiratory depression is probably the most clinically significant effect and is dose-related. It may be severe enough to be life-threatening. Respiratory rate, tidal and minute volume are all reduced. The mechanism of action involves a decrease in the sensitivity of the respiratory centre within the brain stem to increased levels of circulating carbon dioxide in the blood stream. In patients without pre-existing respiratory disease in whom the dose is carefully titrated against the pain, respiratory depression is rarely a problem.

Drowsiness and *lethargy* may be a problem during the initial stages of opioid administration but usually resolve within a few days when the dose has been stabilised. *Euphoria* or *dysphoria* may be experienced and in normal subjects there can be marked *mental clouding*. These effects may become more pronounced as the dose is increased. Effects on the sensorium following therapeutic doses of opioids are usually less than following therapeutic doses of other drugs that affect the central nervous system, such as barbiturates.

Difficulty in concentration, a feeling of *heaviness in the limbs*, and a *sensation of warmth*, may also be noted.

Myosis, or constriction of the pupils is characteristic of opioid ingestion. Tolerance to this effect does not occur.

Nausea and *vomiting* result from direct stimulation by opioids of a section within the area postrema of the medulla known as the chemoreceptor trigger zone. This area contains a high density of dopamine and $5HT_3$ receptors. Drugs such as haloperidol and metoclopramide which block the action of these neurotransmitters are effective antiemetics for opioid-induced vomiting. Although ondansetron is a specific $5HT_3$ inhibitor, the exorbitant cost of this agent generally precludes its use other than for chemotherapy-induced vomiting due to cis-platinum (Editorial, 1991).

True opioid-induced vomiting is rarely a problem after 4 or 5 days of therapy; continuation beyond this time warrants a search for an alternative cause. Individuals vary in their susceptibility to the nausea and vomiting produced by opioids, which is more marked in ambulant patients. In most cases these effects diminish with successive doses.

Increased release of antidiuretic hormone from the hypothalamus can follow opioid administration.

Cardiovascular system

Hypotension results from venous and arterial dilatation. Most opioids can also cause release of histamine which can also cause hypotension. In a healthy cardiovascular system the effect of opioids on cardiac output and cardiac rate are minimal. In patients with coronary heart disease and following myocardial infarction effects may be more pronounced with a decrease in oxygen consumption, a drop in left ventricular diastolic pressure and marked hypotension.

Gastrointestinal system

Delayed gastric emptying and an *increase in tone* in the *first part of the duodenum* can retard the passage of drugs through the proximal part of the gastrointestinal tract for many hours. This can result in a marked decrease in the rate of absorption of drugs given by mouth. The effect will be especially marked after surgery which also has an effect on gastric emptying.

Biliary and pancreatic secretions within the small intestine are *decreased*. Non-propulsive contractions are increased whilst the propulsive contractions are decreased, resulting in an *increased gut transit time*. There is an increase in the viscosity of bowel contents as the increase in gut transit time permits more complete resorption of water from the contents of the intestinal lumen.

A similar situation occurs within the large intestine, where smooth muscle tone can be sufficient to cause spasm and pain. An increase in anal sphincter tone further augments the constipating effects produced throughout the gastrointestinal tract.

Biliary tract pressure rises following *spasm of the sphincter of Oddi* when some patients are given opioids. The effect may be so marked that a dose of morphine may actually precipitate rather than relieve pain.

An increase in tone of the detrusor muscle can cause *urinary urgency*, whilst an increase in tone of the vesical sphincter results in *difficulty in micturition*. These effects are exacerbated by the increased release of antidiuretic hormone. Catheterisation may sometimes be necessary following even therapeutic doses of opioids. Miscellaneous opioid effects include *sweating* and *flushing of the skin*. Histamine release can also cause *urticaria* at injection sites.

What to monitor, when to monitor, how to monitor

The effects of opioids of major clinical importance are summarised in Table 14.3.

The analgesia that results from opioid administration is an obviously beneficial pharmacological effect.

Effects such as undue sedation, constipation and nausea are undesirable and those such as hypotension and respiratory depression may be life-threatening.

Monitoring of all patients receiving opioids is mandatory in order to ensure their continued safety and comfort. Detailed protocols should exist in all areas where opioids are administered. These must include clear outlines of the individual areas of responsibility of doctors, nurses and pharmacists with regard to opioid use together with exact action to be taken when scores are greater or less than a specified value. The monitoring of patients receiving opioids should include the use of pain scores, sedation scores and respiratory rate, as well as routine blood pressure measurement.

An increasing level of sedation may be the first sign of impending respiratory depression, but a drop in respiratory rate to 8 breaths a minute is a clear indication that immediate remedial action may be required. Continuous

Table 14.3 Clinically important effects of opioids

• Itch	• Vomiting
• Nausea	• Analgesia
• Drowsiness	• Hypotension
• Urinary retention	• Constipation
• Respiratory depression	• Suppression of cough reflex

Name _____	Unit No. ___	
Address _____		
_____		
D.O.B.		
Date of Surgery		
Operation		
Circle Methods of Pain Relief Prescribed		
Oral	P.C.A.S.	
IM	Regional Techniques	
IV Bolus	Epidural	
IV Continuous	Tens	
Subcutaneous	Other	

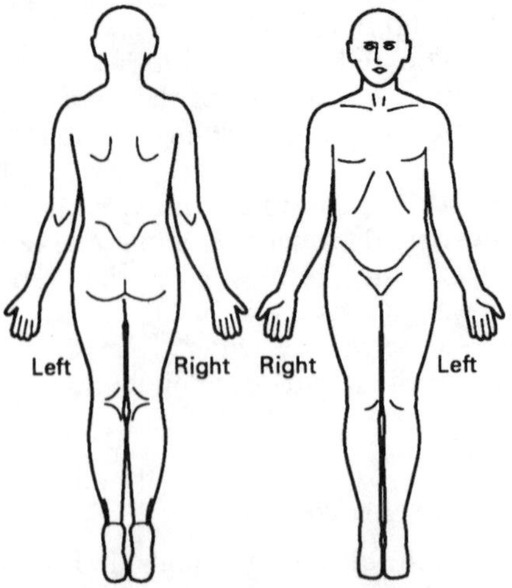

Left   Right   Right   Left

Pain Score			Sedation Score		Body Chart
No pain at rest No pain on movement	0	0	Awake (patient alert)		Shade areas of pain and label 'A' 'B'
No pain at rest Slight pain on movement	1	1	Drowsy (easy to arouse)		Movement =
Intermittent pain at rest Moderate pain on movement	2	2	Very drowsy (difficult to arouse somnolent)		Patient touches the opposite side of bed with hand
Continuous pain at rest Severe pain on movement	3	3	Sleep (normal sleep, easy to arouse)		

Figure 14.2 Acute pain chart

respiratory monitoring using pulse oximetry is highly desirable, as hypoxaemia may occur even when respiratory rate is normal. The recent report 'Pain after Surgery' stresses the importance of patient monitoring.

Individualisation of dosage demands that patients' needs for analgesia should not just be assessed when the next dose is due but also at a time following drug administration when it is judged that the drug is likely to be producing a maximal effect. There is little value in monitoring analgesia if no action is taken when a patient continues to score 3 on a scale of 0 = no pain and 3 = severe pain. This obviously indicates that the amount of pain relief the patient has received is inadequate. Appropriate action would then be to review the prescription and make an appropriate intervention. This may mean giving a supplementary dose immediately, increasing the amount of opioid given when the next regular dose is due if the prescription allows, or calling the prescribing physician straightaway.

Regular and careful assessment of analgesic requirements is especially important during initiation of therapy. Failure to do so may result in patients being in unremitting pain until the next dose is due, or even beyond.

An example of a simple and effective chart for monitoring of patients postoperatively is shown in Figure 14.2. This is currently used in the Derbyshire Royal Infirmary, Derby UK.

Do patients become tolerant to the effects of opioids?

The phenomenon of tolerance reflects the need to take increasing doses of a drug over time, in order to maintain the same therapeutic effect. Generally speaking, tolerance to the analgesic effect of opioids does not occur providing that the drug has been given for an opioid-responsive pain and the patient's underlying pathological condition has not changed. However, patients do become tolerant to some of the pharmacological effects of opioids such as drowsiness and nausea which, although they may be a problem at the beginning of therapy, usually diminish with time.

What is the risk of producing drug dependence in patients receiving opioids?

All drugs that alter mood and feeling have the potential to produce dependence in those who use them. Patients may continue to take these drugs in the absence of a clear medical indication and in spite of adverse medical and social effects. The intensity of the desire or craving for a particular drug varies between agents and individuals. The following discussion centres around the risk of dependence following the legitimate medical use of opioids rather than that following non-medical drug use.

Drug dependence is characterised by a syndrome in which the procurement and use of a particular drug assumes a priority greater than other types of behaviour in an individual's life.

Drug dependence has three components; physical dependence, psychological dependence and pharmacological dependence.

A person who is physically dependent on a drug experiences unpleasant physical symptoms when that drug is withdrawn. The opioid abstinence syndrome includes coldness, irregular respirations, sweating, painful abdominal cramps, vomiting, diarrhoea and sleep disturbance. The time course varies with the agent concerned. If an opioid is stopped abruptly in a patient previously maintained on opioids for more than about 10 days a withdrawal reaction may be precipitated. Opioids may be stopped for many reasons including an inability to take oral drugs because of uncontrolled vomiting. If the opioid is gradually withdrawn over a few days this syndrome should not occur. Patients with malignant disease, who have been previously maintained free of pain by large doses of opioid and who subsequently are given a neurolytic procedure which totally or partially alleviates their pain, may experience marked respiratory depression, drowsiness and nausea if the dose of drug is not rapidly decreased.

In psychological dependence the person feels compelled to take the drug either periodically or continually in order to experience its psychic effects. Psychological dependence almost never occurs in patients who are given opioids for opioid-responsive pain. In these cases it has been suggested that those who prescribe and administer opioids are at greater risk of developing addiction than those who receive them (Royal College of Surgeons of England).

It is very important to remember that opioids have very different effects on different patients groups. Psychic effects such as euphoria and hallucinations are inclined to be more pronounced in pain-free subjects and in those who do not have opioid-responsive pain.

Pharmacological dependence occurs because of changes in the capacity of body tissues to bind drugs (i.e. pharmacological 'receptors'). The body can become 'used to' drugs, so that larger doses are necessary to achieve the same effect; this is notoriously the case with opioids.

What type of pain can be relieved by opioids?

A notable feature of opioids is that analgesia is achieved without a loss of consciousness. Also, patients commonly say that the pain is still present but somehow it no longer distresses them.

Conditions where opioids may be considered first line therapy for relief of pain include

- Acute trauma.
- Early postoperative pain.
- Pain following myocardial infarction.
- Pain due to tumour infiltration of visceral organs.

It is important to remember that not all types of pain can be effectively controlled by opioids.

Potency and duration of action of opioids

The subjective nature of pain makes objective scientific assessment of the relative potencies of analgesics extremely difficult. Much of the early work on the potency ratios of opioid analgesics was done in single dose studies either in human volunteers, or in patients with acute rather than chronic pain. In addition, more sophisticated analytical techniques are now resulting in a reappraisal of our understanding of the importance of some opioid metabolites. Table 14.4 is intended only as a rough guide to indicate the approximate range of doses that may be encountered in pain management. The vast differences between acute and chronic pain are also reflected in the wider range of doses used in chronic pain. Some opioids such as morphine and methadone have a greater analgesic effect

Table 14.4 Dose and duration of action of selected opioids

Drug	Routes	Typical dose range	Duration of action
Morphine	po/im/iv/sc	5 mg upwards	3–4 hours
Buprenorphine	sl/im/iv	0.2–2 mg	6–10 hours
Codeine	po/im	15–60 mg	3–4 hours
Diamorphine	po/im/iv/sc	2.5 mg upwards	3–4 hours
Fentanyl	iv/topical	50–200 μg	10–20 minutes
Meptazinol	po/im/iv	75–200 mg	3–6 hours
Methadone	po/im/sc	5–30 mg	6–8 hours
Papaveretum	im/iv/sc	10–20 mg	3–4 hours
Pentazocine	po/im/iv/sc	30–60 mg	3–4 hours
Pethidine	po/im/iv	25–150 mg	2–3 hours
Phenazocine	sl	5–20 mg	4–6 hours

on chronic dosing. Oral to parenteral potency ratios may also change on chronic dosing. Textbook values can never substitute for the clinical assessment of pain in individual patients (Twycross and Lack, 1990).

Why do different patients need different doses of opioid to produce effective analgesia?

There are many reasons why patients have different analgesic requirements. The importance of ensuring that the type of pain being treated is one that will respond to opioid administration cannot be overemphasised. The rates at which our bodies absorb, distribute, metabolise and excrete drugs are different. Concomitant drugs and pre-existing diseases may influence drug handling. Following intramuscular injection of morphine peak plasma concentrations may be reached between 4 minutes and 1 hour after injection, and the actual concentration may vary by a factor of five.

The subjective nature of pain also profoundly influences the amount of pain and therefore the amount of analgesia an individual patient will require. A patient who is worried about the outcome of her forthcoming operation, is concerned about how her family will manage during her absence and the influence of her time away from work on future promotion is liable to experience more severe pain than a patient who does not have any of these worries undergoing the same procedure.

Drug interactions

Opioids potentiate the effects of other central nervous system depressants, such as tranquillisers, hypnotics, sedatives and anaesthetics.

Potentially fatal reactions can occur following the concomitant use of pethidine (meperidine) and structurally related compounds such as fentanyl with monoamine oxidase inhibitors (MAOIs), or within 14 days of stopping a MAOI. Morphine and other opioids should be used only with extreme caution in patients receiving these drugs.

Contraindications and precautions

Opioids are usually contraindicated in the presence of respiratory depression such as heart failure secondary to chronic obstructive airways disease and during exacerbations of asthma. They are also contraindicated where there is raised intracranial pressure. Elderly or debilitated patients and those with significant renal disease, hypothyroidism, adrenocortical insufficiency, obstructive bowel disorders, hypovolaemic shock or myasthenia gravis should be given opioids with extreme caution.

Although opioid analgesics may be considered broadly similar, some have certain particular properties and traditional uses which should be noted.

Morphine

About 20% of morphine is bound to plasma proteins in the bloodstream. Free morphine distributes to kidney, lung, liver and skeletal muscle. Early work on single doses of oral morphine indicated that 10 mg was approximately equianalgesic with 600 mg aspirin (Beecher *et al.*, 1953) and the oral to parenteral potency ratio was between 1:6 and 1:8. (Honde *et al.*, 1965). However, clinicians have long recognised that following repeated doses morphine exerts a greater analgesic effect. Recent work (Hanks *et al.*, 1987) has suggested an

Table 14.5. A selection of British and North American oral morphine products

Generic name	UK brand name	US brand name	Form	Dose unit
Morphine sulphate	Sevradol	–	Tablet	10,20 mg
Morphine sulphate	–	Statex	Tablet	5,10,25,50 mg
Morphine hydrochloride	–	MOS	Tablet	10,20,40,60 mg
Morphine sulphate	Oramorph	–	Liquid	10 mg/5 ml* 100 mg/5 ml
Morphine hydrochloride	–	MOS	Liquid	1,5,10,20,50 mg per ml
Morphine sulphate	–	Statex	Liquid	1,5,10,15 mg/ml
Morphine sulphate	MST Continus	–	Slow release tablet	10,30,60,100, 200 mg
Morphine sulphate	–	MS Contin	Slow release tablet	15,30,60,90 mg
Morphine hydrochloride	–	MOS.SR	Slow release tablet	30,60 mg

*This strength of Oramorph contains approximately 3 g sugar in 10 ml. The concentrated solution contains no sugar.

explanation for this observation. The two main metabolites of morphine are morphine-3-glucuronide and morphine-6-glucuronide. Morphine-6-glucuronide (M6G) is now known to be a more potent analgesic than morphine (Pasternak *et al.*, 1987). However, penetration of M6G into the central nervous system is slow and may account for the difference in analgesic effects of morphine following single and repeated doses. The oral to parenteral potency ratio of morphine on repeat dosing is now thought to be of the order of 1:3.

Although morphine does undergo enterohepatic circulation, this is not thought to contribute greatly to the increased analgesic effect seen on chronic dosing (Hanks and Ward, 1989).

Unlike unconjugated morphine the glucuronides accumulate in patients with renal impairment which can lead to enhanced opioid effects, due to decreased clearance of the M6G (Sear *et al.*, 1989).

It has been suggested that another metabolite of morphine; normorphine, may be responsible for the neuroexcitatory symptoms occasionally seen in patients on high doses of morphine (Glare *et al.*, 1990). This metabolite was detected in the plasma of two patients receiving high dose morphine who had myoclonus and renal impairment. These findings need to be substantiated in a larger group of patients.

A number of liquid morphine and instant release tablet preparations are now available,

as well as injections and suppositories. The introduction of slow release oral preparations which allow 12-hourly dosing have revolutionised the management of opioid-responsive pain in advanced cancer. Such formulations are not suitable for postoperative use as gastric stasis may result in the dumping of several doses into the intestine when gastric function returns to normal (Brahams, 1984). They are unsuitable for rescue analgesia because of the time taken to reach peak plasma levels. A selection of oral morphine preparations are shown in Table 14.5.

Practical points

- Titrate doses against pain to minimise side effects.
- Monitor for respiratory depression.
- Warn patients that they may be drowsy for a few days whilst dose is titrated, but this effect usually wears off.
- Sedation is unusual in patients with opioid-responsive pain after a few days – look for other causes.
- Watch out for signs of accumulation (drowsiness, respiratory depression) in patients with renal impairment.

Codeine

Codeine is available as the sulphate and phosphate salts. It is about one-twelfth as potent as morphine, to which it is metabolised in the liver, and is about 60% as potent when given by mouth as compared to the intramuscular route. The duration of action is about 3–4 hours. Although employed for the relief of mild to moderate pain, it is more commonly used as an antidiarrhoeal and antitussive. It is traditionally the opioid of choice in cases of head injury and neurosurgery because of its allegedly minimal effect on pupil size, in comparison with other agents. The usual dose is 15–60 mg.

Analgesics such as co-codamol, co-codaprin, Tylenol No. 1, Tylenol No. 1 Forte which may be bought without prescription contain 8 mg codeine per tablet.

Practical points

As for morphine.

Diamorphine

Diamorphine (diacetylmorphine, heroin) is rapidly converted in the body to 6-monoacetyl morphine and subsequently to morphine. Traditionally it has been said that diamorphine has a faster onset of action than morphine, one of the reasons given being its greater degree of lipophilicity and therefore more rapid penetration into the brain (Nimmo and Smith, 1989). This supposition has recently been challenged (Morrison et al., 1991) in a small randomised double-blind cross over study using an ischaemic limb pain model in human volunteers. This study suggested that following intravenous administration the onset of effect of diamorphine was some 50% greater than that of morphine. These results require confirmation in a non-laboratory situation. Early studies suggest the converse may apply to the intramuscular route (Reichie et al., 1962; Beaver et al., 1981). The explanation of these findings is likely to be found in the relative formation and disposition of pharmacologically active metabolites within the brain. The duration of action of diamorphine is generally considered to be somewhat shorter than that of morphine.

The major distinguishing property of diamorphine is that of extreme solubility. One gram diamorphine hydrochloride can be dissolved in 1.6 ml of water to give a volume of 2.4 ml. This compares with 21 ml water needed to dissolve 1 g morphine sulphate. Many patients with advanced cancer are markedly cachexic and therefore diamorphine is the drug of choice for subcutaneous opioid infusions in these patients in the UK. Diamorphine is not routinely available in North America; however morphine acetate is available and this is almost as soluble as diamorphine hydrochloride. Hydromorphone is another suitable alternative (see separate entry).

Practical points

- As for morphine.
- Extremely soluble – opioid of choice for parenteral administration in cachexic cancer patients in UK.

Dihydrocodeine

Dihydrocodeine is about one-tenth as potent as morphine, and is similar to codeine in other respects. The usual dose is 30–60 mg although the combination prescription-only analgesic co-dydramol contains only 10 mg along with 500 mg paracetamol.

Practical points

As for morphine.

Dextromoramide

Dextromoramide is a potent short-acting analgesic which when used sublingually will produce analgesia within about 15 minutes. A single 5 mg dose of dextromoramide is roughly equivalent to 10 mg morphine with regard to peak effect, but the duration of action is only about 2 hours (Twycross, 1984). Although unsuitable for maintenance of continual analgesia, it is useful as a rescue analgesic for short painful procedures such as dressing changes where the patient's baseline analgesia would be insufficient.

Practical points

- As for morphine, plus
- Effective sublingually.
- Excellent 'rescue' analgesic.
- Useful for providing analgesia during short procedures, e.g. dressing changes.

Hydromorphone

Hydromorphone (Dilaudid) is about six to seven times as potent as morphine parenterally. The duration of action is about 4–5 hours (American Pain Society, 1990). It has been successfully used in the management of pain in advanced cancer by continuous and intermittent subcutaneous infusion (Bruera et al., 1988). Hydromorphone is available as tablets (1,2,4,8 mg) oral liquid (1 mg/ml) injection (2,10 mg/ml) and suppositories (3 mg) in North America. It is currently available as an investigational drug in the UK.

Practical points

- As for morphine.
- High potency and extreme solubility (1 g in 3 ml water) allow small volumes to be given parenterally, minimising patient discomfort.

Methadone

Methadone (Physeptone, Dolophine) is well absorbed from the gastrointestinal tract and buccal mucosa (Weinberg et al., 1988). Onset of analgesic effect occurs within 0.5–1 hour following an oral dose and within 10–20 minutes of parenteral administration. Peak plasma concentrations are seen some 4 hours after oral administration, and 1–2 hours after subcutaneous or intramuscular administration (Jaffe and Martin, 1990).

The effects of methadone are very different after single and chronic dosing. The elimination half-life is about 15 hours after a single dose but at least three times that on repeated dosing. Analgesia lasts around 6–8 hours, illustrating that half-life is only one of the factors which influence the duration of action of a drug. Cumulation can produce troublesome sedation. It is more commonly used in the USA than in the UK for the management of severe chronic pain. It is approximately equipotent with morphine in a single dose but about three times more potent on cumulative dosing.

It is available as 5 mg and 10 mg (US only) tablets and 10 mg/ml injection.

Practical points

- As for morphine, plus
- Sedation may occur and persist on cumulative dosing.

Oxycodone

Oxycodone is approximately equipotent with morphine and has an oral to parenteral potency ratio of 1:2 Jaffe and Martin, 1990). It is only available in the UK as 30 mg slow release suppositories. The duration of action is about 3–5 hours but may be about 6–8 hours following use of the slow release suppository. In North America 2.5 and 5 mg tablets of oxycodone alone are available and it is combined with aspirin as Percodan and with paracetamol (acetaminophen) as Percocet.

Practical points

As for morphine.

Papaveretum

Papaveretum (Omnopon, pantopon) is a mixture of a number of opium alkaloids. It contains about 50% morphine as well as approximately 5% codeine, 5% papaverine (a smooth muscle relaxant) and 20% noscapine (a non-analgesic antitussive). Its continuing favour primarily as a postoperative analgesic in the UK marks a triumph of tradition over science. It is only available as a parenteral preparation.

Recent in vitro work suggested a mutagenic effect for papaveretum in mammalian cell lines (Current Problems, 1991). It is currently being reformulated to remove the noscapine, and the Committee on Safety of Medicines do not recommend its use in women of child-bearing age.

Practical points

- As for morphine, plus
- Offers no advantage over morphine.
- Possible teratogenic effect of noscapine currently prohibits use in women of child-bearing age.

Pethidine

Pethidine (meperidine, Demerol, Pethadol) is about one-tenth as potent as morphine. Poor oral biovailability makes it an even weaker analgesic when given by mouth. A duration of action of about 2–3 hours makes it unsuitable for most acute or chronic pain states. It is metabolised to norpethidine (normeperidine) which has a half-life of about 15–22 hours and accumulates in both hepatic and renal failure (Jaffe and Martin, 1990).

Norpethidine (normeperidine) may cause convulsions. It is reputed to cause less spasm of the sphincter of Oddi, making it a suitable analgesic for biliary colic. Although the half-life is only about 3 hours in the adult it is some 22 hours in the neonate which could lead to neonatal respiratory depression.

Pethidine (meperidine) should not be given to patients receiving monoamine oxidase inhibitors (MAOIs) as a hypertensive crisis may result.

Practical points

- As for morphine, plus
- Unsuitable for chronic pain because of low potency and short duration of action.
- Monitor for signs of accumulation and toxicity in patients with hepatic and renal impairment.
- Serious drug interaction with MAOIs.

Phenazocine

Phenazocine is about 5 times as potent as morphine when given sublingually, and may produce analgesia lasting for 6–8 hours. It is reputed to cause less increase in biliary tract pressure than other opioids and be less sedative than morphine. There is no parenteral preparation. It is not available in North America.

Practical points

- As for morphine, plus
- Effective sublingually.
- Analgesia lasts 6–8 hours allowing good night's sleep.
- Disguise bitter taste by administration inside a 'Polo' mint.

Meptazinol

Meptazinol (Meptid) is a unique compound, being a mu agonist and also having central anticholinergic actions which also contribute to its analgesic effect. It is about one-tenth as potent as morphine parenterally, with a duration of action of about 4 hours. It undergoes extensive first pass metabolism which results in an oral bioavailability of about 10%. The incidence of side effects such as nausea, vomiting and dizziness appear higher than with some other opioids whereas the tendency to produce respiratory depression and constipation may be somewhat less. It crosses the placenta but is metabolised by the neonate with a half-life of about 3 hours.

Practical points

- As for morphine, plus
- Incidence of side effects may be higher than morphine.

Nefopam

Nefopam (Acupan) is a centrally-acting drug with a somewhat uncertain mode of action. It is not an opioid and also has no effect on prostaglandin synthesis and therefore has no anti-inflammatory effect. It should not be used following a myocardial infarction or in patients on MAOIs or those with a history of fits, glaucoma or urinary retention. It is used for the relief of moderate acute and chronic pain such as that following trauma, some dental procedures, musculo-skeletal pain and postoperative pain. A major advantage of nefopam is that it does not cause constipation. As it does not cause respiratory depression, unlike opioids, there should be no danger of respiratory arrest if the drug is taken with alcohol. It is not effective for all patients and it is not possible to predict those patients for whom it will provide good pain relief. Elderly patients should start on a dose of 30 mg every 8 hours due to possible decreased clearance. Healthy adults should begin with 60 mg and increase to 90 mg if required. The oral to parenteral potency ratio is about 1:3 and following intramuscular injection the onset of effect is about 15 minutes with maximum analgesia being achieved in approximately 90 minutes. It is only available in the UK.

Practical points

- Does not cause constipation.
- Does not cause respiratory depression.
- Not effective for all patients.
- Contraindicated in patients with glaucoma, urinary retention, history of fits or those taking MAOIs.

Nalbuphine

Nalbuphine (Nubain) is a mu antagonist and kappa partial agonist (like pentazocine and butorphanol). It is only available for parenteral administration because of a significant first pass effect, and therefore of limited application in chronic pain. Drowsiness is the most commonly reported side effect, otherwise the incidence of side effects is similar to morphine. It has been shown to be an effective analgesic in pain following myocardial infarction.

Practical points

• No oral preparation, therefore unsuitable for chronic pain.
• May cause more drowsiness than morphine.

Pentazocine (30–60 mg 3–4 hourly by injection)

Pentazocine (Fortral, Talwin) was the first of the nalorphine-like agonist-antagonist analgesics to be used in clinical practice. It has a low oral bioavailability, and is a weak and unpredictable analgesic when given by mouth. It is best given by injection in doses of 30–60 mg, every 3–4 h. It is difficult to demonstrate any advantages over morphine in either acute or chronic pain states. It is potentially hazardous if used to relieve pain following myocardial infarction as it increases pressure in the left ventricle and pulmonary artery (Alderman et al., 1972). It has been shown to be less effective than two cocodaprin tablets in patients with rheumatoid arthritis and cancer. The incidence of psychotomimetic side effects such as hallucinations, dysphoria and depersonalisation approaches 20% in some patients and is dose-related and more prevalent on long term use.

Practical points

• Contraindicated in myocardial infarction.
• Low oral bioavailability and dose dependent side effects.

Buprenorphine

Buprenorphine is the only synthetic opioid partial agonist used to any great extent in current clinical practice in the UK and is about 50 times more potent than morphine. It is available for parenteral and sublingual use. As it has a high affinity for the mu receptor the duration of action may be some 8–10 hours. It has the usual opioid side effect profile but nausea and vomiting appear more marked in ambulant patients, and when they occur can be severe. A clinical dose range of 0.2–10 mg has been demonstrated (Budd, 1981) but the availability of only 0.2 and 0.4 mg tablets means that from a practical standpoint the dose range is more limited.

It is recognised that whilst some patients respond well to buprenorphine others experience intense nausea and vomiting necessitating withdrawal of the drug.

Practical points

• Long duration of action.
• Effective sublingually.
• Some patients experience intense nausea and vomiting.

It is a strong analgesic drug to be used for moderate to severe pain.

Naloxone

Naloxone is an opioid antagonist which is usually used in clinical practice to reverse the respiratory depressant effects of opioid analgesics. The duration of action of naloxone is dose-related and much shorter than that of the majority of opioids. The rate and depth of respiration must be closely monitored in patients in whom naloxone has been used so that any recurrence of respiratory depression can be quickly treated. In cases of deliberate opioid overdose up to 10 mg may be occasionally needed to reverse the respiratory depressant effects of the ingested opioid. Naloxone is currently available in vials of 400 µg/ml for intravenous, intramuscular or subcutaneous injection. It is only partially effective in reversing the effects of partial agonists, but respiratory depression is rarely a problem with the agents in current use. It has been used in the treatment of central post-stroke pain, (thalamic pain) (Budd, 1985).

Practical points

• Very high doses may be needed to reverse respiratory depression due to opioid overdose.

- Only partially effective in reversing the effects of partial agonists.
- May precipitate a withdrawal reaction in patients dependent on opioids.
- Side effects very rarely a problem.
- Ventricular tachycardia and fibrillation reported in patients with ventricular irritability (very rare).

Combination analgesics

Fixed combinations of drugs offer little flexibility in terms of dosing. A need to increase the dose of one of the constituents leads to an inevitable and often undesirable increase in the other contents.

There are several generic and a plethora of branded preparations of combination analgesics available in the UK and North America. These usually comprise a small dose of a weak opioid together with either paracetamol or aspirin. Some are available without prescription. The low dose of opioid contained in many preparations makes it difficult to see how they could provide any greater degree of pain relief than paracetamol or aspirin alone. However, they remain popular with physicians and patients alike. Many branded combination analgesics are no longer prescribable in the UK within the National Health Service. The combination analgesic co-proxamol is notable for its lethality in overdose. Ingestion of only a small quantity of tablets when taken in conjunction with alcohol can cause rapid and fatal respiratory depression due to the synergistic action of alcohol and dextro-propoxyphene.

The constituents of generic combination analgesics and those with a higher opioid content in the U.K. are shown in Table 14.6.

It is becoming more common to see two different analgesic drugs prescribed together. Examples are codeine and NSAIDs in dental pain and the addition of NSAIDs to morphine to control bone pain in cancer.

Paracetamol (acetaminophen)

Paracetamol (acetaminophen) is a mild analgesic and antipyretic with some anti-inflammatory activity. It is only a weak inhibitor of prostaglandin synthesis, but may be more effective against enzymes in the CNS than those in the periphery. It is rapidly and almost completely

Table 14.6 Combination analgesics available on NHS prescriptions

Generic name	Constituents	Available without prescription?
Co-codamol	codeine 8 mg paracetamol 500 mg	yes
Co-codaprin	codeine 8 mg aspirin 400 mg	yes
Co-dydramol	dihydrocodeine 10 mg paracetamol 500 mg	no
Co-proxamol	d-propoxyphene 32.5 mg paracetamol 325 mg	no
Aspav	papaveretum 10 mg aspirin 500 mg	no
Solpadol/Tylex	codeine 30 mg paracetamol 500 mg	no
Benorylate	aspirin/paracetamol ester 2 g benorylate is approx. equivalent to: aspirin 1150 mg & paracetamol 970 mg	yes

absorbed from the gut with peak plasma levels occurring 30–60 minutes after oral ingestion. Given 0.5–1 g, every 4–6 h max 4 g daily (adults). Following therapeutic doses the plasma half-life is between 1 and 4 h, but may be many times this following acute overdose. The majority is conjugated in the liver to the sulphate and glucuronide metabolites; very little is excreted unchanged. Following an overdose of paracetamol a toxic metabolite called N-acetyl-p-benzoquinone is formed when hepatic glutathione stores are depleted. This causes hepatic necrosis and renal tubular necrosis. Hepatic and renal damage can be prevented by the administration of N-aceyl cysteine, a glutathione precursor. In other respects paracetamol is considered to be of low toxicity.

Practical points

- Well tolerated in therapeutic doses.
- Severe hepatotoxicity may develop following overdose.

Aspirin

Aspirin or acetylsalicylic acid is a mild analgesic, antipyretic and anti-inflammatory agent. It inhibits the production of prostaglandins both in the CNS and in the periphery. Aspirin inhibits the production of thromboxane A_2, a potent aggregating agent, normally found in platelets. This property accounts for the pro-

Table 14.7 Chemical classification of NSAIDs

Drug class	Generic name	Unit dose	Tab Cap	Sol Tab	E/C Tab	S/R Tab	Liq Susp	Inj	Sup	Typical adult dose
Salicylate and derivatives	Aspirin	300 mg	*	*	*					300–900 mg
		600 mg		*						4-hourly
	Aloxiprin	=500 mg aspirin		*						250–1000 mg up to 4 × daily
	Benorylate	750 mg	*							1500 mg twice daily
	(Aspirin/ paracetamol ester)	2 g					*			2–4 g twice daily
	Choline magnesium trisalicylate	= 500 mg	*							500–1500 mg twice daily
	Diflunisal	250 mg								500 mg
		500 mg	*							daily or twice daily
	Salsalate	500 mg	*							500 mg–1 g 3–4 × daily
Propionic acid derivatives	Ibuprofen	100 mg					*			200–600 mg
		200 mg	*							3 or 4 times
		300 mg			*					daily
		400 mg	*							
		600 mg	*							S/R 300–900 mg twice daily
	Fenbufen	300 mg	*							300 mg mane
		450 mg	*	*						600 mg nocte or 450 mg twice daily
	Fenoprofen	200 mg	*							200 mg–600 mg
		300 mg	*							3–4 × daily
		600 mg	*							
	Flurbiprofen	50 mg	*							up to 300 mg
		100 mg	*						*	daily in
		200 mg			*					divided doses
	Ketoprofen	50 mg	*							50–100 mg
		100 mg	*						*	once daily
		200 mg				*				
	Naproxen	250 mg	*				*			250–500 mg
		500 mg	*						*	twice daily
	Tiaprofenic acid	200 mg	*							600 mg daily,
		300 mg	*			*				2–3 divided doses
Acetic acids	Diclofenac	25 mg			*					up to 150 mg daily
		50 mg		*	*					in divided doses
		100 mg				*			*	
		75 mg						*		
	Indomethacin	25 mg	*				*			200 mg daily in
		50 mg	*							divided doses
		75 mg				*				
		100 mg							*	
	Sulindac	100 mg	*							200 mg twice
		200 mg	*							daily
	Tolmetin	200 mg	*							up to 1800 mg daily
		400 mg	*							in 3 or 4 divided doses
	Ketorolac	10 mg	*						*	10–30 mg every 4–6 h up to 90 mg daily for 2 days only
		30 mg					*	*		
Enolic Acid	Phenylbutazone	100 mg	*		*					up to 300 mg daily in 3 divided doses
	Azapropazone	300 mg	*							1200 mg daily in
		600 mg	*							2–4 divided doses

Table 14.7 *continued*

Drug class	Generic name	Unit dose	Tab Cap	Sol Tab	E/C Tab	S/R Tab	Liq Susp	Inj	Sup	Typical adult dose
Fenemates	Mefenamic acid	250 mg	*	*			*			500 mg 3 times
		500 mg	*							daily
Oxicams	Piroxicams	10 mg	*	*						10–30 mg daily in
		20 mg	*	*					*	single or divided doses.
	Tenoxicam	20 mg	*							20 mg daily
Miscellaneous	etodolac	200 mg	*							up to 600 mg daily
		300 mg	*							in 1–2 divided doses
	Nabumetone	500 mg	*			*				1 g nocte
Topical	Felbinac	3% gel								massage lightly 2–4 times daily
	Ibuprofen	5% cream								4–10 cm cream 3–4 times daily
	Piroxicam	0.5% gel								3 cm 3–4 times daily

longation of bleeding time following use of aspirin. Many factors affect the absorption of aspirin, which occurs partly in the stomach but largely in the upper part of the small intestine. Following oral therapeutic doses aspirin is rapidly hydrolysed to salicylate, peak plasma levels occurring about 2 hours after ingestion. The drug is widely distributed in body tissues.

Rectal absorption is unreliable, but salicylic acid is rapidly absorbed from the intact skin following topical application. Salicylates are highly bound to plasma proteins. Salicylate is mainly metabolised by enzymes in the liver. After high doses these enzymatic systems become saturated leading to an increase in the plasma half-life of salicylate from 2 or 3 hours to between 15 and 30 hours. The metabolic products are excreted by the kidneys.

Aspirin has a dose-dependent effect on the excretion of uric acid, causing inhibition at low doses and an increase in elimination at high doses.

Gastrointestinal side effects are common following use of aspirin even at therapeutic doses. Nausea, vomiting and gastric ulceration can occur. As aspirin is highly bound to plasma proteins it may displace other highly bound drugs such as anticoagulants and methotrexate resulting in an enhanced therapeutic effect. Up to 5% of asthmatic patients find that aspirin may precipitate a severe asthmatic attack. There is a high degree of cross-reactivity with NSAIDs and other agents such as tartrazine which inhibit prostaglandin synthesis.

Aspirin should not be given to children under 12 years of age as it is associated with a high incidence of Reye's syndrome which culminates in encephalopathy and fatty degeneration of the liver.

Following overdose salicylates may cause respiratory stimulation, respiratory alkalosis, metabolic acidosis, acute renal failure, pulmonary oedema, convulsions and cardiac arrest.

Practical points

- Gastrointestinal side effects may be a problem – minimise by using soluble tablets administered with food.
- May precipitate severe asthmatic attack in some patients.

Non-steroidal anti-inflammatory agents (NSAIDs) (Table 14.7)

Within the group of drugs known as the non-steroidal anti-inflammatory agents there are more than 20 different chemical compounds which are available in a bewildering variety of formulations and presentations. They account for about 5% of all prescriptions in the UK and are responsible for about 25% of the adverse reactions reported to the Committee on Safety of Medicines (CSM) each year.

Mechanism of action

The four cardinal signs of inflammation are:

- Rubor (redness)
- Calor (heat)

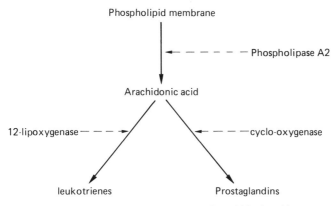

Figure 14.3 Metabolic pathway of arachidonic acid

- Tubor (dolor)
- Dolor (pain)

are mediated by the action of prostaglandins and substances such as senotonin (5-HT), histamine and bradykinin. Prostaglandins are produced in body tissues following a variety of physical, chemical and neurohumoral stimuli. Following stimulation, the enzyme phospholipase A_2 releases arachidonic acid from membrane phospholipids (Figure 14.3).

Two groups of compounds, prostaglandins and leukotrienes, are formed by the action of cyclo-oxygenase and lipoxygenases on arachidonic acid. Both are mediators of inflammation. Leukotrienes are involved in such diseases as asthma and psoriasis. Prostaglandins refers to a vast family of compounds which are involved in a variety of body processes as well as inflammation.

NSAIDs inhibit the production of prostaglandins by reversibly inhibiting the enzyme cyclo-oxygenase. Aspirin is slightly different from other NSAIDs in that it irreversibly inhibits the enzyme.

Although all NSAIDs reduce inflammation by the same mechanism of inhibition of prostaglandin synthesis they differ in the incidence and type of side effects they produce. There is also a considerable variation in the therapeutic response of different patients to any single agent, and in the response of individual patients to a variety of NSAIDs. These factors partly justify the plethora of compounds currently available.

Although broadly similar in many respects, a chemical classification of NSAIDs helps the clinician to make an informed choice when changing from one agent to another.

Indications for use

NSAIDs are indicated for the relief of pain and inflammation in gout, rheumatoid arthritis and osteoarthritis, soft tissue injuries such as frozen shoulder, some sports injuries and sprains and strains, dysmenorrhoea and postoperative pain, including gynaecological procedures. Over 50% of patients will respond to the first NSAID prescribed whilst a resistant 5% may be unresponsive to all NSAIDs. It is advisable to become familiar with one compound from each chemical group so that, if necessary, the side effects specific to each group can be avoided. Dosage should be increased until relief is obtained or the maximum tolerated dosage has been reached. If an increase in dosage is necessary, it should not be done more frequently than every five half-lives, so that the plasma level of drug has been allowed to reach a plateau. If a patient's symptoms are only intermittent a compound with a short half-life is preferable, whilst for cases of chronic pain a drug with a long half-life allowing once daily dosing may be better. However, these must be used with caution in elderly patients where cumulation of drug can cause problems.

Side effects

Gastrointestinal upset manifest as nausea, bleeding from the gut and diarrhoea may be produced by any of the NSAIDs. The most common site of ulceration is the stomach.

Gastrointestinal bleeding is partly due to a direct local irritant effect and partly to a systemic effect.

The acidic nature of most NSAIDs means that they are well absorbed from the acid medium of the stomach. However, should gastrointestinal upset be a problem the drug should be taken after food.

Ibuprofen is probably the least likely of all NSAIDs to produce gastrointestinal upset. Skin rashes can be caused by many NSAIDs. Some asthmatic patients find that they are hypersensitive to aspirin and other NSAIDs and their use can precipitate a severe asthmatic attack.

These drugs may cause fluid retention which can lead to hypertension, heart failure and oedema in susceptible patients. Renal function may be adversely affected by NSAIDs, although severe renal toxicity is rare. Likewise, hyperkalaemia and blood dyscrasias are rare but can be life-threatening. The incidence of blood dyscrasias with phenylbutazone means that this drug is now only available for the treatment of ankylosing spondylitis. Occasional NSAIDs, especially indomethacin, can cause side effects such as dizziness, headache and hallucinations.

There are few absolute contraindications to the use of NSAIDs but they should be used with caution in patients with pre-existing renal and hepatic disease, hypertension and cardiac failure.

Formulation factors

Prostaglandins are present in the stomach where they have a protective effect on the gastric mucosa. Pharmaceutical manufacturers have produced oral NSAIDs with an enteric-coating or in a slow-release formulation in an effort to overcome the problems of gastrointestinal side effects. However, only a small proportion of these effects are due to local irritation; the majority are caused by systemic metabolites. Therefore the use of enteric-coated, slow-release or rectal formulations will only partly alleviate this problem.

Fenbufen, sulindac, nalbumetone and benorylate are examples of pro-drugs which are promoted as being useful for patients in whom gastrointestinal side effects are a problem. A pro-drug is one that is absorbed in a pharmacologically inactive form and then metabolised,

usually in the liver, to pharmacologically active metabolites. Thus although the protective influence of the prostaglandins normally found in the stomach will be unaffected by such preparations, as this mechanism is only partly responsible for gastric side effects, some patients taking these preparations may find only partial relief of their problems. All such preparations are more expensive than conventional oral dosage forms and a clear need, and demonstrable benefit must be shown before the expense of such preparations can be justified. Some patients given an enteric-coated preparation do notice an improvement in gastrointestinal tolerance. This may be because less drug is absorbed. Slow-release preparations will result in a more gradual climb to peak blood levels and therefore perhaps fewer side effects.

Sometimes, when other analgesics have failed, it is necessary to give NSAIDs to patients who have had a peptic ulcer in the past. Ibuprofen is probably the drug of choice in these cases. If symptoms occur an H_2 blocker such as ranitidine or cimetidine may be given concomitantly to protect the gastric mucosa. Recently an oral prostaglandin analogue called misoprostol has become available for use in this situation. However, the prophylactic use of misoprostol has yet to be proved cost effective.

Drug interactions

There are a small but significant number of drug interactions associated with NSAIDs. Some but not all, e.g. diflunisal, prolong bleeding time and therefore should not be used by patients taking oral anticoagulants.

As NSAIDs can cause a rise in blood pressure, they antagonise the effects of antihypertensive agents. Particular care is needed in patients taking ACE inhibitors such as captopril.

The risk of renal failure is increased in patients taking NSAIDs and diuretics. Patients taking potassium-sparing diuretics such as spironolactone should be carefully monitored for hyperkalaemia. Anticoagulants, methotrexate and oral hypoglycaemic drugs are highly bound to plasma proteins. NSAIDs can compete for these binding sites and thus potentiate the effects of these agents with possible disastrous results. Careful monitoring of such patients is mandatory.

Topical preparations

Some NSAIDs are available in a topical formulation, the contention being that there should be reduced incidence of side effects following the use of such preparations. Application over the affected area, such as an inflamed joint, is advocated. In theory this should result in a therapeutic concentration of drug in the affected tissue or synovial fluid but minimal levels elsewhere. However, some experimental data have shown that drug levels in distant joints are not markedly lower than those over which the preparation was applied. Thus it appears that once the drug is systemically absorbed it is widely distributed. Application is messy and these products are many times the cost of oral generic NSAIDs. Widespread use seems difficult to justify.

The various non-steroidal anti-inflammatory agents are compared and contrasted in Table 14.7.

Practical points

- Gastrointestinal symptoms are common, e.g. nausea, diarrhoea.
- Gastrointestinal bleeding is only partly due to a direct irritant effect.
- If GI effects are a problem, give drug after food.
- NSAIDs may precipitate an asthma attack in about 5% of asthmatics.
- Fluid retention caused by NSAIDs may exacerbate heart failure, hypertension and oedema.
- Use with caution in elderly patients and those with renal and hepatic impairment.
- Psychosis and hallucinations reported with indomethacin (rare).
- Most NSAIDs prolong bleeding time.
- NSAIDs should not be given concurrently with methotrexate, anticoagulants or oral hypoglycaemic agents.
- NSAIDs may antagonise the effects of antihypertensive agents.

Local anaesthetics

The first local anaesthetic to be used in clinical practice was cocaine. This was isolated in 1860 from the leaves of a shrub called *Erythroxylon coca* which grows high up in the Andes mountains in Peru. However, it was not until 1884 that it was used in medicine to produce local anaesthesia in dentistry. A search for synthetic substitutes for cocaine resulted in the production of procaine in 1905. Today the most widely used local anaesthetics are lignocaine, bupivacaine and prilocaine.

Local anaesthetics act on the cell membrane and block the increase in the permeability of the sodium channels in the membrane which usually follows depolarisation.

The duration of action of local anaesthetics depends on the length of time the drug is in contact with a nerve or nerve plexus, before absorption into the systemic circulation and metabolism by plasma esterases. To prolong the duration of action, vasoconstrictors such as adrenaline are often incorporated with local anaesthetics. These keep the anaesthetic in the vicinity of the nerve for a longer period. However, vasoconstrictors should not be used when local anaesthetic is injected into digits, hands or feet as prolonged arterial constriction can lead to irreversible hypoxic damage, tissue necrosis and gangrene.

Adverse effects

Following absorption into the circulation, local anaesthetics can affect all structures in which there is a potential for nerve conduction. They can produce marked effects within the central nervous system (CNS) due to a depression of neuronal activity. Drowsiness is relatively common, and lignocaine may produce euphoria or dysphoria. Restlessness and tremor can progress to clonic convulsions and finally CNS depression and respiratory arrest.

High concentrations of local anaesthetics may adversely affect the myocardium with decreases in conduction, cardiac contractility and arteriolar dilatation.

Hypersensitivity to local anaesthetics is a rare but serious occurrence and is more common with the ester-type agents such as amethocaine, benzocaine, cocaine and procaine. Allergic dermatitis or asthma attacks are frequent manifestations.

Practical points (general)

- Duration of action of local anaesthetics is increased by concurrent use of vasoconstrictor agents such as adrenaline.

- Adrenaline cannot be injected into digits, hands, feet, ear or penis.
- High concentrations of local anaesthetics can cause cardiac arrhythmias and CNS toxicity manifest as drowsiness, blurred vision, paraesthesiae, restlessness, tremors, dysphoria and respiratory arrest.
- Hypersensitivity to local anaesthetics is rare.

Lignocaine (lidocaine)

Lignocaine (lidocaine, Xylocaine etc) was introduced into clinical practice in 1948 and is now the most widely used local anaesthetic. It has a fast onset of action and when given in conjunction with a vasoconstrictor the duration of local anaesthesia is about one and a half hours. Side effects mainly result from its actions on the CNS. Drowsiness, dizziness, paraesthesiae, convulsions and coma may occur, and more rarely ventricular fibrillation and cardiac arrest at high doses. It is an amide-type agent and therefore suitable for individuals who are sensitive to ester-type local anaesthetics. It is also used in cardiology as an anti-arrhythmic agent. The practical points below refer to the use of lignocaine as a local anaesthetic agent.

Practical points

- As for local anaesthetics (general) plus.
- Rapid onset of action.
- Duration of action (with adrenaline) – 1–2 hours.
- Maximum single dose – without adrenaline approx. 200 mg.
- Maximum single dose – with adrenaline approx. 500 mg.

Bupivacaine

Bupivacaine (Marcaine, Sensorcaine) is a potent agent with a duration of action of up to 8 hours but it may take 30 minutes to achieve the maximal effect. Even at low concentrations it can decrease cardiac conduction and contractility. It is contra-indicated in intravenous regional anaesthesia such as Bier's block. Bupivacaine is widely used in spinal and epidural anaesthesia. Bupivacaine, which is highly lipid soluble, is not as extensively absorbed into the systemic circulation as the less lipid soluble lignocaine. This makes it preferable for obstetric analgesia as less drug will be liable to cross the placenta into the fetal circulation.

Practical points

- As for local anaesthetics (general) plus:
- Slow onset of action – up to 30 minutes.
- Used for epidural blockade in labour – effects last 2–3 hours.
- Effects may last up to 8 hours.
- Contra-indicated in intravenous regional anaesthesia.
- May cause cardiotoxicity.

Prilocaine

Prilocaine (Citanest) is an amide-type anaesthetic with similar pharmacological properties to lignocaine but a longer onset and duration of action. A unique toxic effect is the production of methaemoglobinaemia due to its metabolites.

Practical points

- Slow onset of effect.
- Duration of effect – 1–2 hours.
- Metabolites can cause methaemoglobinaemia.
- Mainly used in dental practice.

Amethocaine

Amethocaine is rapidly absorbed from mucous membranes, its use is now restricted to ophthalmic practice. It is unsuitable for highly vascular, traumatised or inflamed surfaces and is contra-indicated in bronchoscopy and cystoscopy where safer alternatives are available.

Benoxinate

This local anaesthetic is used in ophthalmic practice where it produces minimal mydriasis and corneal injury.

Benzocaine

Benzocaine is poorly water soluble and therefore not extensively absorbed. It is incorporated into many topical preparations where application can result in prolonged superficial anaesthesia.

Anticonvulsant drugs

Anticonvulsant drugs are used in the relief of chronic pain following certain types of nerve injury. When a nerve is damaged but not totally denervated, it fires in a disordered and unpredictable manner. This causes a characteristic burning pain with paroxysms of shooting pain superimposed. This pattern of neuronal firing is analogous to the aberrant neuronal discharges within the brain which herald an epileptic seizure. Therefore it would seem logical to use the same type of drug to treat both conditions, the aim of which is to stabilise neuronal discharge.

There are three anticonvulsant drugs commonly used in the management of chronic pain due to nerve injury. These are phenytoin, carbamazepine and valproic acid.

Phenytoin

Phenytoin stabilises excitable cell membranes by inhibiting depolarisation in the sodium channels and in this respect resembles the action of local anaesthetics. It suppresses episodes of repetitive neuronal firing caused by passage of intracellular current.

Two factors strongly influence the way the body handles phenytoin. The first is limited aqueous solubility and the second is dose-dependent elimination.

Poor solubility in water means that absorption after oral ingestion is slow and unpredictable, with the time to peak plasma levels being anything from 3 to 12 hours after a single dose.

Following intramuscular administration the drug is precipitated at the site of injection and absorption is again slow and unpredictable. In order to keep the drug in solution in the parenteral formulation, propylene glycol is used as a vehicle. This means that the preparation is markedly alkaline and therefore very irritating to tissues. Propylene glycol can also cause cardiac arrhythmias and when administered intravenously the drug must be either given slowly or diluted in saline so that the rate of administration does not exceed 50 mg per minute. Hypotension may also occur.

The major metabolites of phenytoin are pharmacologically inactive and the rate at which an individual excretes phenytoin is genetically determined. The capacity to metabolise phenytoin differs between individuals and the hepatic enzyme system becomes saturated at a certain unpredictable point. This means that if the dose is increased above this critical level there will be a disproportionate increase in the

plasma level as the enzyme system is already working at maximum capacity and can only metabolise a fixed amount of drug over a given time. Clinical toxicity may be seen with gait disturbance, ataxia, drowsiness and nystagmus. Megaloblastic anaemia, gingival hyperplasia and hirsutism may be a problem at any dosage.

Any patient taking phenytoin should have their plasma levels checked if clinical toxicity is suspected. Although there is a therapeutic range for phenytoin when it is used for the treatment of epilepsy, this is not necessarily applicable to its use in the management of chronic pain. Clinical observation would seem to suggest that the beneficial effects in terms of pain relief occur at plasma levels below the epileptic therapeutic range.

The non-linear relationship between dose and plasma concentration also means that phenytoin dosage can only be increased slowly. An appropriate starting dose would be 100 mg at night, increasing until pain relief is achieved or clinical toxicity supervenes.

Phenytoin is more than 90% bound to plasma proteins and therefore is susceptible to displacement by other highly bound drugs, causing an increased free phenytoin plasma level with possible attendant toxicity. Salicylate and tolbutamide exhibit this effect. Other drugs affect plasma levels of phenytoin either by increasing or decreasing the rate of metabolism. Doses range from 150 to 400 mg daily, orally.

Phenytoin metabolism occurs in the hepatic endoplasmic reticulum and can be induced or inhibited by drugs that influence microsomal enzyme activity. The metabolism of phenytoin is increased by carbamazepine and theophylline but decreased by sodium valproate. The effect of phenobarbitone is variable.

Practical points

- Toxic effects depend upon route of administration, dose and duration of exposure.
- Minimise acute oral toxicity by introducing drug slowly; e.g. start with 100 mg nocte, and titrate upwards according to side effects and therapeutic response.
- In most patients phenytoin may be given as a single dose at night thus minimising daytime sedation.
- Ataxia, drowsiness, confusion, nystagmus and blurred vision are common signs of acute toxicity.

- Rapid intravenous administration produces cardiac arrhythmias, CNS depression and hypotension.
- Toxic effects associated with chronic dosing include gingival hyperplasia, hirsuitism and gastrointestinal symptoms.

Carbamazepine

Carbamazepine is the usual drug of choice for the treatment of trigeminal neuralgia. It has the same effect as phenytoin on sodium channels in cell membranes. Like phenytoin, it is only partially soluble in water and therefore only slowly and unpredictably absorbed after oral administration. Peak plasma levels may occur 4–8 hours after a single dose but may be delayed by as much as 24 hours.

It is metabolised to the 10,11 epoxide which also has anticonvulsant activity. Carbamazepine induces its own hepatic metabolism, a phenomenon known as auto-induction. This means that the half-life is shorter after multiple dosing than after a single dose. The dose of carbamazepine should be increased slowly to minimise the incidence of CNS side effects such as ataxia, drowsiness, dizziness, diplopia, blurred vision, nausea and vomiting. A starting dose of 100 mg twice daily is usually well tolerated. This can be increased according to the patient's tolerance and therapeutic response about every 3–5 days. Up to 2 g daily in two or three divided doses may be required.

Although there is a therapeutic range for carbamazepine in the treatment of epilepsy, plasma level monitoring does not appear to be of value when the drug is used to treat chronic pain except in the confirmation of clinical toxicity.

A long list of side effects have been attributed to this drug. Skin rashes including Stevens–Johnson syndrome, exfoliative dermatitis, and photosensitivity occur in up to 3% of patients. Death has resulted from the haematological and cardiovascular effects such as aplastic anaemia and left ventricular failure. Long term therapy with carbamazepine can be accompanied by water retention. This is known as the syndrome of inappropriate anti-diuretic hormone secretion. However, with careful monitoring it remains a valuable agent for the relief of neuralgias.

As carbamazepine is metabolised by microsomal enzymes in the liver, the clearance of the active drug from the plasma can be influenced by other drugs which either inhibit or induce these enzymes. This can result in either a diminished therapeutic effect or clinical toxicity. Table 14.8 summarises these effects.

Table 14.8 Effect of various drugs on carbamazepine clearance

Drugs which increase clearance	Drugs which decrease Clearance
• Haloperidol	• Erythromycin
• Phenobarbitone	• Dextropropoxyphene
• Clonazepam	• Diltiazem
• Sodium valproate	• Tricyclic antidepressants
• Phenytoin	• Cimetidine

Practical points

- Drug must be introduced slowly starting with, e.g. 100 mg nocte; because of long initial half-life and to minimise side effects.
- Initial side effects include ataxia, drowsiness, dizziness, nausea, vomiting, blurred vision.
- Auto-induction reduces half-life on chronic dosing to 10–20 hours.
- Metabolism of carbamazepine is affected by some concurrent drug therapy.
- Regular blood counts necessary to monitor haematological effects.

Sodium valproate

The mechanism of action of sodium valproate (Epilim, Epival, Depakene) is incompletely understood but most probably involves an effect on the metabolism of gamma amino butyric acid (GABA) in the brain.

Valproate is rapidly and almost completely absorbed by mouth with peak levels occurring about 1 to 4 hours after ingestion. The half-life is about 15 hours and metabolism is largely by conjungation in the liver.

Nearly 20% of patients may experience some degree of gastric intolerance and the drug is presented in an enteric coated formulation to minimise this effect. Anorexia, nausea and vomiting may occur. Unlike phenytoin and carbamazepine, CNS effects such as sedation and ataxia are rare. Valproate has been shown to be hepatotoxic in a small number of patients, with occasional fatalities reported. It inhibits platelet aggregation and may cause transient hair loss. The hair that regrows is often curlier than before. There is no indication for the monitoring of plasma levels. Aspirin enhances the effect of valproate, whereas antidepressants and antipsychotics antagonise the anticonvulsant effect. This latter interaction is probably of no relevance to the use of valproate in the management of chronic pain. Doses used range from 600 to over 2 g daily in two or three divided doses.

Practical points

- Up to 20% of patients may experience nausea, vomiting or anorexia.
- Use enteric-coated preparation if gastrointestinal effects are a problem or administer after food.
- Causes minimal sedation or ataxia.

Psychotropic agents

The antidepressant effects of tricyclic antidepressant drugs (TCADs) such as amitriptyline, imipramine and doxepin were discovered during the 1950s, and the beneficial effect of these drugs in chronic pain states was observed a decade later.

Many chronic pain patients are clinically depressed and certain pain states may be masked depressive illness. Where there is co-existing chronic pain and depression relief of both disorders may often be obtained following the use of TCADs. They are used in neuropathic pain, diabetic neuropathy and central post-stroke pain (Watson *et al.*, 1982; Krinsdahl *et al.*, 1984).

However, certain evidence suggests that the analgesic effect of TCADs is not mediated simply by an antidepressant action. Following the use of TCADs, onset of relief of pain may occur within 3–7 days whereas the antidepressant effects are not usually seen until 2 or 3 weeks after treatment is started. In addition, relief of pain is not necessarily accompanied by relief of depression where those two states coexist.

Table 14.9 Summary of typical anti-muscarinic effects

dry mouth	metallic taste	dizziness
blurred vision	constipation	tachycardia
palpitations	urinary retention	

The mechanism whereby TCADs relieve pain is unclear.

Traditionally tertiary amine TCADs such as amitrptyline have been used in pain relief. However some patients are unable to tolerate the anticholinergic and hypotensive side effects produced by these agents.

Side effects of tricyclic antidepressant drugs

The side effects of TCADs are considered as a group. Broadly speaking, agents vary only in the degree to which they are liable to produce these side effects.

The following rhyme is often helpful in remembering the anti-muscarinic effects:

red as a beet
blind as a bat
dry as a bone
hot as a hare
mad as a hatter

Elderly patients are particularly susceptible to certain side effects of TCADs such as drowsiness, confusion, agitation, urinary retention and postural hypotension. To minimise these risks patients should be started on a low dose which is increased gradually according to tolerance and therapeutic response. The daily requirement may be given as a single dose at night. This makes the patient less aware of the dry mouth produced by this group of drugs. It also minimises day time drowsiness which can also be a problem and helps to ensure a good night's sleep; something which many chronic pain patients may well have not experienced for a considerable time.

Because of the pronounced anticholinergic action of this group of drugs their use in certain conditions is usually precluded. These conditions include prostatic hypertrophy, narrow-angle glaucoma and cardiovascular disorders.

Table 14.10 Summary of non-antimuscarinic side effects

arrhythmias	confusion	postural hypotension
black tongue	paralytic ileus	tremor
rashes	convulsions	agranulocytosis
leucopenia	thrombocytopenia	jaundice

Practical points

- Give as single dose at night to minimise effects of dry mouth and daytime drowsiness and promote good sleep pattern.
- Caution in elderly patients – increased likelihood of side effects.
- Warn patients about possibility of dry mouth, blurred vision and postural hypotension.
- Artificial saliva can be useful in controlling dry mouth commonly caused by these drugs.

Amitriptyline

Amitriptyline is well absorbed after oral administration. Doses start at 10–25 mg increased gradually to a maximum of 150 mg at night. Pronounced anti-muscarinic effects result in delayed gastric emptying and consequently the time to peak plasma levels may vary from 2 to 12 hours. Once absorbed, the lipophilicity of these drugs means that they are widely distributed in body tissues. They are strongly bound to plasma proteins and to constituents of tissues.

Amitriptyline is metabolised in the liver by hepatic microsomal enzymes. Some of the metabolites are pharmacologically active. The marked sedative action and long half-life of amitriptyline favour once daily night time dosing. Patients' tolerance and dosage requirements vary widely. Care must be taken in elderly patients where a starting dose of 10 mg daily should not be exceeded. Amitriptyline has an impressive list of side effects but anti-muscarinic and cardiovascular effects dominate the clinical picture. Side effects of TCADs are summarised in Tables 14.9 and 14.10. Paradoxically, patients taking amitriptyline often complain of profuse sweating. Amitriptyline should not be used following recent myocardial infarction, or in the presence of heart block, mania or porphyria. Use with caution in patients with diabetes, heart disease, glaucoma, hepatic or thyroid disease.

Miscellaneous drugs used in the management of pain

A variety of miscellaneous drugs have been used in the management of pain. The pharmacology of these agents is briefly discussed here and their uses are detailed under the section on the management of chronic pain.

Baclofen

Gamma-aminobutyric acid (GABA) is an inhibitory transmitter which is found in the spinal cord. Baclofen (Lioresal) is a derivative of GABA and exerts an antispasmodic effect by depressing monosynaptic and polysynaptic transmission within the spinal cord. The use of baclofen is limited by the adverse effects produced by the large oral doses that are required to decrease spasticity. These include ataxia, dizziness, weakness, drowsiness and mental confusion. Adverse effects are prominent in the elderly. The drug should be introduced slowly starting with 5 mg twice daily and increasing according to patient tolerance about every 3 or 4 days to around 20 mg four times daily. Intrathecal baclofen is currently under investigation for the long-term treatment of spasticity (Penn et al., 1989; Ochs et al., 1989). This route bypasses the blood-brain barrier allowing therapeutic efficacy without accompanying toxicity.

Practical points

- Start with 5 mg twice daily and titrate upwards as tolerated.
- Take with food or milk to minimise nausea.
- Counsel patient on expected initial side effects.
- Monitor for ataxia, drowsiness, dizziness, weakness and confusion.
- Side effects more pronounced in the elderly.
- Abrupt withdrawal may precipitate hallucinations, fits or cardiac arrhythmias.

Benzodiazepines

Over 2000 benzodiazepines have been synthesised but only about 10 are used in clinical practice as anxiolytics and anticonvulsants. They include agents such as diazepam (Valium), alprazolam (Xanax), lorazepam (Ativan) and clonazepam (Rivotril, Klonopin). The central depressant effects of benzodiazepines are mediated via the reticular formation. These drugs modulate neurotransmission mediated by GABA. A specific benzodiazepine receptor has been isolated in the brain. The effects of these agents can be reversed by the benzodiazepine antagonist flumazenil (Anexate). The duration of effect of flumazenil is much shorter than that of benzodiazepines. The potent addictive potential of this group of drugs has now severely curtailed their use in clinical practice, including pain management.

Clonidine

Clonidine is an alpha-2 agonist and produces analgesia by a non-opioid spinal mechanism which involves modulation of nociceptive processing within the dorsal horn via stimulation of an alpha-2 receptor. In the relief of pain in cancer it is given epidurally in a dose of approximately 150 μg.

Practical points

- Hypotension may occur following intraspinal use.
- Hypotension more pronounced in patients with pre-existing hypertension.
- Theoretical possibility of rebound hypertension on cessation of chronic therapy.
- May produce cardiac dysrhythmias in patients with pre-existing cardiac disturbances.
- No commercially available preparation for epidural use.

Guanethidine

Guanethidine is selectively taken up by the noradrenergic nerve endings of postganglionic neurones where it releases noradrenaline (norepinephrine) from storage sites. The concentration of guanethidine builds up within the nerve endings, preventing release of any remaining transmitter and stopping the reuptake of noradrenaline from the synaptic cleft. Postganglionic neurones depend on the recapture of the majority of the transmitter to maintain sympathetic tone. In summary a biphasic effect is produced with initial release of noradrenaline and subsequent sympathetic blockade. Guanethidine is used in various regional intravenous blocks to produce sympathetic blockade and thereby relieve pain. The clinical effects of the block are dose-dependent and develop over time. A dose of 10 mg of guanethidine diluted to 25 ml with sodium chloride 0.9% will produce sympathetic blockade in the hand. The use of intravenous regional blocks is discussed

under nerve blocks in chronic pain. Side effects are minimal as the drug is given into an isolated limb. Addition of an alpha adrenergic blocking drug such as thymoxamine or phenoxybenzamine to the solution prevents the clinical effects from the released noradrenaline and allows early vasodilatation.

Practical points

- Minimal side effects as drug is 'fixed' to tissues in an isolated limb.
- Unlike sympathetic ganglion blocks, a guanethidine-induced sympathetic block may be performed on patients who are taking anticoagulants.

Mexiletine

Mexiletine (Mexitil) is a potent antiarrhythmic agent in the same class as lignocaine. However, unlike lignocaine it is effective by mouth with a systemic bioavailability of about 90%. It is metabolised in the liver and has an elimination half-life of about 11 hours. It has been used in doses of 200–300 mg daily for pain relief in various chronic pain states.

Practical points

- Contra-indicated in bradycardia or heart block.
- Side effects are dose-related and include gastrointestinal upset, hypotension, drowsiness, ataxia and confusion.

Nifedipine

Nifedipine (Adalat) relaxes vascular smooth muscle at lower plasma concentrations than are required to dilate coronary and peripheral arteries. It is this ability to smooth muscle and increase peripheral blood flow that have led to its use in pain management at doses of 10–20 mg three times daily.

Practical points

- Effects are potentiated by cimetidine.
- If used in diabetic patients readjustment of diabetic control may be necessary.
- Vasodilatation may cause headache, flushing and lightheadedness.

Neurolytic agents

Neurolytic agents have an indiscriminate action when injected into nerves. As they destroy both small and large fibres they interfere irreversibly with both motor and sensory function.

Chlorocresol (chloromethylphenol) has now been almost completely superceded by phenol as a neurolytic agent. *Phenol* is a virtually colourless solid which is only poorly soluble in water: 6.7% phenol in water represents a saturated solution. It is most destructive when formulated in an aqueous solution, and rather less so if mixed with glycerin or contrast media. However, solutions in glycerin are very viscous and difficult to inject down a fine needle. Injection of phenol is usually painless and there is a gradual feeling of warmth followed by pain relief and numbness. There is a build-up of effect over 24–48 hours. Solutions of phenol are hyperbaric with respect to cerebrospinal fluid and therefore when patients are positioned for intrathecal injection the painful site must be lower than the point of entry of the needle.

Absolute alcohol (dehydrated alcohol) is more easily injected than phenolic preparations and is hypobaric; therefore patients should lie with the painful part uppermost. Injection of alcohol is followed by immediate and progressive burning paraesthesiae which peaks in about 10 minutes and fades after a few hours. This initial intense pain can be prevented if local anaesthetic is injected prior to the alcohol.

10% ammonium sulphate and *glycerin* injection have also been used as neurolytic agents. None of these preparations are readily available from a commercial source and they are usually specially prepared by hospital pharmacy departments.

Acute and chronic pain

Acute and chronic pain are two very different entities and must be managed as such. If acute pain is not effectively treated it may progress to a chronic pain state.

Acute pain

Acute pain is defined as that which follows an acute injury or disease and persists only as long as the tissue pathology itself. Acute pain has a diagnostic function, acting as a warning sign to indicate that an injury or other acute insult has occurred. The patient is therefore alerted to take the appropriate action. Putting a hand on a hot object results in pain: we then take our hand away minimising further tissue damage, and institute appropriate first aid measures. An inflamed appendix causes pain which leads us to seek medical help. If the body was unable to feel pain our life expectancy would be much reduced because of a lack of attention to injury and disease.

When acute pain has fulfilled this diagnostic function, it is important that it is effectively controlled. If the pain is allowed to persist, reflex responses become abnormal and can compromise the patient's recovery. Those with hypertension, hypoxia, hypercapnia, hypovolaemia or heart disease would be especially at risk.

Acute pain is usually transient and self-limiting, resulting from a readily identifiable cause. It is often accompanied by autonomic signs such as an increase in heart rate, respiratory rate and blood pressure. There may also be a marked emotional response.

Chronic pain

Chronic pain may be divided into four different types:

1. Pain from an acute injury or disease that persists beyond the normal healing time (example – development of adhesions after surgery).
2. Pain related to a chronic degenerative disease or persisting neurological condition (example – osteoarthritis, post-stroke syndrome).
3. Pain that emerges without an identifiable organic cause and persists episodically for months or even years (example – persistent pain resulting from an accident where there was no discernible injury).
4. Pain associated with malignant disease.

Chronic pain is a very distressing experience. It has no diagnostic value and may be thought of as the end product of various physiological, psychological and social processes. Factors which contribute to the onset of pain are often very different from those which maintain it. These various processes interact with each other to produce the final chronic pain state. The predominance of one or other of these determinants varies with each patient. The

Table 14.11 Psychological and social features found in patients with chronic pain

• reinforcement of sick role	• pending litigation with potential for financial gain
• abnormal illness behaviour	
• existence within family of social model for chronic illness	• manipulation for self gain of family and friends
• past or present drug abuse	• depression or grief
• hypochondriasis	• inadequate personality

initial injury or disease may be a relatively minor contribution to the final pain state. Some psychological and social features that may be found in patients with chronic pain are shown in Table 14.11. Multifactorial complaints and the invalid state of many patients make it all too tempting to label chronic pain as a primarily psychological complaint. However, occurrence of pain in the complete absence of organic injury or disease is not very common. A patient should only be labelled as having psychogenic pain following a positive psychiatric diagnosis rather than by a diagnosis of exclusion.

The transition from acute to chronic pain is a gradual process in which the character of the pain changes until it bears almost no relation to that which followed the initial injury. Chronic pain is similar to other chronic medical conditions in that it may profoundly influence a patient's well-being and personality.

What are the differences between acute and chronic pain?

The outward manifestations of acute and chronic pain are very different and if those caring for the patient are unaware of these differences the patient may continue to suffer unrelieved pain.

Acute pain is accompanied by autonomic, physical and emotional signals. Characteristically the patient is sweating, anxious and vocalises his complaints of pain. Heart and respiratory rate are increased.

In contrast, the patient in chronic pain may appear quiet, depressed and withdrawn with none of the physical manifestations that we commonly associate with pain. An unwary observer may wrongly assume that the patient is not in pain and therefore not offer any relief.

Patients suffering pain as a result of cancer exhibit a mixture of both acute and chronic pain characteristics.

The differing nature of acute and chronic pain states demands different management strategies. However, there is no place for standardised drug regimes in either situation. The dose and dosage interval of each drug must be individualised to the needs of each patient. Here again the need for assessment of pain must be emphasised. If pain is to be effectively controlled, it must also be adequately assessed. Whenever possible, this assessment must be undertaken by the patient themselves rather than a third party. Lest we forget, the patient is the one with the pain!

Some of the factors which differentiate acute and chronic pain are outlined in Table 14.12.

The subjective nature of pain coupled with the placebo response, which may account for up to 30% of the pain relief seen in some patients, make critical evaluation of pharmacological treatment extremely problematic. Thus a prospective randomised double-blind controlled trial against the accepted gold standard for that particular condition provides the only true test of the value of any individual therapy. Any extrapolation of the results to other populations, disease states or symptoms must be viewed with caution. However, not all conditions, and malignancies in particular lend themselves to such stringent trial protocols and we must retain a critical but open mind when assessing the value of non-controlled open studies in these situations.

The vast differences between acute and chronic pain are also reflected in the wider range of doses used in chronic pain. A typical dose of morphine for the relief of postoperative pain or

Table 14.12 Some factors which differentiate acute and chronic pain

- Acute pain is transient whereas chronic pain is constant or recurring.
- Acute pain is self-limiting whereas chronic pain tends to increase rather than decrease.
- Acute pain serves a diagnostic function whereas chronic pain has no such role.
- Chronic pain is the result of a developmental process whereas acute pain is not.
- Psychological factors play a greater role in the suffering of the chronic pain patient than they do in the patient with acute pain.
- Environmental and social factors are more influential in chronic pain than in acute pain.
- The association between the initial tissue damage and the complaint of pain becomes weaker as the developmental process proceeds.

that following trauma would be 10–20 mg by intramuscular injection repeated every 4 hours. This is in marked contrast to the doses of morphine that are often necessary to control chronic pain of malignant origin. These may easily range from 10 mg to 300 mg or more every 4 hours. Combinations of different drugs are often used.

The management of acute pain

There is accumulating evidence that pain following acute injuries or disorders is inadequately treated. A recent report (Seers, 1989) revealed that 43% of patients undergoing abdominal surgery complained of at least quite a lot of pain and 22% rated the pain as 'very bad' on the first postoperative day. One week after the operation altogether 86% of patients had experienced at least 'quite a lot of pain'. Until recently, early postopertive pain has usually been exclusively managed using opioids; with a nurse assessing the severity of the patient's pain and then deciding on the amount of analgesia the patient should receive. Donovan et al. (1987) found that less than 50% of patients were asked about their postoperative pain by any member of the health care team. In a study of 221 nurse-patient pairs (Seers, 1989) the mean ratings for pain when assessed by the nurse were consistently and significantly lower than the patients' ratings. These studies emphasise the importance of direct patient participation in pain assessment. Such deficiencies are added to by the lack of knowledge on the part of doctors regarding the principles of pain control and the pharmacology of analgesics, especially that of opioids. Coupled with this is an unrealistic fear held by many doctors and nurses about the risks of producing respiratory depression and addiction in patients who are given opioids for pain relief.

However, although opioids do depress respiration, pain itself is a respiratory stimulant and antagonises the depressant effects of the drug. It has also been estimated that the likelihood of addiction in these circumstances is about 1 in 3000 (Royal College of Surgeons of England, 1990) and those prescribing or administering the drug are at greater risk of developing addiction than those who receive them. Ultimately this leads to conservative prescribing and administration with resultant inadequate relief of pain.

The transient nature of acute pain means that 'as required' dosing is usually considered acceptable. However, this does not mean that the patient should be made to earn their analgesia by having moderate to severe pain before they receive the next dose. Such a schedule results in more rather than less analgesia being necessary to relieve the pain. The question of whether or not to give prophylactic analgesia to a patient who is not in pain, and the time lag between administration of analgesic and onset of effect are rarely considered.

The theoretical dosage interval should be based on the known duration of action of each particular drug, which for opioids will commonly be 3 or 4 hours and 4–6 hours for non-steroidal anti-inflammatory agents.

As well as postoperative pain, severe acute pain encompasses conditions such as trauma, myocardial infarction and labour pain. In these situations the onset of analgesia needs to be as fast as possible and therefore parenteral administration is the usual preferred route; with intravenous administration providing the speediest relief. Speed of onset of analgesia may also go hand in hand with rapid emergence of side effects. This makes patient monitoring especially important.

The various therapeutic modalities available for the relief of acute pain fall into six categories:

a) Nerve blocks.
b) Non-opioid analgesics.
c) Systemically administered opioids.
d) Epidural and intrathecal administered agents.
e) Stimulation therapies.
f) Psychological therapies.

The last two fall outside the scope of this chapter and will be considered elsewhere.

Nerve blocks

Nerve blocks may be done with local anaesthetics, neurolytic solutions, and occasionally with steroids.

Local anaesthetic agents block the conduction of impulses along nerves. All types of nerves are affected in a reversible manner with smaller, non-myelinated fibres being more readily susceptible than larger myelinated fibres. Thus sensory and autonomic nerves succumb before motor nerves. These agents can provide very effective analgesia in a variety of acute and chronic situations either when used alone or in combination with corticosteroids or opioids.

The use of local anaesthetic blocks falls into three categories

a) Diagnostic
  – to map out individual pain pathways in the body.
  – to help determine the exact site and cause of the pain.
  – determine a patient's response to pain relief.
b) Prognostic
  – mimic the areas of analgesia that would be produced by an irreversible neurolytic block given in the same place.
  – allow the patient to experience the side effects such as sensory loss that would result from a permanent block and thus decide whether or not they wish to have the block.
c) Therapeutic
  – Control severe acute pain.
  – Break the vicious circle or aberrant impulses which is thought to perpetuate certain chronic painful conditions.
  – Act as a holding action until more definitive analgesic procedures can be performed.
  – To be used in combination with other analgesic measures in order to provide relief of pain.

When used alone they can produce analgesia without the troublesome side effects such as respiratory depression, sedation, nausea and vomiting which can accompany opioid use. The use of local anaesthesia is limited by the fact that not all pain arises from areas innervated by superficial nerves, especially when major surgery has been performed. However, this problem can sometimes be solved by the use of an epidural technique. Even if local anaesthesia does not result in total analgesia it usually allows a reduction in the amount of opioid necessary to achieve good pain control.

Topical application and local infiltration of anaesthetic agents are commonly used to relieve pain.

Surface anaesthesia of nose, mouth, throat, respiratory tract, oesophagus and genito-urinary tract is commonly achieved with solutions, creams or ointments of lignocaine (lidocaine), cocaine, tetracaine or benzocaine. Most local anaesthetics are rapidly absorbed through mucous membranes, so the amounts used should be carefully measured. After topical administration of lignocaine (lidocaine) the peak effect is seen in about 3–5 minutes and lasts for half to three-quarters of an hour. Topical application of local anaesthetic provides useful anaesthesia following circumcision and donor grafting.

Infiltration anaesthesia achieves good analgesia by injecting local anaesthetic solution into superficial or deeper tissues without disruption of body functions. However, large amounts of drug may be needed to produce anaesthesia in a small area. Increasing the risk of systemic toxicity. In the absence of adrenaline approximately 3 mg/kg lignocaine (lidocaine) can be used in healthy adults. When adrenaline is used these amounts may be increased by one-third. Infiltration of local anaesthetic into peripheral nerves or nerve plexuses produces temporary sensory and motor loss for a few centimetres distal to the injection site.

Use of nerve blocks for postoperative pain relief

Individual or groups of peripheral nerves can be blocked to provide postoperative analgesia. The duration of effect of most local anaesthetics is only a few hours. Infiltration of a long acting agent such as bupivacaine into the wound incision prior to closure provides analgesia for many hours and the effect can be prolonged by inserting a catheter through which local anaesthetic can be given either by continuous or intermittent infusion. Other catheter techniques provide analgesia following fracture of the femor, skin grafts and varicose vein surgery.

Infusion of local anaesthetic via a catheter into the intrapleural space produces good postoperative analgesia following thoracotomy, upper abdominal and breast surgery. Complications include pneumothorax, and injury to the lung and intercostal vessels.

Paravertebral thoracic block of spinal nerves using bupivacaine 0.5% with adrenaline provides good analgesia in patients who have undergone a thoracotomy. Lumbar thoracic block achieves good analgesia post-nephrectomy.

Intercostal blocks require multiple injections which are usually given posteriorly, at the angle of the ribs. For an adult each injection would typically comprise 3–5 ml 0.25–0.5% bupiva-caine with adrenaline 5 μg/ml, at each site. These blocks provide good analgesia following cholecystectomy, gastrectomy, mastectomy, thoracotomy and sternotomy. The advantages of this block in comparison to systemic analge-sia include an improvement in forced expira-tory volume in 1 second (FEV1) and peak expiratory flow rate (PEFR). There is also a reduction in severity and duration of hypoxae-mia. The major complications are pneumo-thorax and hypotension as a result of posterior spread of anaesthetic to the sympathetic chain.

Blockade of the brachial plexus is achieved by infiltration of local anaesthetic into the fascial sheath which surrounds the brachial plexus and extends from the neck to the axilla. It provides good anaesthesia after surgery to the upper limb, especially following implan-tation of digits or severed upper limb or other situations in which blood supply to extremities is reduced.

Caudal block is relatively simple to perform and is a popular method of obtaining postoper-ative pain relief in children following surgery below the umbilicus. Weakness of the lower limbs and urinary retention can occasionally be a problem. Penile block relieves pain after a circumcision.

Other indications for the use of nerve blocks to relieve acute pain

Paravertebral cervical block can relieve severe pain due to musculoskeletal conditions. Para-vertebral thoracic block is effective in providing pain relief for fractured ribs, acute herpes zoster and pleurisy. Repeated paravertebral somatic block may reduce the incidence of post herpetic neuralgia. Lumbar paravertebral block will reduce the pain of fractured lumbar vertebrae. Intercostal block can relieve post-traumatic pain such as fractured ribs or sternum, and chest pain that follows contusion and acute herpes zoster.

Blockade of the suprascapular nerve, which is a branch of the brachial plexus and the major sensory nerve supply to the shoulder joint, is useful for the control of pain arising from acute bursitis or periarthritis which is refractory to periarticular or intra-articular block.

Myofascial trigger points are a frequent cause of pain. If there is mechanical overload in an isolated muscle or its associated fascia hyperac-tivity in a trigger point causes acute pain. If this acute pain syndrome is not relieved chronic multiple myofascial pain may result. Following topical application of an anaesthetic spray such as chlorofluoromethane the trigger point can be inactivated either by mechanical passive stretch of the affected muscle to its full length or injection of the trigger point with local anaes-thetic such as bupivacaine 0.05%. Injections may need to be repeated over a few days. In cases of severe muscle spasm such as low back pain (lumbago) due to sudden lumbosacral muscle spasm, injection of local anaesthetic is complementary to other measures such as heat and massage. Sometimes relief may be ob-tained by injecting trigger points with steroid alone. A combination of long-acting local anaesthetic such as 10–15 ml bupivacaine 0.25% with 40 mg methylprednisolone in-filtrated around the area will relieve the pain of acute bursitis. Onset of analgesia occurs in 10–15 minutes and lasts 4–8 hours. A series of injections are necessary for prolongation of effect. A similar treatment works well for relief of lateral humeral epicondylitis (tennis elbow) and medial humeral epicondylitis (golfer's elbow).

b) Non-opioid analgesics

This group of drugs encompasses agents which have anti-inflammatory, analgesic and anti-pyr-etic actions. It includes paracetamol and all the non-steroidal anti-inflammatory drugs (NSAIDs). The pharmacology of these agents was discussed earlier in the chapter. They are effective in relieving pain caused by inflam-mation where sensitization of pain receptors has resulted in pain following a usually non-noxious chemical or mechanical stimulus. This sensitization is caused by the action of prosta-glandins. As well as being effective at relieving pain due to inflammation such as gout, rheuma-toid arthritis and osteoarthritis, soft tissue injuries, some sports injuries sprains, strains and toothache they also relieve headaches which may be mediated by prostaglandins. Over 50% of patients will respond to the first NSAID prescribed whilst a resistant 5% may be unresponsive to all NSAIDs. The analgesic action of these drugs occurs across quite a narrow dose range, which supports the view that the action of these drugs is predominantly peripheral. NSAIDs also reduce fever mediated by enhanced production of prostaglandins. This includes fever resulting from infection, inflammation, tissue damage, graft rejection and malignancy.

With a dramatic increase in the number of patients undergoing day case surgery, the analgesic needs of these patients warrant special attention. Local anaesthesia is used for many day cases and this confers some relief of pain postoperatively. Although regional anaesthesia techniques may well result in even greater benefits with regard to postoperative pain, they require time and considerable skill to perform and are not without their problems. General anaesthesia usually means that additional pain relief is needed within a few hours of the operation and the common drugs used are opioids and non-steroidal anti-inflammatory agents. The problems of opioid side effects are discussed elsewhere in this chapter.

Investigators who have studied patients undergoing oral surgery (Campbell, 1990) who were given 600 mg ibuprofen preoperatively found that reduced the need for postoperative analgesia ($p<0.01$). In patients undergoing minor orthopaedic surgery 80% of those who had either periopertive opioid or perioperative paracetamol 1 g with codeine 16 mg had no need for postoperative analgesia. The overnight admission rate was four times higher in patients who were given perioperative opioids than in those who received no perioperative analgesia. This confirms the investigations of earlier workers (McQuay et al., 1988). Wall and Woolf (1988) suggested that these findings may be due to the fact that preoperative analgesia provided protection from the afferent stimulation of the spinal cord which usually causes hyperexcitability of the spinal cord. The benefit conferred by NSAIDs may result from inhibition of prostaglandin synthesis prior to tissue damage. These observations call for further large scale studies into the role of preoperative analgesia as well as more frequent use of local anaesthetic techniques.

Nefopam (Acupan) is a centrally-acting non-opioid analgesic. Although cost may preclude widespread routine use its novel mode of action, non-constipating effects and reputed lack of interaction with alcohol mean that it may well have a useful role in day case and outpatient management of acute pain.

Nerve blocks

Severe muscle spasm can occur following accidental or surgical trauma. Infiltration of dilute solutions of local anaesthetic can result in good pain relief. This technique is also beneficial in patients who experience severe low back pain due to sudden lumbosacral muscle strain. Such procedures should be viewed as adjuncts to other corrective therapy such as exercise, heat and massage.

A series of injections of dilute bupivacaine given every 3–5 days will relieve the pain in scars which can occur following trauma or surgical operation. A similar procedure is effective in neuromas which develop following mastectomy, neck dissection and in stumps and phantom lambs after amputation.

Patients with painful chronic arthritis in major joints can obtain significant pain relief following intra-articular injection of local anaesthetic and corticosteroid. In these patients it is important to ensure that they have a supply of systemic analgesics to relieve the pain after the analgesia from the local anaesthetic has worn off and before the corticosteroid takes effect.

Blockade of various spinal nerves will relieve pain in a range of chronic pain states. Occipital nerve blocks may be used diagnostically, prognostically and therapeutically for management of occipital headache, neuralgia, and other painful conditions of the posterior portion of the head.

Prognostic paravertebral cervical blocks are useful in the management of cancer pain, and for temporary relief of severe pain due to musculoskeletal pathology.

Blockade of the brachial plexus can relieve pain due to reflex sympathetic dystrophy, phantom limb pain and other types of causalgia and post-amputation pain.

Paravertebral thoracic block can be used for the relief of chronic pain persisting after thoracotomy, trauma and infectious neuralgia. It is also beneficial in relieving segmental neuralgia due to osteoporosis and compression of nerves from vertebral pathology. Paravertebral lumbar block is a useful diagnostic tool prior to the use of neurolytic agents to relieve intractable perineal and bladder pain in advanced cancer.

The trigeminal nerve supplies sensory fibres to all of the face and the anterior two-thirds of the head. Tic douloureux (trigeminal neuralgia) is an exquisitely painful condition where severe lancinating pains are experienced in the distribution of one or more divisions of the trigmenial nerve.

Carbamazepine is now considered first line treatment in the management of the condition, but when the pain proves refractory to treatment destruction of the gasserian ganglion with alcohol, glycerol or via a radio-frequency lesion will usually result in pain relief, though at the expense of sensory loss.

Blockade of maxillary nerve alone may also relieve pain from trigeminal neuralgia, certain neoplastic pain syndromes and atypical facial pain.

Blockade of either the glossopharyngeal and/or vagus nerve may be used diagnostically or prognostically to provide pain relief in regions served by the glossopharyngeal nerve and for relief of pain following throat cancer.

So-called target blocks enable a high concentration of a drug to be delivered to a specific area of the body. The restriction of the drug to an isolated area minimises the chances of systemic toxicity. In the limbs the regional circulation can be isolated using an arterial tourniquet. The only real potential problem with this procedure is the accidental release of the tourniquet, which must be kept inflated for a minimum of 20 minutes to allow the drug to become fixed in the tissues. The drug is injected in a vein and from there perfuses back to the tissues. The use of guanethidine in this way produces a safe and effective sympathetic block. It is used for the relief of pain in reflex sympathetic dystrophy and in some cases of vascular insufficiency for the relief of ischaemic pain at rest. Intravenous regional sympathetic blockade has also proved useful following traumatic degloving injuries. In these cases a prolonged increase in local blood supply will increase the chances of survival of threatened tissues. This also applies to the reimplantation of digits and to facilitate angiograms by ensuring optimum visualisation of the vascular bed such as prior to thumb reconstruction from toe transplantation.

Peripheral sympathetic blockade can also be achieved by injection of local anaesthetic into sympathetic ganglions. The sympathetic supply to the head, neck and arm can be blocked by injection of the stellate ganglion with local anaesthetic. The usual indications are for relief of pain such as Sudeck's atrophy, post-herpetic neuralgia, and post-amputation pain as well as vascular insufficiency such as seen in Raynaud's disease. Lumbar sympathetic block will relieve pain due to frostbite, ischaemia and is also effective in the management of hyperhydrosis.

Epidural local anaesthetics with or without corticosteroids are frequently used in the management of chronic non-malignant pain to reduce oedema and decrease pressure on spinal nerve roots. Occasionally combinations of opioids and steroids are used in severe low back pain, where they provide pain relief for several days, thus buying time until a more definitive treatment can be given. Prolonged pruritus may be a problem but some success has been reported with cimetidine in alleviating this condition.

In patients with pain due to malignancy epidural opioids are more frequently used as they enable smaller doses to be used with the decreased chance of side effects. Where long-term use is contemplated a catheter attached to a subcutaneous reservoir can be implanted under the skin and topped up as necessary. Patients at home must be alerted to the signs and symptoms of infection which can occur with long-term use of epidural catheters. Epidural blockade with opioids produces powerful analgesia that is limited to discrete segments without the accompanying locomotor or vasomotor blockade seen when local anaesthetics are used. Fentanyl is sometimes favoured for continual epidural block. It is very lipid soluble and short-acting with effects persisting for between 90 minutes and 3 hours. Highly segmental analgesia is produced and an infusion of about 20–50 μg per hour is often sufficient to provide continual analgesia.

Local anaesthetics are sometimes used in the relief of pain due to malignancy in conjunction with opioids. The decision as to whether or not to use a local anaesthetic will partially depend on the desirability or otherwise of producing a sympathetic block. As the life expectancy of the patient with cancer diminishes and if the pain is less and less successfully managed with opioids and co-analgesics, the time for consideration of a neurolytic may well have arrived. Intrathecal neurolytics can provide relief from otherwise intractable pain. Such procedures are rarely indicated in patients with a life expectancy of more than about a year or those with chronic benign pain where the risks of producing muscle weakness, faecal and urinary incontinence are considered too great. Epidural neurolytic blocks are not as accurate as intrathecal blocks.

The coeliac plexus block is one of the most useful neurolytic blocks and effectively relieves severe abdominal pain emanating from carcinoma of the pancreas. Injections of phenol or alcohol under X-ray control are used.

Perineal pain in cancer can be abolished using a bilateral phenol block of S4 roots accessed via the S4 foramen. Using this approach bladder function should remain intact.

The analgesics of the future

Since the introduction of morphine into clinical practice scientists have been striving to produce a synthetic opioid which will combine analgesic efficacy with safety and absence of side effects. The majority of synthetic opioids developed to date fall far short of this target. Morphine remains the gold standard. As our understanding of the role of the individual opioid receptor types increases, this may be paralleled by the development of pure agonists and antagonists specific for these receptors. This should allow the clinician to more carefully select an agent for a particular patient and predict with more accuracy the likelihood of some side effects as well as enhancing the production of analgesia – in theory!

The synthesis of a long-acting non-toxic local anaesthetic agent would be a valuable addition to the therapeutic armamentarium. N-butyl-*p*-aminobenzoate (BAB) is a highly lipid soluble congener of benzocaine. It has been shown to produce long lasting sensory blockade following epidural administration in cancer patients whose pain was refractory to radiotherapy, opioid and non-opioid analgesics (Korsten, 1991). Further studies are needed to establish the efficacy and safety of this new agent in clinical practice.

Our understanding of the neurophysiological mechanisms and in particular, the role of the various neurotransmitters involved in pain modulation, is still in its infancy. We must await further information from the neurophysiologists before the scientists can work towards producing the designer drugs predicted by an increased understanding of these mechanisms.

The role of excitatory amino acids such as glutamate and aspartate in central nociceptive processing is an example of such research. The receptors for these two amino acids can be approximately divided into those activated by N-methyl-D-aspartate (NMDA) and the non-NMDA receptors. The NMDA receptor is thought to be involved in the modulation of nociception within the spinal cord. Constant intensity stimulation of C fibres results in some neurones within the dorsal horn exhibiting an exaggerated response after the first few initial stimuli. This phenomenon is known as wind-up. It is dependent on frequency and is also sensitive to antagonists at the receptor. Such agents do not modulate cell afferent input but abolish wind-up so that the neurones respond to C-fibre stimulation in the normal way. As the NMDA receptor-channel complex is concerned with the amplification and prolongation of nociceptive afferent inputs within the spinal cord, it is likely that it is involved in chronic pain. It may be that NMDA antagonists could be utilised as analgesics by virtue of their ability to reduce central amplification of nociception by reason of their ability to reduce 'wind-up'.

In the meantime much can be achieved by teaching everyone involved in the relief of pain all that is currently known about the pharmacology of conventional and co-analgesics. The time allocated in undergraduate and postgraduate teaching programmes for the study of pain and the pharmacology of analgesics still remains woefully inadequate.

References

Aitkenhead, A. R., Vater, M., Achola *et al.* (1984) Pharmacokinetics of single-dose intravenous morphine in normal volunteers and patients with end-stage renal failure. *British Journal of Anaesthesia.* 56:813–9

Alderman, E. L., Barry, W. L., Graham, A. F. (1991) Genotoxicity of papavertum and noscapine. *Current Problems*, No. 31

Awerbach, G. I., Sandyk, R. (1990) Mexilitine for thalamic pain syndrome. *International Journal of Neuroscience*, **55**, 129–133

Beaver, W. T., Schein, P. S., Hekt, M. (1981) Comparison of the analgesic effect of intramuscular heroin and morphine in patients with cancer pain. *Clinical Pharmacology and Therapy*, **29**, 232–236

Beecher, H. K., Keats, A. S., Mosteller, F., Lasagna, L. (1953) The effectiveness of oral analgesics (morphine, codeine, acetyl salicylic acid) and the problem of placebo 'reactors' and 'non-reactors'. *J. Pharmacol. Exp. Ther.* **103**, 393–400

Bernstein, J. E., Bickers, D. R., Dahl, M. V., Roshal, J. Y. (1987) Treatment of chronic post herpetic neuralgia with topical capsaicin. *Journal of American Acad. Dermatol.*, **17**, 93–96

Bernstein, J. E., Korman, N. J., Bickers, D. R. *et al.* (1989) Topical capsaicin treatment of chronic herpetic neuralgia. *Acad. Dermatol*, **21**, 265–270

Brahams, D. (1984) Death of a patient participating in a trial of oral morphine for relief of post operative pain. *Lancet*, 1083–1084

Bruera, E., Brenneis, C., Michaud, M. *et al.* (1988) Patient-controlled subcutaneous hydromorphine versus continuous subcutaneous infusion for the treatment of cancer pain. *Journal of National Cancer Institute*, **80**, 1152–1154

Budd, K. (1981)High dose buprenorphine for postoperative analgesia. *Anaesthesia*, **36**, 900–903

Budd, K. (1985) The use of the opioid antagonist naloxone in the treatment of thalamic pain. *Neuropeptides*, **5**, 419–422

Campbell, F. G., Graham, J. G., Zilkha, K. J. (1966) Clinical trial of carbamazepine in trigeminal neuralgia. *Journal of Neurology, Neurosurgery and Psychiatry*, **29**, 265–267

Campbell, W. I. (1990) Analgesic side effects and minor surgery: which analgesic for minor and day case surgery? *British Journal of Anaesthesia*, **64**, 617–620

Couch, J. R., Ziegler, D. K., Hassanein, R. (1976) Amitriptyline in the prophylaxis of migraine: effectiveness and relationship of antimigraine and antidepressant effects. *Neurology*, **26**, 121–127

Deigard, A., Petersen, P., Kastrup, J. (1988) Mexilitine for treatment of chronic painful diabetic neuropathy. *Lancet*, **i**, 9–11

DeMoragas, J. M., Kierland, R. R. (1957) The outcome of patients with herpes zoster. *Archives of Dermatol.*, **75**, 193–196

Donovan, M., Dillon, P., McGuire, L. (1987) Incidence and characteristics of pain in a sample of medical and surgical patients. *Pain*, **30**, 69–78

Dunlop, R., Davies, R. J., Hockley, J., Turner, P. (1988) Analgesic effect of oral flecainide. *Lancet*, **i**, 420–421

Editorial (1991). Ondansetron versus dexamethasone for chemotherapy-induced emesis. *Lancet*, **338**, 478–479

Fishbain, D. A., Goldberg, M., Rosomoff, R. S., Rosomoff, A. (1991) Completed suicide in chronic pain. *Clinical Journal of Pain*, **7**, 29–36

Glare, P. A., Walsh, T. D., Pippenger, C. E. (1990) Normorphine, a neurotoxic metabolite? *British Medical Journal* 355.725 (letter)

Hanks, G. W., Hoskin, P. J., Aherne, G. W. *et al.* (1987) Explanation for potency of repeated oral doses of morphine? *Lancet*, **ii**, 723–725

Hanks, G. W., Ward, P. J. (1989) Enterohepatic circulation of opioid drugs. Is it clinically relevant in the treatment of cancer patients? *Clin. Pharmacokinetics*, **17**, (2) 65–68

Hardy, P. A. J. (1991) Editorial. Use of opiates in treating chronic benign pain. *British Journal of Hospital Medicine*, **45**, 257

Harrison, D. C. (1972) Haemodynamic effects of morphine and pentazocine differ in cardiac patients. *New England Journal of Medicine*, **287**, 623–627

Honde, R. W., Wallenstein, S. L., Beaver, W. T. (1965) Clinical measurement of pain. In: de Stevens G. (ed). *Analgetics* Academic Press, New York: 75–122

Jaffe, J. H., Martin, W. R. (1990)Opioid analgesics and antagonists. In: *The pharmacological basis of therapeutics*, 8th edn. Eds. Goodman Gilman, A. G., Rall, T. W., Nies, A. S., Taylor, P. Pergamon Press

Jones, R. F., Anthony, M., Torda, T. A., Poulos, C. (1988) Epidural baclofen for intractable spasticity. *Lancet*, **i**, 527

Killian, J. M., Fromm, G. H. (1968) Carbamazepine in the treatment of neuralgia: use and side effects. *Archives of Neurology*, **19**, 129–136

King, S. A., Strain, J. J. (1990) Benzodiazepine use by chronic pain patients. *Clinical Journal of Pain*, **6**, 143–147

Korsten, H. H. H. (1991) Long-lasting epidural sensory blockade by n-butyl-p-amino benzoate in the terminally ill intractable cancer pain patient. Paper presented at the joint annual meeting of the British and Dutch Pain Societies, London, April

Kyinsdahl, B., Molin, J., Froland, A., Gram, L. F. (1984) Imipramine treatment of painful diabetic neuropathy. *J.A.M.A.*, **251**, 1727–1730

Martindale 29th edition p. 729 1989

Mever, M. B. Zelechkowski, K. (1971) Intramuscular lignocaine in normal subjects. In: Scott & Julian (eds) *Lignocaine in the treatment of ventricular arrhythmias.* Livingstone Edinburgh, p 161

McQuay, H. J., Caroll, D., Moore, R. A. (1988) Postoperative orthopaedic pain – the effect of opiate premedication and local anaesthetic blocks. *Pain*, **33**, (3) 291–295

McQuay, H., Moore, R. A. (1984) Be aware of renal function when prescribing morphine. *Lancet*, **ii**, 284–285

Morrison, L. M., Payne, M., Drummond, G. B. (1991) Comparison of speed of onset of analgesic effect of diamorphine and morphine. *British Journal of Anaesthesia* **66**, 656–659

Nimmo, W. S., Smith, G. (1989) *Anaesthesia: Volume 1.* Oxford: Blackwell Scientific Publications

Ochs, G., Struppler, A., Meyerson, B. A. *et al.* (1989) Intrathecal baclofen for long-term treatment of spasticity: a multicentre study. *Journal of Neurology, Neurosurgery and Psychiatry*, **52**, 933–939

Pasternak, G. W., Bodnar, R. J., Clark, J. A., Inturissi, C. E. (1987) Morphine-6-glucuronide, a potent mu agonist. *Life Science* **41**, 2845–2849

Penn, R. D., Savoy, S. M., Corcos, D. *et al.* (1989) Intrathecal baclofen for severe spinal spasticity. *New England Journal of Medicine*, **320**, 1517–1521

Petersen, P., Kastrup, J. (1987) Dercum's disease (adiposis dolorosa). Treatment of severe pain with intravenous lignocaine. *Pain*, **28**, 77–80

Petersen, P., Kastrup, J., Zeeburg, I., Boysen, G. (1986) Chronic pain treatment with intravenous lignocaine. *Neur. Res.*, **8**, 189–190

Plummer, J. L., Cherry, D. A., Cousins, M. J. *et al.* (1991) Long-term spinal administration of morphine in cancer and non-cancer patients: a retrospective study. *Pain*, **44**, 215–220

Portenoy, R. K. (1990) Pharmacological management of chronic pain. In: *Pain syndromes in Neurology* (ed.) Field, H. L. Butterworths

Ralcliff, B. W., Davies, E. H. (1968) Controlled sequential trials of carbamazepine in trigeminal neuralgia. *Archives of Neurology*, **15**, 129–136

Reichle, C. W., Smith, G. M., Gravenstein, J. S. *et al.* (1962) Comparative analgesic potency of heroin and morphine in post operative pain. *Journal of Pharmacology and Exp. Therapy*, **136**, 43–46

Sawe, J., Syensson, J. O., Odar-Cederlof, I. (1985) Kinetics of morphine in patients with renal failure. *Lancet*, **ii**, 211

Sear, J. W., Hand, C. W., Moore, R. A., McQuay, H. J. (1989) Studies on morphine disposition; influence of renal failure on the kinetics of morphine and its metabolites. *British Journal of Anaesthesia* **62**, 28–32

Seers, K. (1989) Patients perceptions of acute pain. In: Wilson Barnett, J., Robinson, S. (eds) *Directions in nursing research*, p 107–116. Scutari Press, London

Sinnott, C., Edmonds, P., Cropley, I., Hanks, G. (1991) Flecainide in cancer nerve pain. *Lancet*, **337**, 1347

The Royal College of Surgeons of England. The College of Anaesthetists. Commission on the provision of surgical services. Report on the Working Party on Pain after Surgery, 1990

Twycross, R. G. (1984) Relief of pain. In: *Management of Terminal Malignant Disease*. Saunders, C. 2nd Ed. Edward Arnold

Twycross, R. G. and Lack, S. A. (1990) *Therapeutics in Terminal Cancer* 2nd edn, Churchill Livingstone

Watson, C. P. N., Evans, R. J., Reed, K. *et al.* (1982) Amitriptyline versus placebo in post herpetic neuralgia. *Neurology*, **32**, 671–673

Watson, C. P. N., Evans, R. J., Watt, V. R. (1988) Post herpetic neuralgia and topical capsaicin. *Pain*, **33**, 333–340

Weinberg, D. S., Inturissi, C. E., Reidenberg, B. *et al.* (1988) Sublingual absorption of selected opioid analgesics. *Clinical Pharmacology Therapy*, **44**, 335–342

Westbrook, L., Cicala, R. S., Wright, H. (1990) Effectiveness of alprazolam in the treatment of chronic pain: results of a preliminary survey. *Clinical Journal of Pain*, **6**, 32–36

Yosselson-Superstine, S., Lipman, A. G. Sanders, S. H. (1955) Adjunctive antianxiety agents in the management of chronic pain. Israel. *Journal of Medical Science*, **21**, 113–117

Zeisat, H. A., Gentry, W. D., Angle, H. V., Ellinwood, C. H. (1979) Drug use and misuse in operant pain patients. *Addictive Behaviour*, **4**, 263–266

15

Special procedures

Valerie M. F. King and Patricia A. Jacob

Introduction

The pharmacological, sensory and psychological methods of pain management cannot exclude each other; indeed a combination may be necessary to provide satisfactory pain relief.

In this chapter a description is given of procedures which interrupt pathways by which painful sensations are perceived. Procedures commonly used are described in detail. Most often they are carried out in pain clinics which have developed in response to the challenge of those patients with intractable pain. The clinic setting provides the means to examine the pain syndrome itself, with specialists working together, interchanging ideas and emerging from this, new therapies which can be implemented and evaluated.

The methods include the blocking of the conduction of nerve impulses and the interruption of pain pathways with the use of local anaesthesia and other drugs which provide an analgesic effect. Neurolytic agents, which are drugs capable of destroying nerve fibres, are also used. These are specialist treatments usually carried out by anaesthetists with a special interest in the pain syndrome.

In managing chronic pain patients the long term benefits of these procedures have to be the main consideration. With regard to this it should be stated that some procedures are conducted routinely without a sound research base to support their long term pain relieving effects.

The nurse's role

The nurse involved with procedures for the alleviation of pain is in the unique position to assess, assist in treatments, measure and evalu-

ate their outcome, in this challenging and developing field. This has implications both for the patient and nurse, with growth of new ideas and research-based practice to benefit the patient and for the nurse's development.

Pain, by its subjective nature, has to be approached in a holistic way. Each patient is individual with varying concepts of their particular pain problems. Skills in interviewing and counselling are essential for an exchange of information and to gain the active cooperation and confidence of the patient.

Chronic pain sufferers are often seen repeatedly, either on an inpatient or outpatient basis or a combination. It is therefore conducive to the continuity of their care to have a named nurse who will attend them on subsequent visits.

It cannot be overemphasised that the role of the nurse in the pain clinic setting is primarily to assist the patient in overcoming a pain problem. Pain, particularly when protracted, can cause disturbance in normal physical and psychological functioning which at times can be overwhelming. Within the multidisciplinary team the nurse can play a major part in helping a patient to regain their normal functioning.

Nursing actions and rationale common to all procedures

Preparation

The nurse should provide a quiet, calm atmosphere in which the patient can discuss their particular pain problem. Individual need should be assessed with regard to any difficulty or disability which may affect the performance of the procedure. Any relevant medical history such as diabetes or allergies should be ascertained and current medications noted, e.g.

warfarin, which may contraindicate performance of the procedure.

Although the doctor will have discussed the procedure with the patient prior to their giving consent it is helpful for the nurse to give a clear, step-by-step description of the nature of the treatment, including the common side effects and complications that can arise. The patient's expectations should be discussed as they may be falsely optimistic. To allay this the expected level of pain relief and duration of action of the procedure should be fully explained. Raising these issues will provide the patient with the opportunity to ask questions and to gain reassurance without which the patient may be unnecessarily anxious. It will also ensure that informed consent has been given to the particular procedure.

During procedure

The nurse's prime responsibility is for the comfort and reassurance of the patient, the secondary role being to assist the doctor to perform the procedure under aseptic conditions. A calm, relaxed atmosphere should be provided throughout its duration and may be helped by the use of background relaxation music. If monitoring of the patient's vital signs is required during and following the procedure baseline observations should be recorded at the outset.

Post-procedure

The procedure should be recorded in a book accessible to all staff, stating patient's name, doctor and nurse present, drugs used and any complications. This will provide quick and easy access to information if any later queries or complications arise, when the patient's individual notes may not be readily available.

The image intensifier

The image intensifier is an X-ray machine with instant screen image. It is used to enable precise location of landmarks for nerve blockade. Modern image intensifiers also have a freeze-frame facility which minimises exposure time.

When in use patients must be positioned on an X-ray table. Female patients should be asked if they are pregnant or trying to conceive, in order to prevent accidental exposure of the fetus.

All staff present during its use should wear protective lead aprons, neck collars and film badges for radiation monitoring. These are usually read monthly and returned to the department. Lead aprons should be stored on hangers after use to prevent damage and inspected regularly for signs of wear.

The image intensifier would be used for the following procedures:

Facet block
Facet freeze
Caudal epidural
Caudal freeze
Coeliac plexus block
Splanchnic block
Lumbar sympathetic block
Infra-dental blocks
Intercostal nerve block if the patient is obese
Intercostal freeze
Epidural with insertion of a radio-opaque catheter
Trigeminal nerve root blockade
Percutaneous anterolateral cordotomy

Whilst the image intensifier is in use a radiographer or trained anaesthetist should be in attendance. The nurse should be able to operate the machine and record the readings in the procedure book regarding time and amount of exposure for each patient.

When in use there should be a warning indicator positioned outside the room to prevent other staff from entering without protective clothing.

Cryoanalgesia and radiofrequency

Nerves and nerve ganglia may be inactivated or destroyed by two methods which are more or less opposite to one another. One is by *freezing* (cryoanalgesia) and the other is by *heating* (thermocoagulation). Freezing has the advantage that it is usually reversible – that is, function returns. When cryoanalgesia is used for pain relief, nerve function sometimes returns without the return of pain.

Heat coagulation, on the other hand, usually results in more permanent destruction, so must be approached very cautiously. The most commonly used method employs the use of an electric current alternating at extremely high (radio-) frequency, so that while heat is produced, no electricity passes into the tissues.

Indications

They have distinct advantages over other methods of pain relief. Nerve blocks are not usually effective for such prolonged periods and the use of neurolytic drugs such as alcohol and phenol can be unpredictable and irreversible.

Cryoanalgesia has been used in the management of postoperative pain, for example following thoracotomy. Freezing of the relevant intercostal nerve reduces the need for strong analgesics which may depress respiration. It has also been used successfully in the management of facial neuralgia, providing relief for many months and in some cases, long after normal facial skin sensations have returned. In many instances this has proved to be much more effective and less drastic than cutting nerves which may only give short term pain relief with prolonged sensory loss. Other chronic pains such as low back pain, painful scar tissue, and malignant pain have been treated successfully with the use of the cryoprobe.

Equipment and technique

RF coagulator

This essentially consists of a needle electrode which can be sterilised and passed into the appropriate tissues. A cable connects it to an electronic box, which can be set to deliver the radiofrequency current for set periods of time, usually varying from 20 or 30 seconds to 2 minutes. A thermocouple attached to the probe enables the tissue temperature at the tip of the electrode to be measured, and read off on the box. To ensure that the electrode is correctly placed, stimulation is first delivered; it should result in tingling in the affected area. The usual procedure is then to see how long it takes, with the needle in place, to reach a certain tempera-

ture, say 65° or 70°, and then to coagulate at this temperature for periods of 30 or 60 seconds until the desired result is achieved in the locally anaesthetised patient. The end-point in trigeminal ganglion coagulation, for instance, is a subjective feeling of numbness and loss of pinprick sensation in the area affected by pain, similar feelings and sensations are sought in the painful area in cases of percutaneous cordotomy.

Cryoprobe

A modern cryoprobe or cryoneedle consists of an inner tube with a very fine nozzle through which nitrous oxide or carbon dioxide is delivered under pressure within an outer tube which is sealed at the end. As the gas is delivered under pressure through the nozzle, it expands, and in so doing cools. A lower temperature can be obtained with nitrous oxide which cools to around −70°C at the centre of the iceball (−20°C is the minimum temperature at which nerve destruction will take place). Heat is absorbed from surrounding tissues and the warm exhaust gas is passed back along the tube and vented. An iceball forms, encompassing the end of the probe (Figure 15.1).

Various mechanisms are involved in the nerve damage brought about by the use of cryoanalgesia. There is physical disruption by the ice crystals and rupture of cell membrane takes place. Osmotic damage is caused by hyptertonia on membrane function. Ischaemic necrosis by thrombosis occurs and it is thought that auto-antibody formation may take place.

An example of the apparatus used is the Spembly-Lloyd cryoprobe which incorporates a peripheral nerve stimulator by which the position of the probe can be elicited.

The cryoprobe can be used under direct vision where a nerve is accessible and can be exposed surgically. Alternatively, it can be used percutaneously by making a track through the tissues with an introducer, under local anaesthetic. The probe can then be passed through it

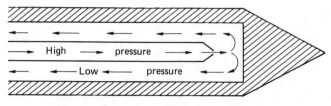

Figure 15.1 Cross section of cryoprobe tip.

in the direction of the nerve and its position checked with the aid of an image intensifier and/or the nerve stimulator.

Clinical application

This can be considered under the following three headings:

Superficial   e.g. for skin cooling, glosso-pharyngeal nerve, painful fungating tumour.

Percutaneous e.g. intercostal nerve, sacral roots, facetal, caudal, occipital nerves, neuroma, trigger points, lateral cutaneous nerve of thigh.

Open   e.g. intercostal nerve, ilioinguinal nerve, supra-orbital nerve, supra-trochlear nerve, infra-orbital nerve, mental nerve and lingual nerve.

Facet block

Indication

As the spine gets older the intervertebral discs become drier and thinner. One of the results of disc degeneration is that the facet joints, which link the vertebrae together, come under much greater pressure and are prone to wear and tear. This can lead to irritation and inflammation of the facet joints themselves, resulting in the symptoms of both back and leg pain, with acute episodes.

Although degeneration of the vertebral discs and the facet joints is an inevitable part of the ageing process, only certain people will present with the symptoms of pain. There are many factors which may predispose some people to back pain. These include poor posture, obesity, high risk occupations, incorrect lifting techniques and insufficient exercise.

Description

The intervertebral discs separate the main body of each vertebra. The vertebrae connect with one another by means of articular facets situated on articular processes. These processes are linked by a cartilaginous joint, allowing movement of the spine. These joints are known as facet joints because the articular processes have flat, smooth surfaces that bear resemb-lance to the facets of a diamond (Figures 15.2 and 15.3).

Pain caused by inflammation of a facet joint can be relieved by the injection of local anaesthetic and steroid into or around the affected joint, with the aid of an image intensifier. Injections are an effective and relatively simple way of delivering treatment to a localised area without possible side effects associated with the use of oral analgesia and oral anti-inflammatory drugs. They can be performed on an outpatient basis and can provide relief for several months.

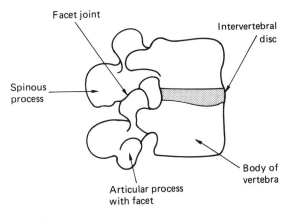

Figure 15.2 Diagram of facet joint.

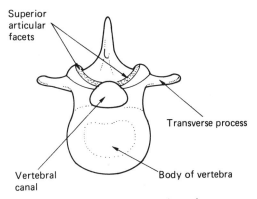

Figure 15.3 Lumbar vertebra as seen from above.

Facet block continued on p.210

Equipment for facet block

Sterile dressing pack
Sterile gloves
1 × 10 ml syringe
1 × 5 ml syringe
20 gauge 3.5 in spinal needle
21 gauge needle
25 gauge needle
Local anaesthetic for skin infiltration, e.g. 2% lignocaine

Long acting local anaesthetic, e.g. bupivicaine 0.5%
Steroid, e.g. methylprednisolone
Antiseptic to clean skin prior to procedure, e.g. betadine
Antiseptic to clean skin post-procedure, e.g. chlorhexidine
Small dressing, e.g. waterproof plaster
Image intensifier

Preparation for facet block

Nursing action	Rationale
1. Position the patient in the prone position on a low X-ray table.	This is the most effective position to allow location of the facet joints with the aid of the image intensifier.
2. Position the patient's arms in front of them, supported by a pillow. An additional pillow may be placed under the chest.	To ensure the comfort of the patient.
3. Drape the patient's legs with a sheet.	To minimise exposure and to help keep the patient warm.
4. Open dressing pack, deposit sterile gloves, syringes and needles onto sterile area, ensuring area is not contaminated.	To minimise the risk of infection.
5. Provide and check with doctor drugs to be administered.	To ensure correct drugs, dosage and that they have not expired.
6. Remain with the patient throughout the procedure and reassure them. Advise against any sudden movements.	To reduce anxiety and fear. To avoid trauma which could complicate the procedure.

During procedure

Doctor/nurse action	Rationale
1. The procedure is performed using an aseptic technique. Skin is prepared with antiseptic solution.	To minimise risk of infection.
2. The skin is infiltrated with local anaesthetic. Encourage patient to state if local anaesthetic is ineffective.	To reduce discomfort. To ascertain if more local anaesthetic is required.
3. The spinal needle is introduced and the affected joint is located with the aid of the image intensifier.	To help provide accurate location of the joint.
4. The long acting local anaesthetic and steroid are injected into or around the affected joint. Additional joints may be located and injected.	More than one joint may give symptoms of pain.

5. The area is cleaned and a small dressing applied.
6. Assist patient whilst getting up and off the table.   To ensure the safety of the patient.

Post-procedure

Nursing action

1. Advise patient that immediate relief may be obtained from the local anaesthetic but they may experience some return of pain symptoms before the steroid becomes effective which could take several days.

Facet freeze

Indication

The indications for performing a facet freeze are the same as for facet block. However, a freeze may provide longer relief of pain symptoms. A diagnostic facet block would have been carried out at a previous visit to prove effectiveness of block before proceeding to using cryoanalgesia. (See section on cryoanalgesia.)

Description

As for facet block.

The nerve supplying the affected joint would be located with the aid of the image intensifier and frozen. This would lead to the blocking of nerve impulses which give rise to the pain symptoms. The procedure is normally performed using local anaesthetic in an outpatient setting.

Equipment for facet freeze

Sterile dressing pack
Sterile gloves
1 x 5 ml syringe
21 gauge needle
25 gauge needle
12 gauge cannula (medicut)
Antiseptic solutions, e.g. betadine and chlorhexidine

Iodine spray
Cryoprobe and machine
Substantial sterile pressure dressing
Image intensifier
Local anaesthetic for skin, e.g. lignocaine 2%

Preparation

Nursing action	*Rationale*
1.–6. Same as for facet block.	
7. Cryoprobe and machine are assembled according to specific instructions for the apparatus used.	
8. Purge the cryoprobe.	To remove water vapour from the system and therefore avoid blockages inside the probe.

During procedure

Doctor/nurse action	*Rationale*
1.–2. Same as for facet block.	
3. The cannula is introduced into the skin at the identified level.	To create a track through which the cryoprobe can be inserted.
4. The cryoprobe is inserted through the cannula and advanced to the estimated site of the nerve with the aid of the image intensifier.	To ensure accurate placement of the probe.
5. The gas is switched on. Two freeze-thaw cycles of two minutes are used at a steady temperature of —70°C at the centre of the iceball (if nitrous oxide is used).	Repetition of cycle increases size of iceball thus increasing time of loss of nerve function.
6. The indicator on the apparatus should be checked to ensure the correct temperature and gas pressure are maintained.	To maintain size of iceball.
7. Observe for increasing anxiety, pallor, convulsions or syncope. (Complications are rare with this procedure.)	Shock may occur due to accidental intravascular injection of local anaesthetic or toxic reaction to local anaesthetic.
8. When the probe is fully defrosted as shown by the indicator on the apparatus, and freely moveable within the tissues, it is removed.	Avoidance of trauma.
9. The area is cleaned. Iodine spray is applied and a sterile pressure dressing. Advise the patient to leave this in situ for at least 24 hours. It can then be replaced with a smaller dressing which should cover the wound for a week.	To minimize the risk of infection. Some bleeding may occur due to depth and diameter of track in the tissues. There may be slight discharge.
10.The patient is assisted to assume a sitting position. When the patient is ready he/she may be assisted off the table.	To ensure the safety of the patient.

Post procedure

Nursing action	*Rationale*
1. Advise patient to seek medical assistance if discharge from wound is persistant, fever develops, or if there is swelling, discomfort or inflammation around the wound site.	Potential risk of infection or haematoma from invasive procedure.

Epidural analgesia

Epidural blockade, a major conduction block, has seen a rapid increase in its clinical application in the past 30 years, for alleviation of both acute and chronic pain. This has largely been brought about by the development of local anaesthesia and intensive research by anaesthetists exploring pain management.

Indications for epidural analgesia

These can be divided into acute and chronic pain, also for diagnostic and prognostic blockade.

Acute pain	in surgery	• particularly useful for thoracic and abdominal operations, vaginal and perineal, urological and lower limb surgery.
	in obstetrics	• most effective way of relieving pain during labour and allows for caesarian section with the mother remaining conscious.
	post-operative pain	• block can be prolonged after surgery using bolus or continuous infusion.
	acute painful states	• effective analgesia for conditions such as; ureteric colic, acute pancreatitis, following trauma, multiple rib fractures, herpes zoster, ischaemic vascular pain.
Chronic pain	back pain	• local anaesthetic agent with long-acting corticosteroid to reduce inflammatory changes.
	chronic non-malignant pain	• single bolus injections or epidural catheter can be inserted to try different drugs. This may involve daily bolus injections for 3–4 days with detailed monitoring of pain relief achieved for each particular drug used.
	malignant pain	• use of local anaesthetic and other analgesic drugs, e.g. opiates. Epidural can remain in situ for remainder of patient's life.

Relevant anatomy and physiology

The epidural space is located between the spinal dura and the vertebral canal. In reality it is a potential space, a capillary interval occupied by the internal vertebral venous plexus, epidural fat, segmental blood supply and lymphatics. It extends the length of the vertebral column from the foramen magnum superiorly to the sacral hiatus caudally. It varies in size, being largest in the mid-lumbar region. The distance between the ligamentum flavum and lamina and the dura in the midline is approximately 1.5–2 mm in cervical and upper thoracic regions, 3–5 mm in the mid-thoracic and lower thoracic regions and 5–6 mm in the lumbar region. The epidural space is limited laterally owing to the attachment of the dura to the connective tissue covering the vertebrae and the ligamenta flava. It can thus be considered as a closed compartment.

Adjacent vertebrae are held together posteriorly by short, tough ligaments and it is through these ligaments that access to the spinal canal is gained. The laminae of the vertebrae are connected by the ligamentum flavum while the shafts of the spinous processes are connected by the intraspinous ligament. The supraspinous ligament runs superficial to the tips of the spinous processes. To insert a needle into the spinal canal between two vertebrae, these ligaments have to be traversed, the ligamentum flavum being the toughest and is obvious by its resistance to the needle.

In the sacrum, there are no ligamenta flava, the laminae being fused together, except for the

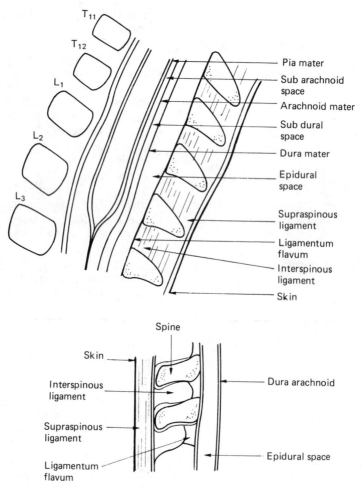

Figure 15.4 Diagrammatic sagittal cross-section of lower vertebrae and spinal cord to show the position of the epidural space and related structures.

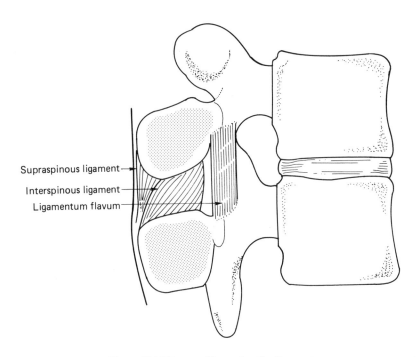

Supraspinous ligament
Interspinous ligament
Ligamentum flavum

Figure 15.5 Diagram illustrating the ligaments.

fifth sacral vertebra, which forms the sacral hiatus, having no laminae. It is through this hiatus that a caudal block is performed (Figures 15.4, 15.5).

Epidural blockade can be performed at four levels; cervical, thoracic, lumbar and caudal, having varying physiological effects involving respiratory, cardiovascular and neuroendocrine function dependent on the level used.

Administration of local anaesthetic drugs in sufficient volume will interrupt the passage of sensory, motor and autonomic impulses in both dorsal and ventral spinal roots and to some extent, in the spinal cord itself. Loss of sensation is usually the first indication of successful epidural blockade. Injection of local anaesthetic relieves pain in most cases for the duration of its action but by adding a long acting corticosteroid any inflammation present may be reduced. This can produce prolonged improvement, e.g. in chronic back pain. A single injection may be given, intermittent bolus injections, or continuous infusion with the use of a syringe driver. If frequent intermittent injection or the continuous method is indicated, this will require the use of an epidural catheter.

Identification of the epidural space

Loss of resistance technique is the most commonly used. As previously mentioned, it relies on the fact that there is marked resistance to injection through the epidural needle, providing the needle lies in the ligamentum flavum. When the needle enters the epidural space, resistance almost completely disappears. A freely moveable plunger to the syringe used is essential and most often a glass syringe or a plastic syringe with a loss of resistance device is employed. Pressure is exerted manually onto the plunger of the syringe containing air or normal saline solution, until loss of resistance is felt. Only a small amount is injected, which is harmless.

Another method is the 'hanging drop' technique. The basis for this is the negative pressure often found within the epidural space. A winged needle is used and it is advanced with both hands. A drop of fluid is placed at the hub of the needle when the interspinous ligament has been engaged. It is advanced carefully forward through the ligamentum flavum. On entering the epidural space it is suddenly sucked into the needle. It is not wholly reliable due to the fact that negative pressure may not always be present, for example, if expiration is forced or breathholding takes place.

Epidural top-up procedure – the extended role of the nurse

An extended role can be described as one which is not included in basic training. With a specialist unit such as a pain clinic the role of the specialist nurse may encompass procedures which have previously been carried out by the medical staff. If it arises from the need to ensure continuing comfort for the patient, it would seem reasonable for the nurse to extend his/her role, given that it is carried out with a high level of theoretical knowledge and practical skill. Since each nurse is individually responsible and accountable for his/her actions, nurses who wish to give epidural drugs will need to maintain and update their knowledge and competence.

The aim in giving epidural drugs is to relieve pain in the most effective manner for an individual patient, whilst taking all reasonable precautions to see that the patient comes to no harm as a result. To this end it is advisable for the unit's nursing and medical staff to have an agreed policy, with a formal assessment of the nurse wishing to undertake epidural administration.

A doctor will always give the first dose of an epidural drug to a patient. This will allow for ensuring that the epidural catheter is correctly placed and effectiveness and any side effects have been noted. The doctor must record certain details on the patient's drug chart; the insertion date of the epidural line, the name and dose of the drug, and the date and time of administration. Where indicated, the appropriate antidote and the circumstances under which it should be given must also be documented. The doctor will ensure that medical assistance is easily summoned throughout the period of time a patient is receiving epidural drugs. Medical staff should provide nurses an up-to-date source of information relating to; drugs which may be given epidurally by assessed nursing staff, expected therapeutic effects and criteria for evaluation. Also, an agreed method of administration and possible side effects with appropriate nursing action should be documented. This information should be regularly reviewed and discussed.

Epidural catheterisation

The safety and reliability of this technique allows for long duration relief, even in ambulatory patients. It is a skilled procedure but provides a simple and effective method of pain control. In acute pain management the patient would remain within the unit for the duration of its use. This would also apply to the patient with chronic non-malignant pain where epidural catheterisation may be indicated for a number of reasons, for example, diagnostically, to test the efficacy of varying drugs and doses, or where a single dose has previously proved to be insufficient. Long term epidural catheterisation may also be considered for this group of patients, where conventional analgesic routes have proved unsuccessful or inadequate. For the chronic malignant pain sufferer epidural analgesia can dramatically improve the quality of pain relief for their remaining life. An epidural catheter can be left *in situ* for weeks and in some cases months, the patient being admitted to hospital for insertion of the catheter and until effective pain control is established. This may only require a few days, the patient then being managed at home with medical and nursing support. It is not uncommon for the patient and his/her family to manage epidural administration at home, with the support of the general practitioner and district nurse. Bolus injections may be given, or more commonly a syringe driver is attached via extension tubing to the epidural catheter to provide a continuous infusion. This can be refilled every 24 hours or as required. This method also provides the means by which a 'boost' of the drug can be given for breakthrough pain or preventatively prior to increased activity by the patient which may induce their pain. If frequent 'boosting' becomes necessary the drug regime should be reviewed. Opiates are most commonly used in conjunction with a long acting local anaesthetic agent. Much smaller doses of opiates are required via the epidural route – one tenth of the oral equivalent. The amount of local anaesthetic used will be titrated to the patient's mobility. Higher doses may be considered in the patient whose disease process has rendered him/her bed bound. It may be observed, in patients whose level of pain has rendered them bed bound, rather than the disease process, that epidural infusion allows them to mobilise, thus regaining their independence and self esteem.

The nurse refilling a syringe connected to an epidural infusion requires the same level of expertise as for giving repeat bolus epidural injections and should only undertake this task having had appropriate training. If patients or relatives are to undertake the management they will require adequate training, practice and support both from hospital and community staff. This allows the patient to maintain their independence and measure of control with managing and coping with their particular pain problem.

An epidural catheter can be inserted and taped externally, tunnelled subcutaneously or implanted. Tunnelling or implanting are considered more suitable for long term use, giving the patient more independence. Tunnelling is usually carried out to prevent movement of the catheter and for comfort where the catheter can be positioned more appropriately. Implantation involves the use of an indwelling catheter attached to a subcutaneous reservoir or portal which is surgically positioned. This provides an internal system with less likelihood of infection or movement of the catheter and offers increased comfort for the patient.

Temporary catheterisation with external taping can give rise to problems which the nurse should be aware of. The epidural catheter can migrate either into the subcutaneous tissues or to the skin surface. This is usually discovered by unsuccessful blockade when topping up and the dressing is found to be damp following the attempted epidural injection. Kinking or clotting can occur in the catheter. A change of position may be sufficient to remove a kink, or withdrawal of approximately 1 cm of the catheter, but if a clot is suspected the epidural catheter will have to be removed. On its removal care must be taken. If resistance is felt, probably due to the grip of the overlying vertebral arches, the patient should be asked to flex his/her back. Gentle traction should be applied to the catheter close to the point of entry to the skin. The tip should be inspected following removal. If it is suspected that a piece has broken off the doctor should be informed and the catheter kept for inspection. If the doctor is unable to remove the remaining piece of catheter by superficial probing it is usually left in situ. The plastic used is non-irritant and should not give rise to further complications. On average 3–5 cm of catheter is inserted into the epidural space. If this is exceeded its position becomes unpredictable, with the possibility, albeit rare, of encircling a spinal nerve. This will give rise to severe pain when traction is applied and may damage the nerve, requiring surgery to remove the catheter. Infection is a risk which the nurse must always be alert to. Whilst the patient has a temporary catheter in situ the site must be inspected regularly for any signs of inflammation, the patient's temperature recorded daily and any continuing soreness around the epidural site reported to the doctor. The use of bacterial filters is arguable. If employed they must be changed regularly – usually weekly, which may increase the risk of infection per se, and they are known to filter out such drugs as methylprednisolone.

Equipment for epidural blockade

Sterile epidural block procedure pack containing:

Sterile field sheet
Hand towels
1 × 16 gauge Tuohy needle (usually winged)
1 × 10 ml plastic syringe
1 × 2 ml plastic syringe
1 × kwill filling tube
1 × 23 gauge needle
1 × 26 gauge needle
1 × filter
1 × trocar
1 × 10 ml ampoule sodium chloride injection 0.9%
1 × pair dressing forceps
4 × 3″ × 3″ gauze swabs
3 × sponges
1 × fenestrated patient drape
2 × gallipots
1 × granulated epidural catheter with reconnecting guide

Additional equipment:

Sterile gloves
Local anaesthetic for skin infiltration, e.g. 2% lignocaine
Drug/s to be used for epidural block, e.g. bupivicaine 0.25% or 0.5%, methylprednisolone, clonidine, midazolam, ketamine, morphine
Antiseptic to clean skin prior to procedure, e.g. betadine
Antiseptic to clean skin post-procedure, e.g. chlorhexidine
Iodine spray
Small dressing if single epidural injection given
Close fitting dressing plus tape if epidural catheter inserted
Radio-opaque catheter if X-ray control required to position catheter
Intravenous cannula. This allows for intravenous drugs pre-procedure if patient is very anxious and requires sedation (general anaesthesia is rarely indicated). It is also precautionary, should it be necessary to transfuse the patient post-procedure because of hypotension.

Preparation for epidural blockade

Nursing action	*Rationale*
1. Check pulse and blood pressure	To provide baseline values for later comparison.
For lying position:	
2. Position patient on his/her side with a pillow under their head. Ensure patient is lying on a firm surface (X-ray table if radio-opaque catheter is to be used).	
3. Assist patient to arch his/her back and draw their knees towards abdomen, clasping knees with hands if necessary.	This position opens up the interspinous spaces, thus enabling easier entry into the epidural space.
For sitting position:	
4. Have patient seated on firm surface either on chair with head and arms resting on table or on operating table with legs flexed, feet on chair, bent forward with pillow across chest and hands clasped across pillow with back arched. For cervical epidural – head forward, neck extended, cap to cover hair.	For doctor's operative preference or for obese patients or those unable to assume lying position due to disability, this may afford more accurate identification of interspinous spaces.
5. Drape with sheet.	To keep patient warm and minimise exposure.

6. Open sterile epidural pack and gloves. Pour cleaning solutions. Provide and check local anaesthetic with doctor and any other drugs to be used.

7. Remain with the patient throughout. Help in maintaining position, give reassurance and advise against any sudden movements.

To reduce anxiety and fear.
To avoid trauma which could complicate the procedure.

During procedure

Doctor/nurse action	*Rationale*
1. The procedure is performed using an aseptic technique. Skin is prepared with antiseptic solution.	To minimise risk of infection.
2. The skin is infiltrated with local anaesthetic. Encourage patient to state if local anaesthetic is not working.	To reduce any discomfort. To ascertain if more time is needed or if more local anaesthetic is required.
3. Size introducer is used to puncture skin.	To facilitate passage of Tuohy needle.
4. Tuohy needle is inserted into epidural space usually by technique of 'loss of resistance' to the syringe plunger which occurs when epidural space is reached.	Pressure in the epidural is below atmospheric pressure.
5. Watch for increasing anxiety, pallor or syncope.	Shock may occur.
6. If epidural catheter to be used, inserted through Tuohy needle and threaded into epidural space in direction required for analgesic effect.	Epidural catheter allows for pain free administration of increased quantity of drug or to try different drugs.
7. Pain relieving drugs given in small quantity as test dose either as straight injection through Tuohy needle or via epidural catheter.	To exclude adverse drug reaction or of misplaced catheter – intrathecal or intravascular.
8. Assist patient to more relaxed position.	
9. Area cleaned with antiseptic solution. Sterile dressing applied. If epidural catheter used, secure directly to skin with close-fitting dressing and tape remaining catheter to body either over shoulder or around abdomen.	
10. Full dose of drug given by doctor after appropriate interval following test dose.	
11. Assist patient to assume comfortable position lying flat and transfer to bed for recovery.	

Post-procedure

Nursing action	*Rationale*
1. Position patient appropriately dependent upon level of epidural and pain area.	To facilitate delivery of drug used.
2. Commence monitoring of blood pressure and effect of drug immediately following procedure. Check respirations and size of pupils if opiate used. Continue monitoring every 5 minutes during the first hour.	Detection of possible hypotension caused by drug, e.g. clonidine or bupivicaine. To detect any signs of respiratory depression or effect on central nervous system.

If the patient is showing signs and symptoms of hypotension with/or the mean arterial pressure 25% below baseline:	Profound effect of drug because of peripheral vasodilation and lack of effective intravascular volume
2a. Inform doctor. Ensure patient remains lying flat: legs can be raised (not head down). Doctor may decide to give oxygen and rapid infusion of colloid – Hartman's intravenously. Have ephedrine available and naloxone if opiate used.	
3. Note effect of drug – symptoms such as warmth or numbness and weakness. This will be experienced to some extent in most patients who have had local anaesthesia epidurally.	To gauge efficiency of drug administered and any detrimental effects such as extensive motor blockade which may suggest accidental intrathecal injection.
Any loss of bladder function, fits (uncommon), nausea and vomiting. Note if patient complains of headache.	Suggestive of accidental dural puncture or massive extradural.
If headache persists:	
3a. Keep lying flat. Inform doctor. Increase oral or intravenous fluids. Administration of mild systemic analgesia as prescribed.	To encourage cerebral spinal fluid formation.
4. Monitor pain level during recovery period and inform doctor.	To detect if block ineffective or insufficient analgesic effect.
5. Advise patient to remain immobile until any numbness or weakness has resolved (approximately 2 hours following bolus injection). Provide with call bell.	To prevent patient injuring themselves.
6. On discharge advise to seek medical assistance if any loss of blood or other discharge from injection site, fever, persistent pain or inflammation around injection site.	Potential risk of infection from invasive procedure.
7. If proximal catheter is external advise patient against getting it wet	To avoid risk of dislodging catheter/and or increasing risk of infection.

Caudal (epidural) block

Indications

Caudal block is performed by injecting through the sacral hiatus into the spinal canal. As previously mentioned, the epidural space can be entered via this route, greatly reducing the risk of a dural tap because the subarachnoid space ends at the level of the second sacral vertebra.

In theory, caudal block can be used for the same purposes as lumbar epidural block. However, the local anaesthetic used may not spread high enough and for this reason is usually confined to blockade of the sacral nerves.

Examples of its application are: perineal operations, inguinal and herniorraphy, cystoscopy and urethral surgery. It is less commonly used in obstetrics, with lumbar epidural being the route of choice. In chronic pain management it may be used for conditions such as chronic perineal pain, benign or malignant, coccydynia, chronic pelvic pain. It can be applied diagnostically to demonstrate or isolate any contribution through the sacral and coccygeal nerves towards a particular pain problem.

Relevant anatomy (Figure 15.6)

Considerable individual anatomical variation exists in the sacral area. The size and shape of the sacral hiatus is variable, which can make identification difficult. It is roughly triangular in shape and results from failure of fusion of the fifth sacral vertebra. Its apex can be found at, above or below the lower third of the body of the fourth sacral vertebra. Consequently there is a variation in distance from the apex to a line joining the two sacral cornua. The spinal canal in the caudal region contains the cauda equina in addition to the epidural venous plexus and the loose aereolar tissue generally present in the epidural space.

Description

To create analgesia at the site of the caudal block, local anaesthetic is infiltrated into the skin overlying the sacral hiatus, that is, between the sacral cornua, with deeper infiltration over and around the periosteum of the sacral cornua. The sacral hiatus is then palpated, using the sacral cornuae as landmarks. The needle is then inserted through the skin wheal at right angles to the sacro-coccygeal ligament

which is pierced and the anterior wall of the sacral canal contacted. The needle direction may then be adjusted so that it is more in line with the spinal canal. It is then advanced into the canal. Injection of long-acting local anaesthetic is then made, possibly with the addition of long-acting corticosteroid. To achieve effective spread higher volumes of local anaesthetic are required than those for lumbar epidural. This is due to the fact that injection is being performed at one end of the epidural space, rather than near the middle.

There is often a sensation of loss of resistance followed by the needle being firmly held in place by bone and ligament, when the needle has been advanced into the spinal canal. Nevertheless, it is easy for the needle to be misplaced, in a variety of sites. If the needle is in the subcutaneous tissue it can usually be palpated or there will be a visible swelling. If in doubt, a few millilitres of air will produce localised surgical emphysema. Alternatively, the needle may enter the spinal canal but embed in the periosteal lining. If this should occur resistance

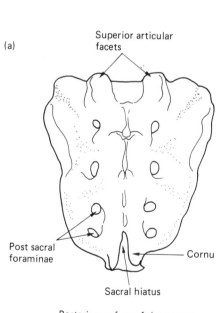

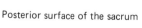

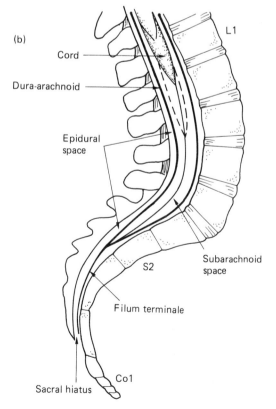

Figure 15.6 (a) Posterior surface of the sacrum; (b) Sagittal section of lumbar and sacral regions of spine

---

Equipment for caudal block

Sterile dressing pack
Sterile gloves
1 × 2 ml syringe
1 × 5 ml syringe
1 × 10 ml or 20 ml syringe (depending on volume of drug to be injected)
1 × 25 gauge needle
1 × 21 or 23 gauge needle
Local anaesthetic for skin infiltration, e.g. 2% lignocaine

Long acting local anaesthetic, e.g. bupivicaine 0.5%
Steroid, e.g. methylprednisolone
Antiseptic to clean skin prior to procedure, e.g. betadine
Antiseptic to clean skin post-procedure, e.g. chlorhexidine
Small sterile dressing, e.g. waterproof plaster
Image intensifier may be required

Preparation for caudal block

Nusing action	*Rationale*
1. Record pulse and blood pressure.	To provide baseline values for later comparison.

For prone position (most commonly used):

2. Position patient in prone position with pillow under lower part of chest. Arms should be brought up, flexed, with hands either side of head. Head positioned to one side on pillow. The lower limbs should be slightly abducted, the feet placed with the big toes in contact and the heels allowed to 'flop' outwards.	Easier for doctor to perform procedure. Prevents tightening of the gluteal muscles which would complicate the identification of landmarks.

For lateral position:

3. Assist patient to arch back and draw knees up in front of abdomen, sacral region should be brought to edge of table.	More comfortable for patient especially if there is any respiratory impairment.
4. Drape patient with sheet.	To minimise exposure and keep patient warm.
5. Open sterile dressing pack and gloves. Pour cleaning solutions. Provide and check local anaesthetic with doctor, and any other drugs to be used.	
6. Remain with patient throughout. Help in maintaining position. Give reassurance and advise against any sudden movements.	To reduce anxiety and fear. To avoid trauma which could complicate the procedure.

During procedure

Doctor/nurse action	*Rationale*
1. The procedure is performed using an aseptic technique. Skin is thoroughly prepared with antiseptic solution.	Special attention to adequate cleansing due to proximity of anus.
2. Skin is infiltrated with local anaesthetic – but large amounts should be avoided.	Landmarks which may be difficult to palpate become more obscure.

3. Needle is inserted and maintained in mid-line of sacral canal whilst injection of drug/s is performed. Test dose used initially followed by full dose.
4. Area cleaned with antiseptic solution. Iodine spray and a small sterile dressing applied.
5. Assist patient to supine position.

To exclude adverse drug reaction or misplaced needle.

Post-procedure

Same as for epidural blockade (see epidural block – post-procedure nos 1–6).

is usually felt. The needle may enter the marrow cavity of a sacral vertebra and any local anaesthetic injected will be rapidly absorbed. Slight withdrawal of the needle and injection of a test dose of local anaesthetic should be carried out (Figure 15.7). The patient should be questioned and observed for any signs of toxicity, such as syncope, drowsiness or convulsions.

An epidural catheter can be inserted into the caudal region but is not commonly used for chronic pain management due to the difficulty of maintaining the position of the catheter and comfort of the patient.

Caudal freeze

A caudal freeze is indicated for relief of intractable pain problems as described for caudal block, where it is hoped to obtain a longer lasting relief of pain symptoms by disrupting nerve conduction in the area treated. This temporary disruption may interrupt the pain cycle, giving weeks to months of pain relief whilst the nerves regenerate. In some cases the pain does not return. A diagnostic block would be carried out at a previous visit to prove effectiveness before proceeding to cryoanalgesia.

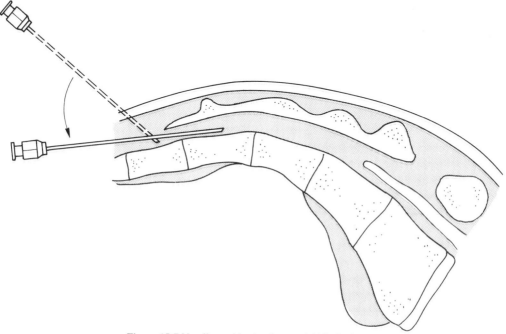

Figure 15.7 Needle positioning for caudal blockade

This procedure is well tolerated by patients and can be performed on an outpatient basis, with repeat treatments if necessary.

The equipment and procedure is the same as that described for facet freeze, excepting that three freeze cycles are used for caudal freezing, each of 2 minutes duration. This involves one in the midline, with slight movement of the probe laterally within the sacral canal, in order to maximise the size of the iceball.

Spinal analgesia

Indications

Spinal (intrathecal) analgesia is performed by injecting analgesic drugs into the subarachnoid space. A very small volume of local anaesthetic, one tenth of the epidural dose, produces effective analgesia, profound muscular relaxation and reduced bleeding. It is useful for operations below the level of the umbilicus, including vaginal and caesarian delivery. It is indicated for those patients with anatomical distortion of the upper airway and is useful for those patients undergoing surgery with a full stomach. Vomiting and aspiration are less likely to occur with a regional block such as spinal analgesia. It is particularly useful for rectal surgery, requiring a smaller area of anaesthesia than general anaesthesia would provide. It also has advantages over other major nerve blocks, for example, when used for lower limb surgery, being simpler, more rapidly induced and more predictable. Spinal analgesia used in surgery can provide pain relief for 2–3 hours from a single bolus injection and a prolonged effect (can be as much as 24 hours) with the use of opioids. It may be of benefit to older and poor risk patients undergoing surgery. This category would include those patients with chronic respiratory disease, renal and some forms of cardiovascular disease. The higher the sensory block the more extensive the sympathetic block will be, therefore the greater the degree of vasodilatation. This is compensated for by vasoconstriction above the level of the block, with an increase in cardiac rate. This may benefit those patients with congestive cardiac failure or ischaemic heart disease, undergoing lower body surgery. In chronic pain states spinal analgesia may be used for assessment and treatment, with neurolytic agents sometimes being indicated, especially with regard to

chronic pain associated with malignancy. This is particularly appropriate in those patients with specific localised pain where alcohol or phenol in glycerin may be used. In these cases it is usual to perform a diagnostic block using local anaesthesia to ascertain the degree of numbness, weakness and pain relief prior to using a neurolytic agent.

Spinal analgesia is usually performed above the level of the cauda equina. Below L_1 it is difficult to block individual nerves, with the increasing danger of denervation of the bladder and/or bowel. The exception to this would be its use in those patients who already have bladder and bowel impairment.

Chronic pain patients who fail to achieve pain relief by other routes and in whom there is a desire to avoid destructive procedures, may benefit from spinal analgesia. Morphine is the most effective spinal analgesic and this may be the route of choice for those who are morphine intolerant – experiencing unpleasant side effects by other administrative routes – or where other routes are impractical, e.g. the patient who is unable to swallow. These patients may also be considered suitable for long term administration of analgesia via an implanted intrathecal device, if demonstrated to be the most effective analgesic route.

There are several contraindications to performing spinal analgesia. It would rarely be used on those patients with pre-existing disease involving the spinal cord or those in any form of shock. It would be contraindicated in those patients undergoing anticoagulant therapy, and those with any localised or systemic infection. If the patient has increased intracranial pressure, sudden reduction in cerebrospinal fluid may lead to pressure and coning of the brain in the foramen magnum. In those patients with chronic or existing severe headache there would be a small but significant risk of increased headache.

Description

Cerebrospinal fluid fills and bathes all the cavities and spaces around the central nervous system. It is the ultrafiltrate of the plasma with which it is in equilibrium. Formation of cerebrospinal fluid takes place in the choroid plexuses, which are small tufts of capillaries in contact with the lining of the lateral ventricles. It is secreted by these plexuses and is passed through the third and fourth ventricles of the brain to reach the subarachnoid space, which lies between the pia and arachnoid mater. In this way the delicate nerve matter of the brain and spinal cord lies between two layers of fluid, which is protective, acting as a buffer and conveying nourishment to the tissues of the central nervous system. It is normally a clear, colourless fluid, the pressure varying from 60 to 100 mm water in the lumbar region when in the lateral position, to 250 mm water in the sitting postion. The volume is variable, but commonly between 120 and 150 ml with approximately 25–35 ml in the subarachnoid space. Its specific gravity is usually 1006–1008. Cerebrospinal fluid is reabsorbed by arachnoid villi and there is some drainage into the connective tissue spaces of the nerves.

The technique is much the same as that used for epidural blockade, excepting that a finer spinal needle is used and is inserted beyond the epidural space into the subarachnoid space. The needle should produce the minimum amount of trauma and the smallest possible puncture in the dura mater. Varying sizes of needle are used from 18 to 29 gauge. The finer needles are more flexible and require an introducer on insertion. Loss of resistance is felt on entering the epidural space and further loss of resistance with sometimes discomfort, as the needle pierces the dura and arachnoid layer to enter the subarachnoid space. Its correct placement is confirmed by the free flow of cerebrospinal fluid. If it is bloodstained time must be taken for it to clear before injecting the solution. If it does not clear another puncture would be necessary.

The commonest complication from this procedure is severe headache. This is due to cerebrospinal fluid leaking from the subarachnoid into the epidural space. This lowering of the cerebrospinal fluid pressure allows descent of the brain. This stretches the dura, cerebral blood vessels and nerve endings. The headache is primarily occipital, radiating to frontal and orbital, and the patient may experience cervical muscle spasm. The headache is postural, being worse when the head is raised and nausea, vomiting, photophobia and dizziness may also be experienced. It may be very severe and last for several days. There is less likelihood of a headache if only one puncture is performed and a fine needle is used.

The patient is treated by being kept fully hydrated with oral or intravenous fluids and a mild systemic analgesic given. Lying flat as routine does not reduce the incidence, but provides relief when headache is present. If it persists, with the patient becoming distressed, an epidural blood patch should be performed to seal the dural pucture site. The patient's own blood is drawn aseptically and sent for culture. Fifteen to 20 ml of blood is injected epidurally, ideally at the interspace where the dural puncture occurred. The patient should remain supine for 30 minutes following the procedure, after which time the headache has usually resolved.

A rare but life threatening complication of rising intercostal paralysis can occur following high spinal anaesthesia. If the phrenic nerves are affected oxygen and artificial ventilation may be necessary.

Procedure

The procedure is the same as for epidural blockade, bearing in mind the difference in technique and site as described.

Sympathetic neural blockade

Sympathetic neural blockade can be useful in the diagnosis and alleviation of some chronic pain syndromes and other conditions, where the autonomic nervous system is involved.

Sympathetic impulses are conducted through a relay of two sympathetic neurones, that is, pre-ganglionic and post-ganglionic, from the central nervous system to the visceral effectors. By definition the sympathetic nervous system is efferent; that is, impulses are conducted away from the brain stem and spinal cord to visceral effectors and therefore should not be involved in the transmission of pain. The exact mechanism whereby pain can be sympathetically mediated or transmitted is not fully understood but many types of pain are influenced by the activity of the sympathetic nervous system and it has been known for many years that certain types of pain can be alleviated by sympathetic blockade.

Relevant anatomy

The sympathetic nervous system is an anatomically distinctive component of the autonomic

226   Pain: Management and Nursing Care

nervous system and comprises autonomic ganglia, nerves and plexuses.

The sympathetic trunk consists of a double chain of nerve fibres and ganglia which lie on either side of the vertebral column, stretching from the base of the skull to the sacrum. Short nerve fibres connect the ganglia to each other, referred to as the 'sympathetic chain ganglia' because they resemble two chains of beads. Each chain usually consists of 22 ganglia. These ganglia, via communicating branches, are connected with the central nervous system through the spinal nerves and cord. Other sympathetic ganglia or collateral ganglia are situated in relation to the double chain of ganglia but lying nearer to the organs they serve. These ganglia and nerves form sympathetic plexuse before fibres are distributed to their respective destinations. The three main plexuses are; the cardiac plexus, the coeliac plexus and the hypogastric plexus.

The anatomical distinctiveness of the sympathetic chain of ganglia allows for sympathetic blockade at the ganglion. The three main levels for ganglionic blockade are; the cervico-thoracic ganglion, which is usually referred to as the stellate ganglion, the coeliac ganglia and the lumbar ganglia (Figure 15.8).

The sympathetic nervous system may also be blocked at the post-ganglionic synapse using a Bier's block technique on the affected limb.

Agents used for sympathetic blockade

Local anaesthetic drugs may be use for short term blockade and also for diagnostic purposes. The therapeutic effect of local anaesthetics can sometimes last longer than their expected duration of action. Neurolytic agents such as phenol or alcohol may be used for more permanent blockade. They are only indicated where the risk of complications is acceptable and where a

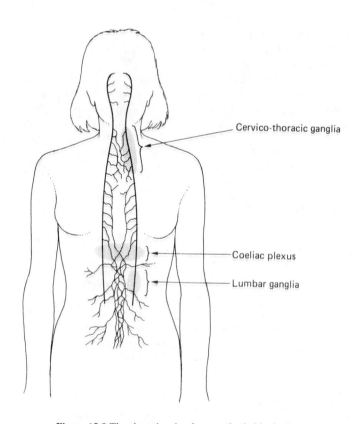

Figure 15.8 The three levels of sympathetic blockade

diagnostic local anaesthetic block has been performed in order to demonstrate that the pain can be alleviated by this method. Guanethidine, which acts as a sympathetic nerve terminal blocker, is one of the drugs frequently used for blocking at the post-ganglionic synapse. Guanethidine prevents the re-uptake of the chemical transmitter noradrenaline, which is produced at the post-ganglionic synapse. As a result normal sympathetic tone is not maintained, producing a sympathetic block. Drugs such as clonidine and atropine may be used in combination with guanethidine. More studies are required to confirm their efficiency.

Stellate ganglion block

Indications

By the injection of local anaesthetic into the vicinity of the stellate ganglion in the neck, the sympathetic nerve supply to the head, neck and arms can be interrupted.

The indications for such a blockade are circulatory insufficiency and pain. The commonest vascular disorder in which this blockade is of value is Raynaud's disease. Painful conditions associated with overactivity of the sympathetic nervous system such as causalgia and reflex sympathetic dystrophy can also be alleviated by this procedure. Post-herpetic neuralgia and

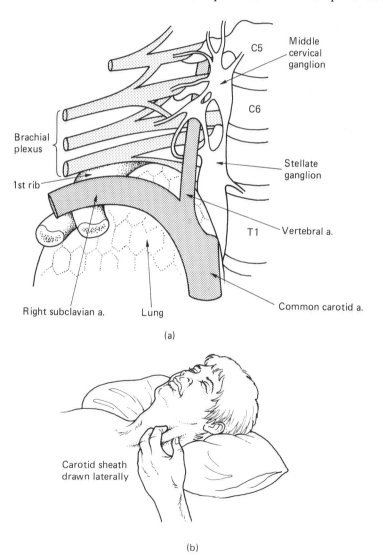

(a)

(b)

Figure 15.9 (a) Position of stellate ganglion; (b) position of patient's head for procedure

pain caused by tumour of the head, neck and arm may be included.

The procedure is usually performed on an out-patient basis, but occasionally a series of blocks my be indicated in order to achieve a therapeutic effect and in this circumstance the patient would be admitted to hospital. Bilateral stellate ganglion blocks are rarely performed on the same day because of increased risk of complications. If indicated, they are usually performed on alternate days.

Description

Fusion of the seventh and eighth cervical sympathetic ganglia and the first thoracic sympathetic ganglia forms the stellate ganglia which lies anteriorly to the base of the seventh cervical vertebra. Several important structures lie close to the ganglion. These include several blood vessels, particularly the vertebral artery, the recurrent laryngeal nerve, the phrenic and vagus nerves, the brachial plexus and the dome of the pleura. Great care must be taken to avoid complications associated with accidental injection into any of these structures. Accidental puncture of the dura is another dangerous complication associated with this procedure.

The anterior approach is usually chosen with the patient lying in the supine position (Figure 15.9).

Equipment for stellate ganglion block

Sterile dressing pack
Sterile gloves
1 × 10 ml syringe
1 × 5 ml syringe
21 gauge or 23 gauge needle
25 gauge needle
Local anaesthetic for skin infiltration, e.g. lignocaine 1%
Long acting local anaesthetic, e.g. bupivicaine 0.25% or 0.5%
Antiseptic to clean skin prior to procedure, e.g. betadine

Antiseptic to clean skin post-procedure, e.g. chlorhexidine
Small sterile dressing, e.g. waterproof plaster.

Because several important structures lie in close proximity to the stellate ganglion, neurolytic agents are rarely used because of the risk of serious complications associated with irreversible damage to the surrounding structures. If neurolytic agents are required very small volumes would be used with the aid of an image intensifier for accurate placement.

Preparation for stellate ganglion block

Nursing action	*Rationale*
1. Warn the patient of possible side effects, e.g. Horner's syndrome – ptosis, face flushed and dry on the injected side, blocked nose and constriction of the pupil are all indicative of a positive Horner's syndrome. This is an inevitable result of a successful block to the sympathetic chain in the neck. Temporary hoarseness and a 'lump' in the throat sensation may also occur. Brachial plexus involvement will result in temporary loss of sensation in the arm.	To reduce fear and anxiety should side effects occur. To reassure the patient that these possible side effects will only be temporary.
2. The patient is assisted into a supine position with the head slightly raised and extended backwards with pillow placed under the neck and shoulders.	To allow easier access to the area to be injected, the anterior approach being the safest.

3. Advise the patient against making any sudden movements during the procedure or from talking or swallowing whilst injection is taking place and the needle is in situ.

To prevent accidental injection into other vital structures.

4. Open the dressing pack. Deposit sterile gloves, syringes and needles onto sterile area, ensuring area is not contaminated.

To minimise the risk of infection.

5. Provide and check with doctor drugs to be administered.

To ensure correct drugs, dosage and that they have not expired.

6. Remain with the patient throughout the procedure and reassure them.

To reduce anxiety and fear.

During procedure

Doctor/nurse action

Rationale

1. The procedure is performed using an aseptic technique. Skin is prepared with antiseptic solution.

To minimise risk of infection.

2. The skin is infiltrated with local anaesthetic. Encourage patient to state if local anaesthetic is ineffective

To reduce discomfort
To ascertain if more local anaesthetic is required.

3. The ganglion is injected at the level of the transverse process of the sixth cervical vertebra.

To avoid puncture of the dome of the pleura.

4. The long acting local anaesthetic is injected slowly.

To minimise the risk of accidental intravenous or intra-arterial injection.

5. The patient must be closely observed for any change in condition, e.g.:

To detect any indication of dangerous complications in order to treat appropriately and promptly.

(a) Signs of central nervous toxicity

Intra-arterial or intravenous injection has occurred.

(b) Sudden chest pain, coughing and/or breathlessness.

Would indicate penetration of the pleura resulting in a pneumothorax.

(c) High spinal anaesthesia and possible respiratory arrest.

Puncture of the dura.

6. The patient should be observed for the signs of a positive Horner's syndrome.

Indicates that the local anaesthetic solution has been injected into the correct tissue plane.

7. The area is cleaned and a small sterile dressing is applied.

8. The patient is assisted to assume a sitting position. When the patient is ready he/she may then be assisted off the table.

To ensure the safety of the patient.

Post-procedure

Nursing action

Rationale

1. The patient should be advised to stay within the unit and recover for a minimum of 1 hour.

To ensure adequate recovery and to observe for any complications.

Coeliac plexus block

Indications

Coeliac plexus block is used for the management of chronic pain due to malignancy of the pancreas, stomach, gall bladder and liver. This block may also be of therapeutic value in alleviating pain caused by chronic pancreatitis, but to a lesser degree.

Intravenous sedation or general anaesthesia would be required for this procedure, to ensure the comfort of the patient. Admission of the patient would therefore be necessary for the recovery period and to assess the effects of the block.

The procedure is usually performed under X-ray control to facilitate accurate location of the plexus and correct placement of the needle. A diagnostic block would be performed using local anaesthetic before carrying out a more permanent block with a neurolytic agent, in order to establish the extent of pain relief which could be produced. Bilateral injections would be required to achieve a block of the whole plexus.

Description

The coeliac plexus is the largest of the three great plexuses of the sympathetic nervous system, and supplies the abdominal viscera. It is situated between the body of the first lumbar vertebra and the twelfth thoracic vertebra and usually exists as two large masses lying anterior to the vertebrae. It is formed by the joining of the greater, lesser and least splanchnic nerves and is composed of the coeliac ganglia and nerve fibres converging at the level of the upper part of the first lumbar vertebra. It surrounds the origin of the coeliac artery, a branch of the abdominal aorta and lies anterior to the crura of the diaphragm. The kidneys are laterally placed on either side and on the right side, the vena cava is anteriorly situated (Figure 15.10).

Important bony landmarks are identified and marked on the skin before the procedure is performed, in order to aid accurate placement of the needle. The identifications made are; the twelfth ribs and the posterior spines of the twelfth thoracic and first lumbar vertebrae.

A 15 cm (6″) needle is inserted at an angle of 45 degrees towards the lateral aspect of the body of the first lumbar vertebra, walked off it anteriorly and then advanced well in front of the vertebra. The injection of a contrast medium will confirm correct needle placement prior to a diagnostic or therapeutic block (Figure 15.11).

Complications associated with coeliac plexus block are the same as for lumbar sympathetic block. Hypotension is quite common, especially in dehydrated and debilitated patients with malignant disease. Other complications include accidental subarachnoid or epidural injection or injection into other vital structures. Misplaced injections are less likely to occur if the important bony landmarks are identified and the procedure is performed under X-ray control.

Equipment for coeliac plexus block

Sterile dressing pack
Sterile gloves
1 × 10 ml syringe
1 × 5 ml syringe
1 × 2 ml syringe
21 gauge needle (and 25 gauge needle plus local anaesthetic for skin and subcutaneous tissue infiltration if a general anaesthetic is not given)
20 gauge 15 cm (6″) spinal needle/s – depending on whether block is unilateral or bilateral
For diagnostic block: local anaesthetic, e.g. bupivicaine 0.25% or 0.5%

For permanent block: alcohol
Contrast medium, e.g. iopamidol
Antiseptic to clean skin prior to procedure, e.g. betadine
Antiseptic to clean skin post procedure, e.g. chlorhexidine
Protective glasses if neurolytic agent is used
Sterile dressing
Image intensifier
Body marker
General anaesthetic equipment
Intravenous infusion equipment

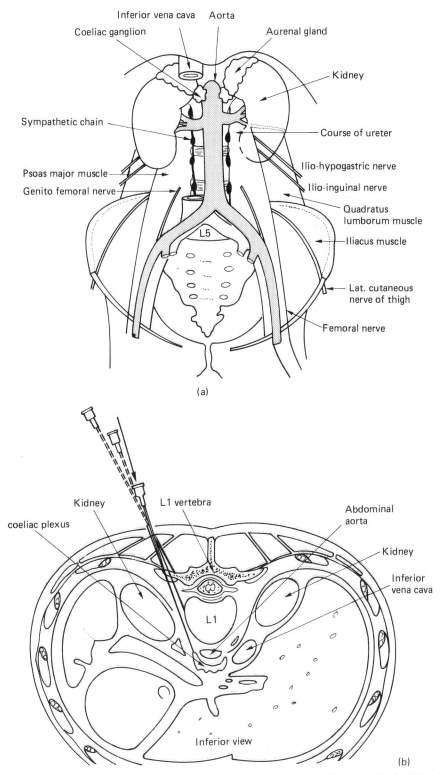

Figure 15.10 (a) Position and relations of lumbar sympathetic chain and coeliac plexus; (b) technique of coeliac plexus block, showing change of alignment

Preparation for coeliac plexus block

Doctor/nurse action	Rationale
1. Check and record pulse and blood pressure.	Provide baseline values for later comparison.
2. Commence intravenous infusion.	Hypotension is likely to occur.
3. Prepare patient for intravenous sedation or general anaesthesia	To ensure the comfort of the patient and facilitate patient cooperation during the procedure.
4. The patient is placed in the prone position on an X-ray table. A pillow is placed under the abdomen. The arms are raised carefully alongside the head, flexed at the elbows.	The posterolateral approach is the easiest. To keep the trunk flat. To ensure the comfort of the patient.
5. Sterile dressing pack is opened. Sterile gloves, needles and syringes deposited onto sterile area ensuring it is not contaminated.	To minimise the risk of infection.
6. Important bony landmarks are identified and marked onto the skin.	To aid accurate location of the plexus and placement of the needle/s.
7. Provide and check drugs to be administered.	To ensure that they are the drugs required and that they have not expired.
8. Remain with the patient throughout the procedure and give reassurance.	To reduce anxiety and fear.

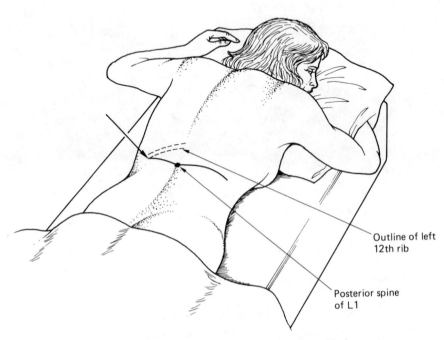

Outline of left
12th rib

Posterior spine
of L1

Figure 15.11 Position of patient for coeliac plexus block.

During procedure

Doctor/nurse action	*Rationale*
1. The procedure is performed using an aseptic technique.	To minimise the risk of infection.
2. The skin is prepared with antiseptic solution. If a general anaesthetic is not given, the skin and subcutaneous tissues are infiltrated with local anaesthetic. Assess effectiveness of local anaesthesia.	To ensure the comfort of the patient on insertion of the needle/s.
3. The needle is inserted at the correct angle.	
4. The position is checked by X-ray in the lateral and antero–posterior planes.	To ensure correct placement of the needle and to give a precise view of its position.
5. The needle is carefully aspirated to check for leakage of blood, urine or cerebrospinal fluid.	To check for misplacement.
6. If the needle has been satisfactorily placed, a small amount of contrast medium is injected and checked by X-ray.	To provide additional confirmation of needle placement.
7. If the block is diagnostic, local anaesthetic is injected, e.g. 20 ml 0.25% bupivicaine on each side. A small test dose may be injected initially.	To minimise the risk of needle misplacement.
8. If a neurolytic agent is used protective glasses would be worn by the doctor and nurse prior to the solution being drawn up and on injection.	To protect the cornea.
9. For a more permanent block a neurolytic agent is used, e.g. 20 ml of 50% alcohol on each side.	
10. Before the needle is withdrawn a small amount of air is injected.	To clear the needle and reduce risk of local irritation of somatic nerve roots caused by neurolytic agent following the path of the needle on removal.
11. On removal of the needle the skin is cleaned and a sterile dressing is applied.	
12. If the patient has had general anaesthesia they would be placed in the semi-prone position prior to being transferred to the recovery area.	

Post-procedure

Nursing action	*Rationale*
1. The appropriate nursing care and observations would be carried out if a general anaesthetic had been administered.	To maintain adequate airway and ensure uneventful recovery.
2. The patient should remain in the recovery area for approximately 1 hour, or until observations are satisfactory and stable.	To provide easy access to resuscitation equipment.

3. The pulse and blood pressure should be recorded at 5 minute intervals, decreasing to every 15 minutes during the first hour post-procedure.

Hypotension may occur.

4. If observations are satisfactory and stable, the patient would be transferred to a bed where they should remain in the supine position for at least 1 hour.

5. Pulse and blood pressure should be recorded for a further hour at 15 minute intervals, or until satisfactory and stable. Intravenous infusion may then be discontinued.

6. The patient would be advised to rest quietly on their bed for 24 hours. They may get up for toilet purposes with supervision. A call bell should be provided.

Postural hypotension can occur.
To ensure the safety of the patient.

7. Advise the patient that mild discomfort may be felt in the back for a few days post-procedure.

Result of bruising due to passage of the needle/s.

8. Advise the patient that they may not feel benefit from the block initially.

Pain relief may not be immediate.

9. Monitor pain level over several days post-procedure.

Splanchnic nerve block

The splanchnic nerves may be blocked, the indications for this procedure being the same as for coeliac plexus block. The technique is similar. The nerves are blocked above the diaphragm at the level of the twelfth thoracic, before they terminate in the coeliac ganglia and finally the coeliac plexus.

The procedure is usually performed under X-ray control and may be performed on an outpatient basis with the use of local anaesthesia. A general anaesthetic is not usually indicated, being less painful to perform than a coeliac plexus block. The same complications can occur but postural hypotension to a lesser degree. However, there is a greater risk of pneumothorax owing to the close proximity of the pleura.

Effective pain relief may be obtained with much smaller amounts of solution compared to coeliac plexus block. The spread of solution around the coeliac plexus may be hindered owing to the presence of malignant tumour and therefore a splanchnic nerve block may be preferable.

Lumbar sympathetic blockade

Indications

The most common indication for lumbar sympathetic block is for the relief of symptoms associated with peripheral vascular disease of the lower limbs. It can be useful in relieving ischaemic rest pain and may aid the healing of areas of ulceration or incipient gangrene. In patients who are assessed to be unfit for general anaesthesia, this procedure may be considered safer than undergoing surgery and can effectively improve the circulation in the affected limb.

Painful conditions associated with overactivity of the sympathetic nervous system, such as causalgia and sympathetic dystrophy, may be alleviated by lumbar sympathetic block. It may also be used in relieving post-amputation pain and pain associated with carcinomatous infiltration of nerves.

Description

The lumbar sympathetic chain lies on the antero–lateral surface of the lumbar vertebral bodies in a fascial compartment, confined within the boundaries of the psoas muscle, the vertebral column and the retro-peritoneal fascia. Drugs that are injected into this compartment will therefore become diffused, bathing the sympathetic chain.

The aorta and inferior vena cava lie anterior to the lumbar sympathetic chain, the kidneys being postero-laterally placed in relation to the chain.

For diagnostic procedures the insertion of one needle only is required at the level of L2 or L3, but in order to achieve a complete block of the sympathetic nerve supply to the lower limb, the second, third and fourth lumbar ganglia are usually blocked.

The procedure is usually performed on an outpatient basis. General anaesthesia is not usually indicated, but intravenous sedation may be required if the patient is particularly anxious. It is performed under X-ray control to aid accurate placement of the needles, which is essential if neurolytic agents are to be used. Radiographic confirmation of the correct placement of the needles can be aided by the injection of a contrast medium, e.g. iopamidol.

For diagnostic purposes local anaesthetic is used, for example, bupivicaine 0.5%. If a more permanent block is required a neurolytic agent such as phenol 6% is used. A bilateral block can be performed if indicated. The second side would usually be blocked several days later.

Serious complications of this procedure such as accidental puncture of a major blood vessel or the kidney are rare, especially if the correct technique is carried out under radiographic control. Owing to the depth that needles have to be passed through the tissues, there is a risk of severe bleeding, especially with patients on anticoagulant therapy or with haemorrhagic disorders and therefore should not be performed if this applies (Figure 15.12).

Equipment for lumbar sympathetic blockade

Sterile dressing pack
Sterile gloves
1 × 10 ml syringe
1 × 5 ml syringe
1 × 2 ml syringe
21 gauge and 25 gauge needles
Up to 3 × 6″ 20 gauge spinal needles (8″ can be used for very obese patient)
Local anaesthetic for skin infiltration, e.g. lignocaine 2%
Long acting local anaesthetic for diagnostic procedure, e.g. bupivicaine 0.5%

Contrast medium, e.g. iopamidol
Neurolytic agent, e.g. phenol 6% in conray for more permanent block
Protective glasses for doctor and nurse if neurolytic agent is used
Antiseptic to clean skin prior to procedure, e.g. betadine
Antiseptic to clean skin post-procedure, e.g. chlohexidine
Sterile dressings
Image intensifier

Preparation for lumbar sympathetic blockade

Nursing action	Rationale
1. Check pulse and blood pressure.	Provide baseline values for later comparison.
2. The patient is assisted onto the X-ray table and placed in the lateral position lying on their unaffected side. The legs should be flexed.	
3. The position of the back should be completely vertical.	To ensure the planes of the X-rays are at right angles. Accurate antero–posterior and lateral views are required.

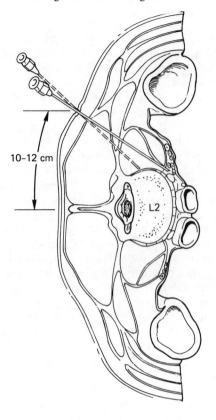

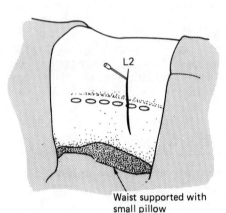

Waist supported with small pillow

Figure 15.12 Lumbar sympathetic block showing technique and patient position

4. The waist is supported with a small pillow.

The vertebral column is curved in a lateral plane offering maximum widening of the spaces between the transverse processes. This affords easier placement of the needles.

5. Advise the patient not to make any sudden movements.

To avoid trauma which may complicate the procedure.

6. Open the dressing pack. Deposit needles, syringes and sterile gloves onto the sterile area ensuring that it is not contaminated.

To minimise the risk of infection.

7. Provide and check drugs to be administered.

To ensure that they are the drugs required and that they have not expired.

8. Remain with the patient throughout the procedure and reassure them.

To reduce anxiety and fear.

During procedure

Doctor/nurse action

Rationale

1. The procedure is performed using an aseptic technique. The skin is prepared with antiseptic solution.

To minimise risk of infection.

2. The skin is infiltrated with local anaesthetic. Encourage patient to state if local anaesthetic is ineffective.

To reduce discomfort felt by the patient on insertion of the spinal needle. To ascertain if more local anaesthetic is needed.

3. The spinal needle is introduced.

4. The position of the needle is checked by X-ray in both the lateral and anteroposterior planes.

To ensure correct placement of the spinal needle and to give a more precise view of needle position.

5. A small amount of contrast medium is injected.

To confirm correct position.

6. For a diagnostic block 10–15 ml of local anaesthetic is injected.

7. If a neurolytic agent is used protective glasses should be used by the doctor and nurse before the solution is drawn up and during injection.

To protect cornea of the eyes.

8. A small amount of neurolytic agent dissolved in a radiographic contrast medium is injected, e.g. phenol in Conray.

To ensure that the neurolytic agent spreads in the correct plane.

9. Patient is kept on side for up to 10 minutes following injection of neurolytic agents which are placed at varying levels.

To restrict lateral spread across the psoas muscle to the genito-femoral nerve which may be damaged by neurolytic agents.

10. Observe for increasing anxiety, pallor, convulsions or syncope.

Shock may occur due to accidental intravascular injection of local anaesthetic or toxic reaction to injection.

11. On removal of the needles the skin is cleaned and a sterile dressing applied.

12. Assist patient into the supine position and transfer to a bed for recovery.

Post-procedure

Nursing action

1. The blood pressure should be recorded at 10 minute intervals during the first 30 minutes. The patient should remain supine for about 1 hour or until blood pressure is satisfactory and stable.

Rationale

Hypotension may occur especially with elderly patients. An intravenous infusion may be required if hypotension occurs.

2. Advise the patient that some mild discomfort may be felt in the back for a few days post-procedure.

As a result of bruising from the passage of the needles.

3. Advise the patient to remain immobile until numbness or weakness is resolved. Provide a call bell. Check that the patient can weightbear when ambulant.

To prevent injuries to patient.

4. Monitor pain level during recovery. With vascular patients assess warmth and colour of affected limb.

To assess effectiveness of the block.

Regional intravenous sympathetic block

Indications

The indications for regional intravenous sympathetic block are pain or circulatory insufficiency which is confined to the limbs. The clinical indications for its use are therefore similar to lumbar sympathetic block and stellate ganglion block, but it is a very safe and much simpler technique to perform. Also, it can safely be used on those patients undergoing anticoagulant therapy.

Description (Figure 15.13)

This procedure involves the intravenous injection of a sympathetic blocking agent such as guanethidine* into the affected limb which has been isolated from the circulation by employing a 'Bier's block' technique. The sympathetic nervous system is therefore blocked at the post-ganglionic synapse by use of this technique. Guanethidine interferes with

---

* In the USA, reserpine is more commonly used.

the re-uptake of the chemical transmitter nor-adrenaline at the sympathetic nerve terminals.

This procedure can be performed on an outpatient basis and can safely be repeated at regular intervals. The disadvantage of this procedure is that it can be very uncomfortable, due to the tightness of the tourniquet and ischaemia which some patients experience difficulty in tolerating. For these patients local anaesthesia, intravenous sedation or entonox may be indicated, more especially if the procedure is to be repeated at intervals.

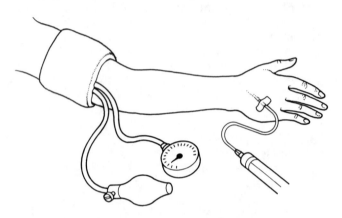

Figure 15.13 Intravenous regional blockade of upper limb

Equipment for regional intravenous sympathetic block

Intravenous cannula
Sterile dressing towel
1 × 10 ml syringe (for upper limb)
1 × 20 ml syringe (for lower limb)
21 gauge or 23 gauge butterfly needle
Tape to secure butterfly needle
Medicated swab
Tourniquet or cuff with three-way tap and pressure gauge

Foam roll
Sympathetic blocking drugs, e.g. guanethidine 20–30 mg mixed with 20 ml 0.9% saline for lower limb, 10 mg guanethidine mixed with 10 ml 0.9% saline for upper limb. Atropine 600 μg can be used in addition or in place of guanethidine. This also applies to clonidine where 150 μg would be used.
Small sterile pressure dressing.

Preparations for regional intravenous sympathetic block

Nursing action	Rationale
1. Record blood pressure.	To determine necessary inflation of tourniquet which should be 50–100 mmHg above the patient's systolic blood pressure to prevent the drug used passing into the general circulation, but allowing it to become fixed in the tissues of the affected limb.

---

2. Advise the patient that some discomfort is inevitable on inflation of the tourniquet and that it will need to remain inflated for 10–15 minutes. — To reduce anxiety and fear.

3. Advise the patient that on inflation of the tourniquet and exsanguination of the limb, the colour of the limb will change and mottled areas of pallor will be observed. A burning sensation may be experienced following injection of guanethidine. On deflation a reductive hyperaemia will be seen as the blood returns to the limb and the colour will change to bright pink and red.

4. Position the patient on a trolley with the affected limb exposed. The patient may need to lie flat immediately after the procedure. — To ensure the comfort and safety of the patient. Hypotension may occur on deflation of the tourniquet.

5. Provide and check with doctor drugs to be administered. — To ensure correct drugs and dosage, and that they have not expired.

6. Remain with the patient throughout the procedure and reassure them. — To reduce anxiety and fear.

During procedure

Doctor/nurse action — *Rationale*

1. A butterfly needle is inserted into a vein in the hand or foot of the affected limb and taped securely.

2. The tourniquet is applied to the affected limb with a foam roll underneath. — For the comfort of the patient.

3. The tourniquet is inflated to a pressure above the patient's systolic blood pressure and securely fastened. — To prevent accidental slippage and release of the tourniquet during the procedure.

4. The diluted drug of choice is injected slowly. — To reduce the likelihood of pain.

5. The tourniquet should remain inflated for 10–15 minutes. Observe the cuff pressure at all times. — To allow the drug to be absorbed into the affected area and prevent it from passing into the general circulation.

6. During this time the patient should be reassured. — To help the patient cope with the discomfort of the tourniquet.

7. The tourniquet is slowly released and removed.

8. Observe for signs of syncope or shock. — Hypotension may occur due to the release of guanethidine, or an adverse reaction to the drug used.

9. If the patient's condition is satisfactory assist them off trolley. — To ensure the safety of the patient.

10. The butterfly needle is removed and a small pressure dressing is applied to the vein.

Post-procedure

Nursing action

1. Advise the patient that they should remain in the unit for a minimum of 1 hour to recover.
2. Monitor pain level, colour and warmth of the affected limb.
3. Advise the patient that relief may not be immediate, and that its effectiveness may depend on repeating the treatment at intervals.

Rationale

To ensure adequate recovery of the patient and to observe for any problems associated with the procedure.

To assess effectiveness of the treatment.

Intercostal nerve blockade

Indications

The use of intercostal nerve blockade is probably most effective for the relief of pain postoperatively in the thoracic and upper abdominal region, but has yet to be widely accepted and practised. For unilateral thoracic procedures it provides better postoperative analgesia than conventional opioid therapy. The nerve block can be performed prior to, during or following the surgical procedure. Intercostal nerve blockade is insufficient by itself for carrying out surgery as it has no effect on visceral structures. Other blocks which provide visceral anaesthesia may be combined with intercostal nerve blockade, e.g. in conjunction with brachial plexus block for operations on breast or upper extremities, stellate ganglion block for intrathoracic surgery and coeliac plexus block for upper abdominal surgery. Intercostal nerve block has been shown to reduce the impairment of respiratory function occurring after thoraco-abdominal surgery. It can improve vital capacity, forced expiratory volume, peak expiratory flow rate and can reduce to some extent the degree of postoperative hypoxaemia. Cryoanalgesia has also proved useful following thoraco-abdominal surgery for alleviation of pain.

Intercostal nerve blockade can also be used for acute painful states such as chest wall trauma, especially fractured ribs, for pain relief and treatment of herpes zoster, and pleuritic pain. It may be used diagnostically, for example differential diagnosis of visceral versus abdominal wall pain. Blocking of intercostal nerves has a place in the treatment of pain associated with

malignancy, where a neurolytic agent may be used, e.g. phenol 6%. Intercostal cryoanalgesia can be used for chronic painful states, usually associated with malignancy.

Description

The intercostal nerves (Figure 15.14) are the primary nerve branches or rami of T_1 to T_{11}. They are typical segmental nerves. T_{12} is unique in that it does not run a course between two ribs but gives off a branch to join the first lumbar nerve before going laterally.

A typical intercostal nerve has four branches; the rami communicantes, the posterior cutaneous branch, the lateral cutaneous branch and the anterior terminal branch. The rami communicantes passes anteriorly to the sympathetic ganglion. The posterior cutaneous branch supplies skin and muscle in the paravertebral region. The lateral cutaneous branch arises in the mid-axillary line and sends subcutaneous fibres anteriorly and posteriorly to a large part of the chest and abdominal wall. The upper five nerves in the anterior terminal branch pierce the external intercostal and pectoralis major muscles to supply the skin of the anterior part of the thorax near the midline. The anterior terminal branch in the lower six intercostal nerves pierces the posterior rectus sheath to supply the rectus muscle and overlying skin.

The intercostal nerve in its most posterior course medial to the angle of the rib, has very little tissue separating it from the pleura. At the angle of the rib it comes to lie in the subcostal groove until it reaches the anterior end of the space. The intercostal nerve is accompanied by the intercostal artery and vein. These lie

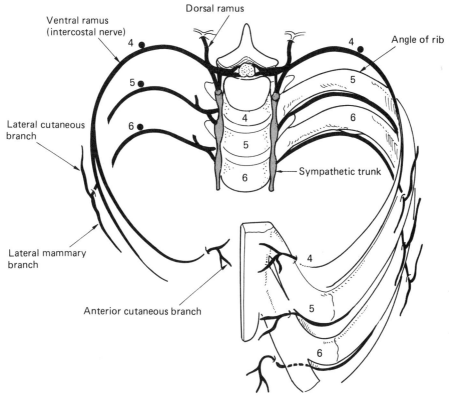

Figure 15.14 The intercostal nerves

superior to the nerve in the inferior groove of each rib. Due to this vascularity absorption of local anaesthetic agents is very rapid, which can produce high blood concentrations. Bupivicaine is most commonly used in combination with adrenaline. The use of adrenaline decreases the rate of absorption of the local anaesthetic and thus reduces peak blood concentration.

Bilateral intercostal blocks (Figure 15.15) can be performed and a series of blocks is usually necessary for surgical application. The intercostal nerve can be blocked at several sites along its course but for optimum analgesia and muscle relaxation the injection is usually performed posteriorly to the mid-axillary line, that is, near to the origin of the lateral branch.

The most feared complication from this procedure is a pneumothorax, but this is in fact rare. If it does occur it is usually small and resolves spontaneously without resorting to the use of an intercostal drain. Dramatic hypotension is another rare complication of this procedure.

Equipment for intercostal nerve blockade

Sterile dressing pack
Sterile gloves
21 gauge needle
23 gauge needle
1 × 5 ml syringe
1 × 10 ml syringe
Local anaesthetic for skin infiltration, e.g. lignocaine 1%
Long-acting anaesthetic, e.g. 0.25% or 0.5% bupivicaine with adrenaline

Neurolytic agent if required, e.g. 6–8% phenol
Protective glasses if neurolytic agent used
Antiseptic to clean skin prior to procedure, e.g. betadine
Antiseptic to clean skin post-procedure, e.g. chlorhexidine
Small sterile dressings.
Skin marker
Image intensifier if using cryoanalgesia

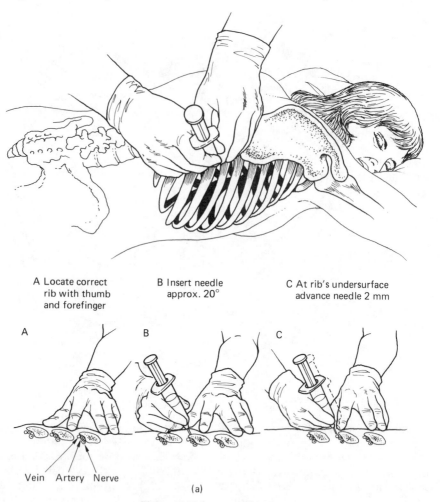

A Locate correct
rib with thumb
and forefinger

B Insert needle
approx. 20°

C At rib's undersurface
advance needle 2 mm

Vein   Artery   Nerve

(a)

Figure 15.15 Intercostal block

Preparation for intercostal nerve blockade

Nursing action	Rationale
1. Check and record pulse and blood pressure.	To provide baseline values for later comparison.

For sitting position:

2. Assist the patient to sit on a chair, leaning forwards over the edge of operating table, head on hands.	Comfortable position for ambulant patient.

For prone position:

3. Assist patient to lie prone with shoulders abducted and arms forward. Small pillow is placed under the mid-abdomen.	Usually indicated for bilateral intercostal blocks. Scapulae move laterally and allow access to the posterior rib angles where the rib is usually easily palpated. Use of pillow straightens the lumbar curve and increases the intercostal spaces posteriorly.

For lateral position:

4. Assist patient to lie in lateral position with affected side uppermost, arm raised above head.

Used for unilateral block at the posterior or midaxillary line.

For supine position:

5. Assist patient to lie supine with arm/s raised and abducted.

For anterior block to the parasternal area.

6. Sterile dressing pack is opened. Sterile gloves, needles and syringes deposited onto sterile areas ensuring it is not contaminated.

To minimise the risk of infection.

7. Important bony landmarks are identified and marked onto the skin.

To aid accurate location of the rib margins and placement of the needle/s.

8. Provide and check drugs to be administered.

To ensure that they are drugs required and that they have not expired.

9. Remain with the patient throughout the procedure and give reassurance.

To reduce anxiety and fear.

During procedure

Doctor/nurse action

Rationale

1. The procedure is performed using an aseptic technique.

To minimise the risk of infection.

2. The skin is prepared with antiseptic solution.
   If a general anaesthetic is not given, the skin and subcutaneous tissues are infiltrated with local anaesthetic. Assess effectiveness of local anaesthetic.

To ensure the comfort of the patient on the insertion of the needle/s.

3. The needle is inserted over the rib selected for the block and directed under the lower edge of the rib directed upwards approximately 2–3 mm.
   The needle is carefully aspirated.

To check for air or blood showing misplacement of the needle.

4. The nerve selected is injected plus the intercostal nerve above and below. Up to 5 ml of local anaesthetic is injected. The patient is asked to hold his/her breath whilst the injection is taking place.

Necessary to block three intercostal nerves to block one intercostal space.
To minimise lung movement over the needle point so that if there has been accidental puncture of the pleura, the risk of serious pneumothorax is reduced.

5. If a neurolytic agent is used protective glasses would be worn by the doctor and nurse prior to the solution being drawn up and on injection.

To protect the cornea of the eyes.

6. Observe the patient for signs of hypotension, nausea and syncope.

Due to fast systemic absorption of the drug injected.

7. On removal of the needle the skin is cleaned and a sterile dressing applied.

Post-procedure

Nursing action	Rationale
1. The patient should remain in the recovery area for aproximately 30 minutes.	To provide easy access to resuscitation equipment.
2. The pulse and blood pressure should be recorded at 10 minute intervals for 30 minutes.	Hypotension may occur.
3. Monitor pain level following procedure.	

Upper limb blocks

Brachial plexus block

A brachial plexus block is useful in both acute and chronic pain states. It can provide anaesthesia of the upper limb during surgery, e.g. dislocation, reduction of fractures and suturing of tendons. Local infiltration, sedation or light general anaesthesia may be required to supplement the brachial plexus block. Postoperative pain in the upper limb may also be alleviated by this method. Patients with chronic painful conditions such as causalgia, reflex sympathetic dystrophy, peripheral neuropathy and Raynaud's disease may benefit from this procedure. A catheter can be used at all sites on the brachial plexus for continuing relief. Neurolytic blocks of the plexus for carcinomatous pain can be conducted – phenol is commonly used, the strength varying between 6 and 10%, using a volume of 10 ml.

The brachial plexus (Figure 15.16) supplies all of the motor and most of the sensory function of the upper limb. It is formed from the anterior primary rami of the C_5–C_8 and the T_1 nerves plus small contributing branches from C_4 and T_2 nerves. The roots form three trunks, each dividing into an anterior and posterior division. The six divisions then join to form cords. Each of these have two terminal branches which supply the greater part of the arm. Emerging from the plexus are small nerves – median, radial and ulnar.

Various sites can be selected for blocking:

Interscalene – this may miss the ulnar aspect of the hand and forearm.

Parascalene
Subclavian perivascular } – these give the most complete limb blocks
Supraclavicular

Infraclavicular
Axillary – this does not block the shoulder but is a simpler method without the risk of pneumothorax.

The local anaesthetic commonly used in blocking the brachial plexus is bupivicaine 0.25% or 0.5%. This is usually combined with adrenaline to minimise the risk of systemic toxicity. This would apply particularly where higher concentrations are indicated. For adults, 30–40 ml of long acting local anaesthetic agent would be usual, no matter which approach used, to ensure maximal spread. Pain relief should be establishes within 20 minutes, a motor block being apparent before a sensory block.

Complications that can arise are intra-arterial or intravenous injection, haematoma and pneumothorax.

Suprascapular block

This can be used for diagnostic purposes and for painful conditions of the shoulder and shoulder joint.

The suprascapular nerve supplies the supraspinous muscle and gives off sensory fibres to the shoulder joint and surrounding structures. It originates from C_4, $_5$ and $_6$ of the upper trunk of the brachial plexus. It descends posteriorly passing through the scapula notch.

The injection is made into the suprascapular

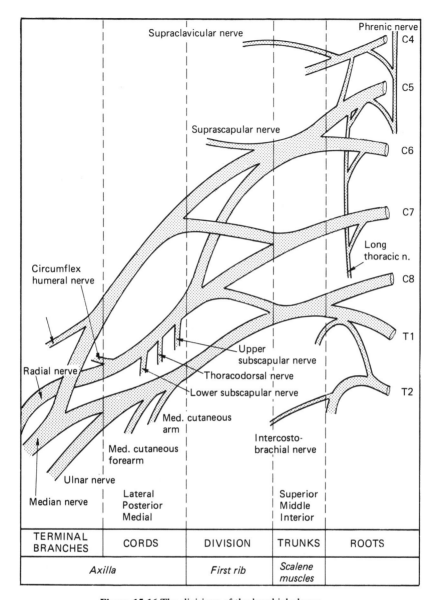

Figure 15.16 The divisions of the brachial plexus

notch with the patient in a sitting position with head flexed forward, arms supported on a surface. A long acting local anaesthetic agent such as bupivicaine 0.5% is used. Complications that can arise are intravascular injection and pneumothorax.

Peripheral nerve blocks

Peripheral nerve blocks may be used to supplement brachial plexus anaesthesia or for short surgical procedures to hands and fingers. They may also be used for specific painful conditions. The nerves involved are:

Elbow blocks – lateral cutaneous nerve of forearm ulnar nerve

Wrist blocks – median nerve radial nerve

Digital blocks – digital nerve

Lower limb blocks

The lumbosacral plexus and its branches can be blocked for operations on the lower extremity and can be useful in the diagnosis and treatment of chronic pain. Their use may also be indicated in accident surgery, in the case of multiple injuries and where shock may be present. In these circumstances a major nerve block higher up may be contraindicated and a combination of lower limb nerve blocking, e.g. sciatic/ femoral block, may be appropriately used. An acute painful hip condition may also be effectively localised in this way. This type of block may also be considered in those patients where an epidural or spinal anaesthetic may be contraindicated. This would include some elderly patients, those with cardiovascular disease, the debilitated and acutely ill.

The lumbosacral plexus (Figure 15.17) is formed from the anterior primary rami of the second lumbar to the third sacral roots. Each root divides both anteriorly and posteriorly and these then join and branch to form the individual nerves. Important branches of the plexus are: the femoral nerve, sciatic nerve, obturator nerve and the lateral femoral cutaneous nerves.

Long acting local anaesthetic such as bupivi-caine 0.5%, with the possible addition of adrenaline, is commonly used for lower limb blocks. Toxicity levels must be considered if bilateral blocks are performed as a volume of 30–40 ml may be required for each limb.

Femoral nerve block

The femoral nerve L_2–L_4 arises from the lumbar plexus and runs downwards in the groove between the psoas major and iliac muscles. It lies lateral to the femoral artery and deep to the inguinal ligament. From here it divides into anterior and posterior divisions. In this procedure the femoral nerve is blocked immediately below the inguinal ligament. Operations such as unilateral removal of varicose veins (with local infiltration of the groin), unilateral below knee surgery and skin grafts from the thigh can be conducted using this block in combination with other nerve blocks.

Sciatic nerve block

This is the largest nerve in the body. It arises from the sacral plexus, passing from the pelvis into the buttock through the greater sciatic foramen. As it leaves the pelvis major it is accompanied by the posterior cutaneous nerve of the thigh. It lies on the muscles around the hip joint and is covered by gluteus maximus. It continues down to the popliteal fossa, dividing here into common peroneal and tibial branches. The sciatic nerve can be blocked in four positions; posterior, anterior, supine and lateral, the posterior being that most commonly used.

Obturator nerve block

The obturator nerve L_2–L_4 passes downwards in the pelvis minor and continues downwards and forwards along its lateral wall to the obturator canal and reaches the medial thigh. It is the motor nerve to adductor muscles to the thigh. An effective block produces a reduction in power of adduction and external rotation of the thigh. It is mainly used in localisation of painful conditions in the hip joint. Due to the close proximity of the obturator vessels, the complications of intravascular injection or haematoma can occur.

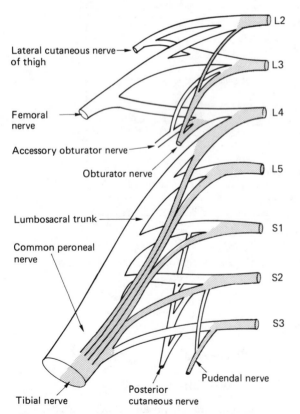

Lateral cutaneous nerve of thigh

Femoral nerve

Accessory obturator nerve

Obturator nerve

Lumbosacral trunk

Common peroneal nerve

Tibial nerve

Posterior cutaneous nerve

Pudendal nerve

L2
L3
L4
L5
S1
S2
S3

Figure 15.17 Lumbosacral plexus

Lateral femoral cutaneous nerve block

The lateral femoral cutaneous nerve arises from L_2–L_3 of the lumbar plexus and lies on the iliac muscle. It runs obliquely downwards and forwards from this muscle on the inner aspect, to pass deep to the inguinal ligament. It emerges on the lateral side of the thigh. It is a sensory nerve, therefore this block does not produce motor weakness.

Peripheral nerve blocks

Nerve blocks can be performed at the level of the knee and ankle. For the knee the saphenous nerve is most commonly blocked. To block at the ankle level, several nerves can be used; the tibial, sural, the superficial peroneal, the deep peroneal and the saphenous nerve.

Facial pain

There are 12 pairs of cranial nerves. The largest of these is the fifth cranial or trigeminal. It is a mixed nerve, but is principally a sensory nerve supplying the face, mouth, teeth, nose, parana-sal sinuses and the anterior two-thirds of the head (Figure 15.18). It has a large ganglion, the trigeminal or gasserian ganglion, which lies in the floor of the middle cranial fossa. From the trigeminal ganglion the nerve divides into three large divisions; the opthalmic, maxillary and mandibular nerves, each with many important branches supplying the respective areas of the face, mouth, teeth and head.

The trigeminal nerve is often involved in pain syndromes and blockade of the nerve and its divisions is used for the management of benign and malignant chronic pain. Some of the most common causes of orofacial pain of non-dental origin which are seen in the pain clinic are: trigeminal neuralgia, atypical facial pain and post herpetic neuralgia affecting the trigeminal division.

Trigeminal neuralgia

This pain syndrome of unknown cause is more common in females than males and generally occurs in the middle-aged. It is characterised by

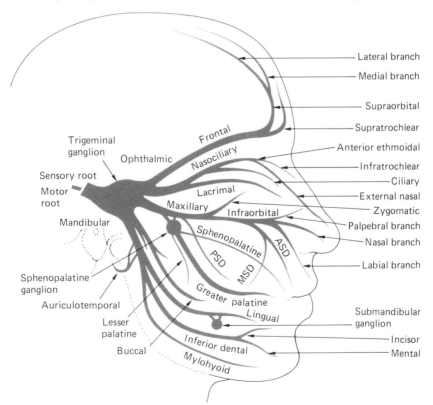

Figure 15.18 The division of the trigeminal nerve

paroxysms of severe stabbing pain lasting no more than a few seconds, but may be repeated rapidly over minutes. The pain may be triggered by gentle stimulation of the face or mouth, for example during washing, eating or talking. The pain is confined to the distribution of the trigeminal nerve, the second and/or third division of the nerve being most commonly affected. The condition is usually unilateral and infrequently crosses from one division to another in an individual bout. Exacerbations and remissions are characteristic, but as time passes the periods of remission become shorter and the severity and frequency of attacks increases. At this stage the patient is in dread of the next paroxysm and afraid of performing actions which may trigger the pain, resulting in both psychological and physical repercussions.

The management of trigeminal neuralgia may vary between different pain clinics. Peripheral nerve blocks may be carried out to provide pain relief when pharmacological management has proved unsuccessful. Individual divisions of the trigeminal nerve may be blocked where they leave the skull and enter the face or mouth. The supra-orbital, infra-orbital, inferior and mental nerves are readily accessible for procedures. The injection of local anaesthetic around the identified division of the nerve is a helpful diagnostic, prognostic and therapeutic aid. The injection of bupivicaine 0.5% in the appropriate peripheral nerve can give temporary pain relief for the duration of the nerve block, but sometimes can last longer than its known duration of action by breaking the cycle of pain. Peripheral nerve blocks using glycerol have also been effectively used to provide relief of pain for long periods. The advantages of glycerol compared to the use of neurolytic agents or rhizotomy are that facial sensations are usually preserved and there is no irreversible damage to surrounding structures.

Cryoanalgesia, which involves freezing the appropriate peripheral nerves under local anaesthetic, can also be used effectively in the management of established trigeminal neuralgia which is not responding to drug therapy. It can provide pain relief for long periods. The advantage of cryoanalgesia compared to surgical or more central procedures is that it does not produce irreversible damage to the nerve or precipitate secondary neuralgia. If the pain returns the patient is no worse off and the procedure may be repeated.

Trigger point injection

A trigger point may present as an acute pain with muscle strain or as a sequel to chronic muscle fatigue. Skeletal muscle comprises almost half of the total body weight and is subject to daily wear and tear. Trigger points may develop in any one of these muscles, causing pain and muscle spasm. They can be acute or latent, are very common and can continue for a long period of time, that is, months to years. The pain is characteristically constant, aching in nature and felt deeply. Latent trigger points may not be interpreted as painful so much as causing limitation of movement and muscle weakness of the affected muscle. Many terms have been used to describe them such as: muscular rheumatism, fibrositis and muscular sciatica.

Injection of trigger points is useful when there are several present and the muscle is unable to stretch due to pain. Using an aseptic technique, the trigger point is located by palpation to find a taut band of muscle. This is carried out with the muscle sufficiently stretched, enabling the point to be held usually between two fingers and relying on feel to then inject perpendicularly. Correct location is confirmed by the patient stating when he/she feels the worst pain. Local anaesthetic, e.g. bupivicaine 0.5%, is commonly used with the possible addition of methylprednisolone for prolonged relief.

Acknowledgements

Thanks are due to Dr Chris Glynn, Dr Alex Jadad, Dr Tim Jack, Chris Lupson, Siobhan Horton and Dr David Bowsher.

Bibliography

Barnard, D., Lloyd, J. W. and Evans J. (1981) Cryoanalgesia in the management of chronic facial pain. *Journal of Maxillofacial Surgery*, **9**, 101–102

Barnard, J. D. W. and Lloyd, J. W. (1977) Cryoanalgesia. *Nursing Times*, **June 16**

Cousins, M. J. and Bridenbaugh, P. O. (1988) *Neural Blockade in Clinical Anaesthesia and Management of Pain*, 2nd Edition, J. B. Lippincott Co., Philadelphia

Covino, B. G. and Scott, D. B. (1989) *Handbook of*

Epidural Anaesthesia and Analgesia, Gene & Stratton Inc.,

Erikkson, E. (ed) (1969) *Illustrated Handbook in Local Anaesthesia*, Munksgaard, Denmark

Evans, P. J. D. (1981) Cryoanalgesia. *Anaesthesia*, **36**, 1003–13

Evans, P. J. D., Lloyd, J. W. and Green, C. J. (1981) Cryoanalgesia: the response to alterations in freeze cycle and temperature. *British Journal of Anaesthesia*, **53**, 1121–1127

Hinchcliff, S. and Montague, S. (eds) (1988) *Physiology for Nursing Practice*, Balliere Tindall, London

Juniper, R. and Parkins, B. J. (1990) *Emergencies in Dental Practice: Diagnosis and Management*, Heinemann Medical Books, Oxford

Katz, J. (1985) *Atlas of Regional Anaesthesia*, Appleton-Century-Crofts (Prentice-Hall Inc.),

Lloyd, J. W., Barnard, J. D. W. and Glynn, C. J. (1976) Cryoanalgesia: a new approach to pain relief. *Lancet*, **2**, 932–924

Nimms, W. S. and Smith, G. (eds) (1989) *Anaesthesia*, Vol 2, Blackwell Scientific Publications, Oxford

Prithvi Raj, P. (1986) *Practical Management of Pain*, Year Book Medical Publishers Inc.

Prithvi Raj, P. (1986) *Practical Pain Management*. Year Book Medical Publishers, pp. 774–782

Thibodeau, G. A. (1987) *Anatomy and Physiology*, Times Mirror/Mosby College Publishing USA, pp. 298–349

Wall, P. D. and Melzack, R. (eds) (1984) *Textbook of Pain*, Churchill Livingstone, Edinburgh

Wildsmith, J. A. W. and Armitage, E. N. (eds) (1987) *Principles and Practice of Regional Anaesthesia*, Churchill Livingstone, Edinburgh

Index